Introduction to
Dental Materials

Introduction to
Dental Materials

Fifth Edition

Richard van Noort BSc, DPhil, DSc
Professor in Dental Materials Science, Department of Restorative Dentistry, University of Sheffield, Sheffield, UK

Michele E. Barbour MPhys, PhD, PGCHE
Senior Lecturer in Dental Biomaterials, School of Oral and Dental Sciences, University of Bristol, Bristol, UK

ELSEVIER   Edinburgh   London   New York   Oxford   Philadelphia   St Louis   Sydney   Toronto   2013

ISBN: 978-0-7020-8108-8

Senior Content Strategist: Robert Edwards
Content Strategist: Alexandra Mortimer
Content Project Manager: Shivani Pal
Design: Bridget Hoette

Printed in India

Last digit is the print number: 9 8 7 6 5 4 3 2 1

Working together to grow libraries in developing countries

www.elsevier.com • www.bookaid.org

CONTENTS

PREFACE

There are very few dental restorative procedures that do not make use of a dental material in one way or another. The dental materials market is competitive and lucrative, and there are strong market forces for the development of new and augmented dental materials, meaning that the typical lifespan of a material before it is modified or replaced can be as little as 3 years. Consequently, many materials in use today will be superseded by new ones within the duration of a typical undergraduate dental degree, and as such dental and dental therapy students must be equipped not only with an understand of *today's* materials, but of the fundamental principles and concepts that *underpin* them, such that they can apply this understanding to new materials as they are developed. A rapid progression of new restorative materials and adhesive products prompted the fourth edition, and now in the fifth edition we again seek to bring the book up to date, still covering the more traditional (but still relevant) materials and supplementing this with coverage of some of the more novel products that clinicians encounter. With all the changes in dental materials since the first edition almost 30 years ago, one thing remains the same: the dentist has ultimate responsibility for what is placed in the patient's mouth and thus needs to have a sound knowledge of the materials used.

The book is set out in three sections, each covering a different aspect of dental materials science.

SECTION ONE: BASIC SCIENCE FOR DENTAL MATERIALS

This section describes the structure of materials, with chapters on atomic bonding, metals, ceramics and polymers. The first chapter has been revised to reflect the growing need to be aware of the safety aspects of dental materials and the care that has to be taken when sourcing materials from across the world. Further chapters explain the necessary terminology used in the description of the physical, chemical and mechanical behaviour of materials. A separate chapter is devoted to the principles of adhesion.

SECTION TWO: CLINICAL DENTAL MATERIALS

This section deals with those materials commonly used in the dental surgery, including dental amalgam, composite resin and compomers, glass–ionomer cements and resin-modified glass–ionomer cements. The composition, chemistry, handling characteristics and properties relevant to their clinical use are discussed. The chapter on lining and base materials considers issues relating to pulpal protection, which is also taken up in the chapter on endodontic materials. Resin bonding to enamel and dentine is covered in a separate chapter, reflecting the high importance of this subject in clinical dentistry. Impression materials are also covered in this section.

SECTION THREE: LABORATORY AND RELATED DENTAL MATERIALS

In this section, the student of dental materials science is introduced to the materials used by dental technicians in the construction of fixed and removable prostheses. A sound knowledge of the materials available and how they are used will help towards developing an understanding of the work of the dental technician and assist in communication with him or her. Also included in this section is a chapter on cementation, describing the wide variety of materials and procedures used in the dental surgery when providing patients with indirect restorations.

The philosophy in the earlier editions of this book was to make dental materials science readily accessible to the dental student, and we have sought in this edition to expand the audience to a growing professional group: the dental hygiene and therapy student. We have endeavored to retain the simplicity and clarity that we feel was the hallmark of the previous editions, but those who are familiar with the previous edition will notice that much has been added to reflect the changes in clinical dental materials. We have retained the comment boxes throughout the text in order to highlight issues of clinical significance, which we hope the reader will continue to find helpful.

It should be appreciated that this book was written on a need-to-know basis and is only the first step towards that process of independent learning and critical appraisal of dental materials. As the title suggests, the book represents only an introduction to dental materials and there is obviously much, much more that can be learnt. The list of suggested further reading at the end of each chapter has again been updated and the reader is urged to take advantage of the better knowledge and understanding that can be gained from reading widely around the subject.

The aim of this textbook is to guide readers down the long road to becoming informed practitioners who not only know what should be done and how it should be done, but also why it should be done. I believe that the student of dental materials science will find this book a useful first step in the right direction.

Michele Barbour and Ric van Noort, 2023

INTRODUCTION

Poor dentition is often thought of as being a modern-day problem, arising as a consequence of overindulgence in all things considered 'naughty, but nice'! At first glance, the diet of years gone by, consisting of raw meat, fish, rye bread and nuts, would be considered better for the dentition than the cooked food and high sugar intake foods consumed today. However, the food was not washed as diligently then as it is now, meaning that it contained grit in the form of sand, flint and shells, which had the effect of wearing away the grinding surfaces of the teeth. The surface protective layer of enamel is only thin, and the underlying dentine is worn away rapidly. Eventually, the pulp is exposed and will be invaded by bacteria, which, before long, will cause the formation of an abscess, leaving no other recourse than to have the offending tooth extracted. The problems this presented were formidable, and we will return to these at a later stage.

Thus, the loss of teeth is by no means a new problem, and has been with man for time for as long as can be remembered.

ETRUSCANS (1000–600 BC)

For some of the earliest records of the treatment of dental disease, one has to go back well before the time of Christ. While much is lost with the passage of time, the Etruscans did leave behind a legacy of some very high-quality dentistry.

The Etruscans were a people that came from the near East and established themselves in the leg of Italy. They were the forebears of the Romans (upon whom they had a great influence) and laid the basis for the formation of the Roman Empire. The quality of their craftsmanship was outstanding. Their skills were put to good use, as they fashioned artificial teeth from cadaver teeth using gold to hold the tooth in place. Gold had the two advantages of being aesthetically acceptable, and of being one of the few metals available to them with the necessary malleability for the production of intricate shapes.

The Romans must have inherited at least some of their interest in teeth, as made evident by one of their articles of law of the Twelve Tables, which states that:

> *To cause the loss of a tooth of a free man will result in a fine of 300 As.*

More remarkable, perhaps, is the fact that the slaves too were offered some protection, but in their case the fine was only 100 As. Although no physical evidence remains that false teeth were worn, it may be inferred from the written records that this was the case. Horace (65 BC), wrote of 'witches being chased and running so fast that one lost her teeth', and later still Martial (AD 40–100), referred to ivory and wooden teeth.

THE DARK AGES

Little is known of what happened in dentistry from Martial's time until the 16th century, and this period must be considered as being the 'Dark Age of Dentistry'. We owe our patron saint of dental diseases, Saint Apollonia, to this period. She was 'encouraged' to speak ungodly words by having her teeth extracted or else be burnt on the pyre. She chose to burn! This did leave the church with somewhat of a dilemma, because suicide was not allowed, but in this case the problem was overcome by considering this as divine will.

There are odd records scattered about throughout this period showing that toothache was a persistent problem. For example, one important person was known to pad out her face with cloth in order to hide the loss of teeth, whenever there was an important function to attend. This was none other than Queen Elizabeth I. Then there was Louis XIV, the 'Sun King', who suffered terribly from toothache and had to make many momentous decisions, such as the revocation of the Edict of Nantes (in 1642), while suffering excruciating pain. Possibly this clouded his judgement.

THE FIRST DENTURES (18TH CENTURY)

In the 18th century, it became possible to produce reasonably accurate models of the mouth by the use of wax. These models were then used as templates from which ivory dentures were carved to the required shape. By the latter part of the 18th century, various craftsmen produced finely carved ivory teeth. They set up in business solely to supply false teeth to the rich. Of course, this type of dentistry was not available for the masses.

Lower dentures made of ivory and inset with cadaver teeth worked reasonably well and managed to stay in place without too much difficulty, especially if weighted with some lead. The difficulties really came to the fore with the upper denture, which refused to stay in place due both to the heavy weight and the poor fit. In order to overcome this problem, upper dentures were fashioned onto the lower denture by means of springs or hinges. This technique would ensure that the upper denture would always be pushed up against the roof of the mouth, but, as can be imagined, they were large, cumbersome and very heavy.

Clearly, the use of cadaver teeth could hardly have been hygienic. Similarly, ivory is slightly porous and thus presented an ideal substrate for the accumulation of bacteria. In fact, George Washington regularly soaked his dentures in port, ostensibly to overcome the bad taste and to mask the smell.

In 1728, Fauchard suggested that dentures should be made from porcelain instead of ivory inset with cadaver teeth, arguing that porcelain would be more attractive (as it could be coloured as required) and would be considerably more hygienic. What made this suggestion possible was the introduction into Europe of the secret of making porcelain by Father d'Entrecolle, a Jesuit priest who had spent many years in China. Given the problems of the high shrinkage of porcelain during firing, it is perhaps not surprising that we had to wait until 1744 for the first recorded case of a porcelain denture, made by a man called Duchateau.

THE VICTORIAN AGE

The Victorians frowned on the wearing of dentures as a terrible vanity, more so because all of these false teeth were absolutely useless for eating with! Nevertheless, false teeth were still worn extensively by the rich. The fact that they were non-functional, combined with Victorian prudishness, is said to lie behind the custom that developed during that time of eating in the bedroom just prior to going to dinner – a custom that insured against any possible disaster at the dinner table as well as making possible the romantic affectation that young ladies lived on air.

A number of important discoveries were made during the 19th century that had a profound effect on the treatment of dental disease. The first of these was made in about 1800 by a 'dentist' from Philadelphia by the name of James Gardette.

He had carved a full set of ivory dentures for a woman patient, and had delivered these to the woman saying that he did not have time to fit the springs there and then, but that he would return to do so as soon as he possibly could. (It was the custom in those days for the dentist to visit the patient!) As it turned out, it was some months before he returned to the woman patient, and he was astonished to find that on asking her to fetch the dentures, the woman replied that she had been wearing them ever since he had delivered them. She had found the dentures a little uncomfortable at first but had persevered, and, after a little while, had found them to be quite comfortable and had no need for the springs.

Upon examination of the dentures, he realized immediately that the retention of the dentures was due to a combination of a suction effect arising from the different pressure of the atmosphere and the fluid film, and the surface tension effects of the fluid. This retention was attained because of the close fit of the denture, so it was possible to do without springs altogether, if only the denture could be made to fit as closely as possible to the contours of the oral structures. Unfortunately, the production of close-fitting dentures still presented a serious problem, which we will return to in a moment.

At this time, the extraction of diseased teeth presented a formidable problem, because there was no painless means of accomplishing the extraction. This situation was to change dramatically in 1844 due to the astuteness of a young dentist called Horace Wells, who discovered the anaesthetic effects of nitrous oxide, more commonly known as 'laughing gas'. One evening, he found himself present at a public entertainment on the amusing effects of laughing gas. A friend who subjected himself to the gas became very violent while under the influence, and in the ensuing fracas stumbled and badly gashed his leg. He had no knowledge of this wound until Wells pointed to the blood-stained leg, upon which his friend responded that he had not felt a thing. Wells realized immediately the importance of this discovery, and the next day subjected himself to the removal of one of his own teeth with the aid of the gas. This turned out to be highly successful, and before long many sufferers of tooth-ache had the offending teeth painlessly extracted.

Unfortunately, Wells did not live to see the benefit of his discovery for long, as he committed suicide 3 years later after becoming addicted to chloroform. As a consequence of Wells's discovery, there were many people who had their teeth painlessly extracted.

At that time, few were in the position of being able to afford dentures of either carved ivory or porcelain. Other techniques had been developed, whereby it was possible to obtain accurate impressions of the oral structures, and much of the ivory was replaced by swaged gold, beaten to a thin plate on a model. The fixing of the artificial teeth to the gold was a difficult and lengthy process, and, like dentures, was also expensive.

This situation was to change dramatically with the invention, by Charles Goodyear (in about 1850), of the process of vulcanization. In this process, rubber was hardened in the presence of sulphur to produce a material called vulcanite. This material was not only cheap but was also easy to work with; it could be moulded to provide an accurate fit to the model and hence to the oral structures. It did not take off as quickly as might have been expected however, because the Goodyear Rubber Company held all the patents on the process and charged dentists up to $100 a year to use it, with a royalty of $2 per denture on top of this. The situation changed when the patent expired in 1881, and cheap dentures could be made available to the masses of people in need of them.

Nowadays, vulcanite has been replaced by acrylic resins, which came with the discovery of synthetic polymers, first made between the two World Wars. Also, wax has been replaced by a wide range of oral impression materials with far superior qualities; this has made possible the construction of very close fitting, complex prostheses.

TOOTH CONSERVATION

If the 19th century was the time for tooth replacement, then the 20th century must be considered the time of tooth preservation. For example, in 1938, 60% of dental treatment was still concerned with the provision of dentures, but by 1976 this had dropped to 7%, with the rest consisting essentially of tooth preservation procedures.

Of course, the idea of preserving a decayed tooth was by no means new. As far back as the 11th century, Rhazes suggested that cavities in teeth could be filled with a mixture of alum, ground mastic and honey. Oil of cloves was promoted by Ambrose Pare (1562) to alleviate toothache, and Giovanni de Vigo (1460–1520) suggested the use of gold leaf to fill cavities. Pierre Fauchard (1728), considered by many to be the father of dentistry, discussed many aspects of dentistry, including operative and prosthetic procedures, and mentioned lead, tin and gold as possible filling materials.

However, there were a number of important gaps in the knowledge of the dentition that held back the development of conservative dental techniques.

There was a lack of understanding of the reasons for tooth decay, which was originally thought to be due to some evil spirit invading the tooth. Some thought it was due to a worm of sorts, and promoted various nasty tinctures with the objective of killing it.

The first serious conservative dental procedures did not come into use until the second half of the 19th century. By then, it was possible to work on people's teeth without causing severe pain and discomfort, thanks to the discovery of anaesthetics. This discovery made the use of the dental drill feasible.

The first such drill only became available in about 1870, but this is not too surprising, given that the drilling of teeth without an anaesthetic would have been unthinkable. Now that the preparation of teeth could be carried out, it was possible to undertake some more adventurous procedures than the wholesale extraction of decayed teeth.

CROWNS AND BRIDGES

By the turn of the century, some highly advanced dental work was carried out in which badly broken-down teeth were reconstructed with porcelain crowns. This procedure was aided by the invention of a cement that would set in the mouth (i.e. zinc phosphate cement), and which is still widely used to this day. That this could give a great deal of satisfaction can be illustrated from the letters of President Roosevelt of the United States of America to his parents when still a young man:

After lunch I went to the dentist, and am now minus my front tooth. He cut it off very neatly and painlessly, took impressions of the root and space, and is having the porcelain tip baked. I hope to have it put in next Friday, and in the meantime I shall avoid all society, as I talk with a lithp and look a thight.

May 19, 1902

This was followed by a letter a week later in which he writes:

My tooth is no longer a dream, it is an accomplished fact. It was put in on Friday and is perfect in form, colour, lustre, texture, etc. I feel like a new person and have already been proposed to by three girls.

Obviously a delighted customer!

As is often the case with these rapid developments, there were to be some problems ahead. One of these was highlighted by an English physician, William Hunter, who accused what was then called 'American Dentistry' of contributing to the ill health of many of his patients. He had a number of patients with ailments he was at a loss to diagnose until he noticed the extensive restorative work in their mouths. These bridges and crowns appeared dirty, and were surrounded by unhealthy looking tissue, which would have been particularly bad, as oral hygiene was virtually non-existent. At that time, root canal treatment was unheard of, so the roots of teeth readily became infected. On many occasions, crowns and bridges would have been constructed on badly diseased teeth. He suggested that these crowns and bridges be removed and the teeth extracted, in response to which he received considerable objection from the patients because of the cost of the dental treatment. But, for those who agreed to have the bridgework removed, a significant number showed an immediate improvement in their health. This led Hunter to describe American Dentistry as 'mausoleums of gold over a mass of sepsis'. Consequently, teeth were blamed for all manner of illnesses that could not be readily diagnosed, and this led to many perfectly sound teeth being extracted unnecessarily.

Eventually, sanity prevailed with the introduction in 1913 of X-ray equipment by C. Edmund Kells. It could now be shown whether a tooth with a dead root was healthy or diseased. If healthy, it could be kept, and only if diseased would it be removed.

These days we take the provision of crowns and bridges for granted. Yet new developments can still excite us such as the introduction of ceramic veneers in the 1980s and the rapid developments in CAD–CAM technology that have opened up new opportunities with new materials such as pure alumina and zirconia, which give the promise of all-ceramic bridges.

FILLING MATERIALS

The middle of the 19th century saw the organization of dentistry into a profession, and many dental societies came into existence, as well as numerous dental journals. One of the first acts of the American Society of Dental Surgeons was to forbid its members to use silver amalgam, resulting in the 'amalgam war'.

Amalgam is a mixture of silver, tin and mercury, and was one of the first filling materials used by the dental profession. However, many problems arose with the use of this material because of a lack of understanding of its qualities. It was not until the work of G. V. Black that some order was created out of the chaos.

He published two volumes on operative dentistry in 1895, which became the world standard for restorative dentistry. Until he had

TABLE 1	Milestones in the History of Dental Materials
600 BC	Etruscan gold bridge work
AD1480	First authentic record of gold fillings in human teeth by Johannes Arculanus, University of Bologna
1500s	Ivory dentures began to be carved from wax models
1728	Fauchard proposed the use of porcelain
1744	Duchateau makes the first recorded porcelain denture
1826	Taveau of Paris suggests the use of silver and mercury to make a paste for filling teeth
1839	The first dental journal is published: *American Journal of Dental Science*
1840s	'Amalgam war' – the use of silver amalgam is forbidden
1850	Charles Goodyear invented vulcanite – sulphur-hardened rubber
1879	The first cement to set in the mouth, zinc phosphate, is introduced
1880s	Silicate cements developed
1895	G.V. Black publishes the first detailed study of the properties of amalgams
1907	W.H. Taggart of Chicago invented a practical method of casting gold inlays
1950s	Introduction of acrylic resin for fillings and dentures
1955	Buonacore discovered the acid-etch technique for bonding to enamel
1970	Composites began to replace silicate cements
1976	Glass ionomer cements are invented by A. Wilson
1978	Light-activated composites appear on the market
1983	Horn introduced the resin-bonded ceramic veneer
1985	Development of dentine-bonding agents
1988	Introduction of resin-modified glass–ionomer cements
1994	First compomer appears on the market

studied both the behaviour of amalgam in detail and how best to use it, amalgam did not have a very good reputation. Since then, however, and up until this very day, amalgam has become one of the most important restorative materials used by the dental profession.

It is a great credit to his intellect and ability that some of his philosophy is only now being challenged; especially in the light of what we know now compared to 1900. It is a lesson the dental profession will have to learn over and over again as new materials are brought onto the market (Table 1).

SUMMARY

As can be noted from the preceding discussion, there are numerous restorative techniques that the dentist needs to learn. In addition, dentists use a wide variety of different materials, some being hard and stiff and others being soft and flexible.

It is important that the dentist fully appreciates the various features of these materials, what it is that makes them so useful for dental applications, and what their limitations are. Only then will the dentist be able to select the most appropriate material for a particular application.

FURTHER READING

Greener EH (1979) Amalgam: yesterday, today and tomorrow. Oper Dent 4: 24

Hyson Jr JM (2003) History of the toothbrush. J Hist Dent 51: 73–80

Irish JDA (2004) 5,500 year old artificial human tooth from Egypt: a historical note. Int J Oral Maxillofac Implants 19: 645–647

Little DA (1982) The relevance of prosthodontics and the science of dental materials to the practice of dentistry. J Dent 10: 300–310

Phillips RW (1976) Future role of biomaterials in dentistry and dental education. J Dent Educ 40: 752–756

van Noort R (1985) In defence of dental materials. Brit Dent J 158: 358–360

Wildgoose DG, Johnson A, Winstanley RB (2004) Glass/ceramic/refractory techniques, their development and introduction into dentistry: a historical literature review. J Prosthet Dent 91: 136–143

Williams HA (1976) The challenge tomorrow in dental care delivery. J Dent Educ 40: 587

Woodforde J (1971) The strange story of false teeth. Universal-Tandom Publ. Co., London

SECTION 1

Basic Science for Dental Materials

Biomaterials, Safety and Biocompatibility

BIOMATERIALS

The dental restorative materials described in this textbook are a special sub-group of what are more generally known as biomaterials. When a material fulfills a function in, or in intimate contact with, the human body, it is referred to as a biomaterial. A biomaterial may be defined as a non-living material designed to interact with biological systems.

There are many different applications of biomaterials. In this book we are concerned with dental restorative materials, such as those used for fillings, fixed prosthetics (such as crowns, bridges, implants), removable prosthetics (such as full and partial dentures), and those materials used in the preparation of these (including impression materials, waxes, laboratory materials). There are many other applications of biomaterials, of course, including in orthopedics, cardiovascular materials and devices, limb prostheses, reconstructive materials following surgery or accidents, and even the humble contact lens, to name but a few.

The latter part of the 20th century saw a remarkable development in new dental materials and technologies. At the beginning of the century, the choice of dental materials on offer was virtually limited to amalgam for posterior teeth, silicate cements for anterior teeth, and vulcanite for dentures, which support the ceramic teeth. Since this time, the situation has evolved considerably, and there is now so much choice and such a vast range of materials available to the clinician that the process of selecting the best materials for a particular clinical situation has become much more complex.

To make matters yet more complicated, there is ever-growing pressure to abide by the principles of evidence-based dentistry and, by corollary, evidence-based dental material selection. However, it is not at all clear what constitutes evidence-based dental material selection, or even what constitutes evidence. If one were to start from the basis that only double-blind, randomized, controlled clinical trials constitute evidence, then with respect to dental materials, we have a serious problem, as such evidence simply does not exist. So the first thing we need to do is to explore our understanding of what constitutes evidence-based dentistry more fully.

EVIDENCE-BASED DENTISTRY

There are many potential definitions of evidence-based medicine, but the one we will use here is *the conscientious, explicit and judicious use of current best research evidence in making decisions about the care of individual patients, taking into account clinical expertise and patient choice.*

What is appealing about this definition is the fact that it encompasses all aspects of the delivery of health care: namely, the evidence of research, the evidence of clinical ability, and the evidence of patient need and choice. The value of clinical ability and patient choice are reasonably easy to understand, whereas the evidence of research requires a more in-depth exploration. This is provided in the supplementary parts of the definition, which state what best research evidence is:

Clinically relevant research, often from the basic sciences of medicine, but especially from patient-centered clinical research, into the accuracy and precision of diagnostic tests (including the clinical examination), the power of prognostic markers, and the efficacy and safety of therapeutic, rehabilitative, and preventive regimens.

New evidence from clinical research both invalidates previously accepted diagnostic tests and treatments and replaces them with new ones that are more powerful, more accurate, more efficacious, and safer.

The important thing to point out here is the recurring theme of safety. In this book we will concern ourselves with dental restorative materials, and a great deal of space is devoted to two important aspects of their use: their composition and their characteristic properties. However, as the evidence-based statement above clearly indicates, we must also consider the safety of patients and of the dental team when handling dental materials.

SAFETY

When a biomaterial is placed in contact with the tissues and fluids of the human body, there is invariably some form of interaction between the material and the biological environment. Thus it is quite reasonable for patients to ask their dental practitioner what evidence there is to show that the material about to be put in their mouth is safe. This does rather pose the question: 'How do we know if a material is safe to use?' Besides, what do we mean by 'safe'? The most straightforward definition of safety in this context is to suggest that dental materials should not cause any local or systemic adverse reactions, either in patients or in the dental personnel handling the materials. How we might seek evidence to support the contention that the dental materials we use will not cause any adverse reactions can be gleaned from two sources, namely:
- basic research using methods of premarket testing
- clinical research via post-market surveillance.

The first of these involves putting the material through a battery of laboratory experiments and testing it for cytotoxicity, mutagenicity, etc., according to well-established ISO 10993 guidelines. But that is not all, as it is important to remember that many materials have the potential to be toxic under unfavorable circumstances and at sufficient doses, and yet can also be beneficial when the appropriate circumstances prevail. Many chemicals used in dental materials in their raw state would be considered highly toxic but might have very different properties when processed and/or combined with other components.

It must be understood that safety testing is not about whether or not a material is toxic; rather, it is about *risk assessment*. Whether or not a material can be used depends on the risk it poses, relative to the benefit it brings. Many dental materials can be shown in the laboratory to be cytotoxic, yet this does not preclude them from being used. For example, zinc oxide–eugenol cements have been used for over 100 years, yet they display substantial cytotoxic and irritant properties. Nevertheless, what makes it effective as a temporary filling material is its ability to kill bacteria, providing its obtunding effect; if allowed to come in contact with the pulp, however, its effect can be highly deleterious. Thus this material carries the risk of killing the pulp but, if used correctly, can save many a pulp from dying by removing the bacterial antagonist and giving the pulp the opportunity to recover from the onslaught. 'Safe' requires careful consideration and definition.

The regulatory controls of dental materials, which are largely classified as medical devices, vary across the world. In Europe once materials have undergone a risk assessment and are considered to carry an acceptable risk, they are eligible for being awarded a CE ('European conformity') mark, assuming the material is also 'fit for purpose'. In the United Kingdom post-'Brexit', this is gradually being replaced by a UKCA (UK Conformity Assessed) certification. 'Fit for purpose' in this context indicates that the material is able to perform the functions for which it has been approved. In effect, all this means is that where a material has been approved for use as, say, an anterior filling material, then it must be able to perform that function. It should be clearly understood that this does not mean that the material is efficacious. Evidence of efficacy is not a requirement for the CE approval process. It also means that the material cannot and must not be employed in situations for which its use has not been approved.

There are many other potentially adverse reactions besides toxicity, such as:

- irritant contact dermatitis
  - acute toxic reaction
  - cumulative insult dermatitis
  - parasthesia
- allergic contact dermatitis
- oral lichenoid reactions
- anaphylactoid reactions
- contact urticaria
- intolerance reactions.

Biological reactions can take place either at a local level or far removed from the site of contact (i.e. systemically). The latter is a very important consideration because it may not always be

readily apparent that clinical symptoms, such as dermatological, rheumatic, or neural reactions, could be associated with a biomaterial. Both the patient and the dental personnel are exposed to these interactions and the potential risks, with the patient being the recipient of the restorative materials and the dental personnel handling many of the materials on a daily basis.

There are therefore many aspects to risk assessment, such as making sure that any unnecessary contact with dental materials that may cause irritant contact dermatitis is avoided (Figure 1.1.1.), especially among members of the dental team who will be working with these materials every day. This is often just a matter of common sense, combined with sensible packaging of the materials to be handled. There is no doubt that manufacturers have become much more aware of these issues over the years, paying a lot more attention to how they present their materials and doing it in such a way as to minimize contact.

It is estimated that there are some 140 ingredients in dental materials that can cause an allergic adverse reaction. The question then is: 'How do we know if the materials used might cause any one of these adverse reactions?' Tests to assess the potential of a dental material to cause an allergic adverse reaction are very difficult since they involve the patient's immune system and we are all different in this respect. Some studies suggest that the frequency of adverse reactions to dental materials can be anything from 1:700 to 1:10 000. Experience tells us that some materials are particularly likely to cause an allergic adverse reaction; these include the poly(methyl methacrylate) used in dentures and latex rubber in surgical gloves. Much of this information is anecdotal, although a limited amount of knowledge has been acquired via post-market surveillance. Many countries and regions have systems in place for the reporting of adverse events associated with dental materials. In the UK and EU this is done via the competent national authority (e.g. the Medicines and Healthcare Products Regulatory Agency [MHRA] in the United Kingdom), while in the USA the reporting procedure is the responsibility of the US Food and Drug Administration (FDA) via the MedWatch program. Despite the wide use of dental materials, information on their clinical safety is not

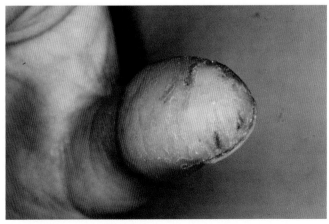

Figure 1.1.1 Irritant contact dermatitis due to resin contact.

particularly abundant, although, from the little evidence that is available, it would appear that adverse reactions to dental materials are fairly rare and that severe adverse reactions are even more so. It should be noted that many compounds potentially cross-react, which means that an allergic sensitization induced by one compound will extend to one or more other similar compounds. Therefore one has to be aware that sensitized individuals are often multi-allergic to a range of compounds.

BIOCOMPATIBILITY

There is a subtle distinction between safety and biocompatibility. Safety is concerned primarily with the fact that materials in contact with the human body should not cause an adverse reaction. A material may be said to be *biocompatible* when it elicits an appropriate hose response, that is to say, that it has the quality of being non-deleterious in the biological environment but must also act or interact in such a way as to benefit the patient. It is important to appreciate that this interaction works both ways. That is, the material may be affected in some way by the biological environment, and equally, the biological environment may be affected by the material. A dental material need not necessarily be inert in order to be biocompatible; that is, it may interact with the environment, for instance, exchanging ions with the saliva; it is biocompatible if it does this to the patient's benefit.

For example, post-operative sensitivity is a local reaction to a restorative procedure. It is often associated with the placement of filling materials, where there is an adverse pulpal reaction following the operative procedure. Although at one time this was thought to be due to a lack of biocompatibility of the restorative material itself, it has now become well accepted that a significant role is played by the ingress of bacteria into the gap between the restorative material and the tooth tissues. If the restorative material were able to provide a hermetic seal, which would prevent bacterial ingress, then post-operative sensitivity from this source would be far less likely. A pulpal reaction could still arise if the restorative material itself were found to be toxic to the pulp. Prevention of bacterial invasion was an important consideration in the development of adhesive restorative materials. Some materials have a distinctly positive effect on the pulp: for example, calcium hydroxide induces tertiary dentine formation by the pulp. This illustrates the above point relating to bioactivity; for a biomaterial to be biocompatible does not mean that it is inert in the biological environment (i.e. that it elicits no reaction) but that it should, ideally, induce a response that is both appropriate and beneficial.

Corrosion is an unwanted interaction between the biological environment and the biomaterial. One of the better-known dental examples is the corrosion of dental amalgams. This corrosion causes discoloration of the tooth tissues and has been implicated in the common observation of marginal breakdown of amalgam restorations. Composite restorative materials can discolor in the mouth due to the corrosive action of the environment, and this causes many to be replaced when the aesthetics become unacceptable. The corrosive effects of the biological environment on the casting alloys used in the construction of fixed and removable intra-oral prostheses can also cause unwanted effects. When a material is susceptible to corrosion in the biological environment, it may release corrosion products into the local biological tissues; this may cause an adverse reaction either locally or systemically. Some patients can develop allergic or hypersensitive reactions to even very small quantities of metals, such as mercury, nickel, and cobalt, that may be released due to the corrosion process. Hence it is important that biomaterials have appropriate corrosion resistance.

From the above, it should be clear that it is very important for the dental clinician to know the composition and chemistry of the materials to be used in the oral cavity and how these materials may interact with the biological environment.

CLINICAL SIGNIFICANCE

Dental practitioners are ultimately responsible for the materials to which a patient will be exposed. They must have a knowledge and understanding of the composition of the materials to be used and how these might affect the patient.

SUMMARY

The main objective of good design in restorative dentistry is to avoid failure of the restoration. However, it is important to appreciate that failure can come in many guises. Some failures may be due to unacceptable aesthetics. A clear example of this is the discoloration of composite restorative materials, which might arise from a lack of chemical stability in the biological environment. A material may need to be removed because it elicits an allergic reaction or corrodes excessively. These are aspects of the biocompatibility of the material. Equally, a restoration may fail mechanically because it fractures or shows excessive wear, possibly because the design was poor or because the material was used in circumstances unsuited for its properties.

Thus the clinical performance of dental restorations depends on:
- appropriate material selection, based on a knowledge of each material's properties
- the optimum design of the restoration
- a knowledge of how the material will interact with the biological environment.

Aspects of the function of dental materials will be covered where appropriate.

FURTHER READING

Hensten-Pettersen A (1998) Skin and mucosal reactions associated with dental materials. *Eur J Oral Sci* 106(2 Pt 2): 707–712.

Kanerva L, Estlander T, Jolanki R (1995) Dental problems. In Guin JD (ed.) *Practical contact dermatitis: a handbook for the practitioner.* McGraw-Hill, New York: 397–432.

Lygre GB, Gjerdet NR, Björkman L (2004) Patients' choice of dental treatment following examination at a specialty unit for adverse reactions to dental materials. *Acta Odontol Scand* 62(5): 258–263.

Scott A, Egner W, Gawkroger DJ et al (2004) The national survey of adverse reactions to dental materials in the UK: a preliminary study by the UK Adverse Reaction Reporting Project. *Brit Dent J* 196(8): 471–477.

Scott A, Gawkroger DJ, Yeoman C et al (2003) Adverse reactions of protective gloves used in the dental profession: experience of the UK Adverse Reaction Reporting Project. *Brit Dent J* 195: 686–690.

Sifakakis I, Eliades T (2017 Mar) Adverse reactions to orthodontic materials. *Aust Dent J* 62(Suppl 1): 20–28.

Syed M, Chopra R, Sachdev V (2015 Oct) Allergic reactions to dental materials – A systematic review. *J Clin Diagn Res* 9(10): ZE04–ZE09.

van Noort R, Gjerdet NR, Schedle A et al (2004) An overview of the current status of national reporting systems for adverse reactions to dental materials. *J Dent* 32(5): 351–358.

Atomic Building Blocks

INTRODUCTION

All materials are built up from atoms and molecules, so it is not really surprising that there is a close relationship between the atomic basis of a material and its properties. Important in this context are the nature of the atoms and the ways in which they are arranged. The atoms combine to determine the microstructure of the solid and, as a consequence, determine its properties. Therefore, if we are to understand the properties of materials, we need to have an understanding of the way atoms can combine to make solids.

JOINING ATOMS TOGETHER

When two atoms are brought together, they may link to form a molecule; any bonds that form are called *primary bonds*. Alternatively, they may move apart and so retain their individual identity. Depending on the degree of interaction between the atoms, one of three states can form, these being gases, liquids, or solids. These are referred to as the three main *phases* of matter, where a phase is defined as a structurally homogeneous part of the system and each phase will have its own distinct structure and associated properties. In the gaseous state there is little or no resistance to the relative movement of atoms or molecules, while in the liquid state the resistance to movement is considerably greater, but molecules can still flow past each other with ease. In solids the movement of atoms and molecules is mostly restricted to local vibrations, although some movement at the atomic level is possible through diffusion.

The controlling factor in bond formation is energy, and a bond will only form if it results in a lowering of the total energy of the atoms being joined. This means that the total energy of the molecule must be less than the sum of the energies of the separate atoms, irrespective of the type of bond being formed. A simple way of visualizing this is the energy-separation diagram, which considers what effect moving two atoms closer together will have on their total energy. A typical energy-separation curve is shown in Figure 1.2.1.

When the two atoms are far apart, the total energy is $2E_a$, where E_a is the total energy of one atom. As they are brought closer together, the total energy begins to fall until it reaches a minimum, E_m, at a distance a_o. Thereafter, as the atoms are brought more closely together, the total energy increases due to repulsion between their clouds of electrons. As the atoms are brought even closer together, their nuclei begin to repel each other as well, but such proximity is not usually achieved in normal circumstances. Thus we have attraction at long ranges and repulsion at short ranges.

The conditions under which two atoms will bond together depend on the atoms' electron configurations, which completely determine their chemical reactivity. The more stable the electron configuration, the less reactive the atom; the extremes of stability are the 'inert gases', such as argon, helium, and neon, which are almost totally non-reactive. Their near-inertness is caused by their having complete outermost electron orbitals, with no opportunity for more electrons to 'join' the atom, and no 'spare' or 'loose' electrons to leave the atom.

All atoms try to reach their lowest energy state, and this is tantamount to having a complete outermost electron orbital, as the inert gases have. The atoms of some elements have 'gaps' for electrons in their outermost orbits, whereas the atoms of other elements have 'spare' electrons in their outermost orbits. By combining with each other, these two different types of atoms can both achieve complete outermost orbitals. The formation of bonds therefore involves only the outermost *valence* electrons.

TYPES OF PRIMARY BONDS

There are three types of primary bonds: *covalent*, *ionic*, and *metallic*.

Covalent Bonds

The covalent bond is the simplest and strongest bond and arises when atoms share their electrons so that each electron shell achieves an inert gas structure. The formation of such a bond for two hydrogen atoms is shown in Figure 1.2.2.

As the two atoms approach one another and the orbitals of the electrons begin to overlap, a molecular orbital is formed where the two electrons are shared between the two nuclei. Since the electrons will spend most of their time in the region where the orbitals overlap, the bond is highly directional.

Ionic Bonds

An atom such as sodium is predisposed to donate its single valence electron, as this would result in a configuration similar to that of neon. Naturally, it cannot do so unless there is another atom to accept the electron.

Elements that can attain an inert gas structure by acquiring a single extra electron are fluorine, chlorine, bromine, and iodine, collectively known as the halogens. Thus, if a sodium

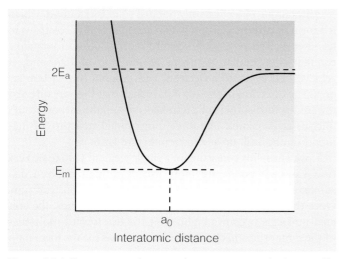

Figure 1.2.1 Energy separation curve for two atoms, each of energy E_a.

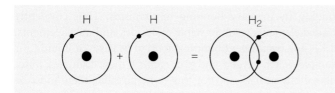

Figure 1.2.2 Two hydrogen atoms combine through covalent bonding to form hydrogen gas.

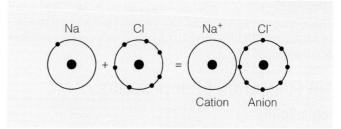

Figure 1.2.3 Formation of an ionic bond between sodium and chlorine.

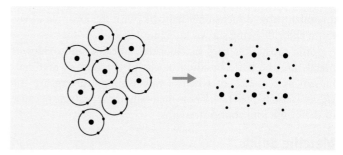

Figure 1.2.4 Formation of a metallic bond, showing a cloud of electrons surrounding the nuclei.

TABLE 1.2.1 **Typical Bond Energies for the Three Bond Types**		
Atoms Bonded	**Bond Type**	**Bond Energy (eV)**
C–C	Covalent	6.3
C–F		5.6
H–H		4.5
H–O		4.4
C–Cl		4.0
Na–Cl	Ionic	4.2
K–Br		3.9
Na–I		3.2
Au–Au	Metallic	2.3
Cu–Cu		2.0
Ag–Ag		1.8
Pb–Pb		0.8
Hg–Hg		0.2

and a chlorine atom are allowed to interact, there is a complete transfer of the valence electron from the sodium atom to the chlorine atom. Both attain an inert gas structure, with sodium having a positive charge due to the loss of a negative electron and chlorine a negative charge due to its acquisition of the extra electron. These two ions will be attracted to one another because of their opposite electrical charges, and there is a reduction in the total energy of the pair as they approach. This is shown in the model in Figure 1.2.3; such bonds are called ionic bonds.

An important difference between the covalent bond and the ionic bond is that the latter is not directional. This is because ionic bonds are a result of the electrostatic fields that surround ions, and these fields will interact with any other ions in the vicinity.

Metallic Bonds

The third primary bond is the metallic bond. It occurs when there is a large aggregate of atoms, usually in a solid, which readily give up the electrons in their valence shells. In such a situation the electrons can move about quite freely through the solid, spending their time moving from atom to atom. The electron orbitals in the metallic bond have a lower energy than the electron orbitals of the individual atoms. This is because the valence electrons are always closer to one or another nucleus than would be the case in an isolated atom. A cloud of electrons, as shown in Figure 1.2.4, surrounds the atoms. Like the ionic bond, this bond is non-directional.

Bond Energies

An important feature of a bond is the *bond energy*. This is the amount of energy that has to be supplied to separate the two atoms and is equal to $2E_a - E_m$, as defined in Figure 1.2.1. Typical bond energies for each of the three types of bonds are given in Table 1.2.1.

A general feature that can be seen from the bond energies is that the covalent bonds tend to be the strongest, followed by the ionic bonds, and then finally the metallic bonds. For the metallic bonds, there is a wide range of bond energies, with some approaching that of ionic bonds, and some being very low.

Mercury has a very low bond energy, giving a bond that is not even strong enough to hold the atoms in place at room temperature, resulting in mercury's liquid state under ambient conditions.

THE FORMATION OF BULK SOLIDS

Ionic Solids

Ions are surrounded by non-directional electrostatic fields, and it is possible that the positively and negatively charged ions can find positional arrangements that are mutually beneficial from the point of view of reaching a lower energy. The ions can form a regular, three-dimensional network, with the example of sodium chloride being shown in Figure 1.2.5.

Ionic substances such as chlorides, nitrides, and oxides of metals are the basic building blocks of a group of materials known as *ceramics*, of which a rather special group are the *glasses* (see Chapter 1.3). These materials are very stable because of their high ionic bond strengths.

Metallic Solids

A similar arrangement to that of the ionic solids is possible with the metallic bond. In this case there is no strong electrostatic attraction between the individual atoms (as there was between the ions in the ionic solids), as they are held together by the cloud of electrons; this cloud forms the basis of the *metals*, which are discussed in Chapter 1.4.

Covalent Solids

There are only a few instances in which atoms of the same element join by covalent bonds to form a solid; these are carbon, silicon, and germanium. It is the directionality of the covalent bond that is the essential difference between it and the other two primary bonds. This directionality places severe constraints on the possible arrangements of the atoms.

An example of a covalently bonded solid is diamond, which is a form of carbon. Carbon has an arrangement of electrons in its outer shell such that it needs four more electrons to obtain a configuration similar to neon; in the case of diamond, it achieves this by sharing electrons with neighboring carbon atoms. The direction of these bonds is such that they are directed toward the four corners of a tetrahedron with the carbon atom's nucleus at its center. The three-dimensional structure of diamond can be built up as shown in Figure 1.2.6.

Covalent solids consisting of a single element tend to be very rare. Covalent bonds are more usually formed between dissimilar elements where each takes up an inert gas configuration. Once the elements have reacted to form these bonds, the created molecule becomes highly non-reactive toward molecules of the same type and does not provide a basis for the formation of a three-dimensional network.

The electron orbitals overlap and the electrons are shared, resulting in a filled orbital that is very stable. In this configuration there are no partially filled orbitals available for further bonding by primary bonding mechanisms. Thus covalently bonded elements result in stable molecules, and most elements, which join by covalent bonding, tend to be gases or liquids, for example, water, oxygen, and hydrogen. Of these examples, water will solidify at 0°C, and for this to be possible, there must be some additional attraction between the water molecules; something must hold these molecules together, but it is not primary bonding.

Secondary Bonding

A consequence of the sharing of electrons by two or more atomic nuclei is that the electrons will spend a disproportionately longer time in one particular position. The effect of this is that one end of the molecule may acquire a slight positive charge and the other end a slight negative charge, resulting in an electrical imbalance known as an *electric dipole*. These

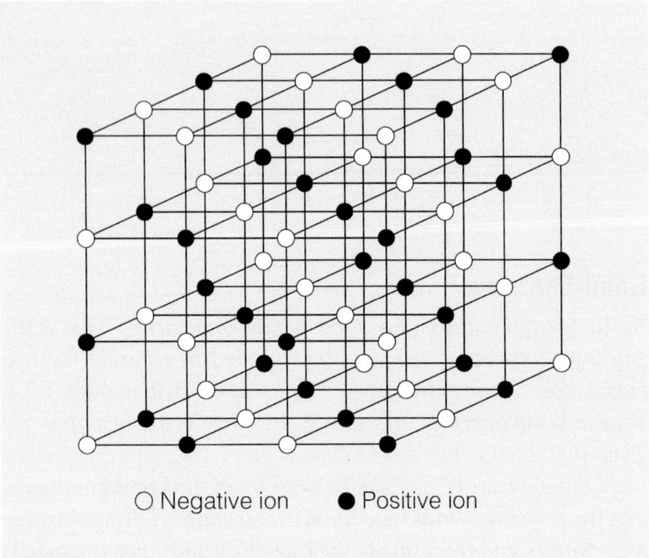

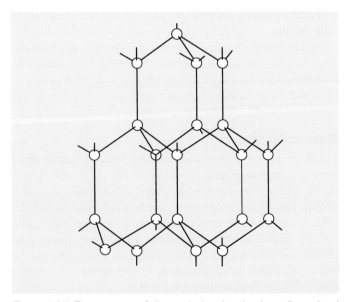

○ Negative ion   ● Positive ion

Figure 1.2.5 Formation of a bulk solid, through the ionic bonding of sodium (●) and chlorine ions (○).

Figure 1.2.6 The structure of diamond, showing the three-dimensional network built up from the tetrahedral arrangement of the carbon bonds.

dipoles allow molecules to interact with one another and to form weak bonds called *van der Waals bonds*. The three main factors that contribute to these relatively weak interactions are:

- interactions between permanent dipoles
- interactions between induced dipoles
- interactions between instantaneous dipoles.

The latter, known as the *London dispersion effect*, is completely general and operates whenever two molecules, ions, or atoms are in close contact. It is the result of an interaction between random motions of the electrons in the two species.

A special case of the dipole–dipole interaction is the hydrogen bond. The hydrogen atom can be imagined as a proton on the end of a covalent bond, but, unlike other atoms, the positive charge of the proton is not shielded by surrounding electrons. Therefore it will have a positive charge and will be attracted to the electrons of atoms in other molecules. A necessary condition for the formation of a hydrogen bond is that an electronegative atom should be in the neighborhood of the hydrogen atom, which is itself bonded to an electronegative atom. An example of this is ice, where there is an interaction between the hydrogen atom in one molecule and the oxygen atom in another molecule, shown schematically in Figure 1.2.7.

The bond strength is only about 0.4 eV and is readily overcome by heating above 0°C. The hydrogen bond is important because it accounts for the extensive adsorption possible by organic molecules, including proteins, and is therefore considered essential to life processes. Secondary bonding forms the basis of molecular attraction in molecular solids.

Molecular Solids

It is possible to create a wide variety of different molecules, some of which can be solid at room temperature. If the molecules are sufficiently large, they are bonded together due to numerous dipole–dipole interactions. The low bond strength means that such solids will have a very low melting temperature and the upper limit for molecular solids is approximately 100°C.

The best way to appreciate how these solids are formed is through a group of molecules known as linear alkanes. These are based on a straight chain of hydrocarbons, with the general formula C_nH_{2n+2}, where n can be any positive integer. The simplest of these is methane (CH_4), which has $n = 1$. If we strip one

Methane (n=1)

Ethane (n=2)

Propane (n=3)

Butane (n=4)

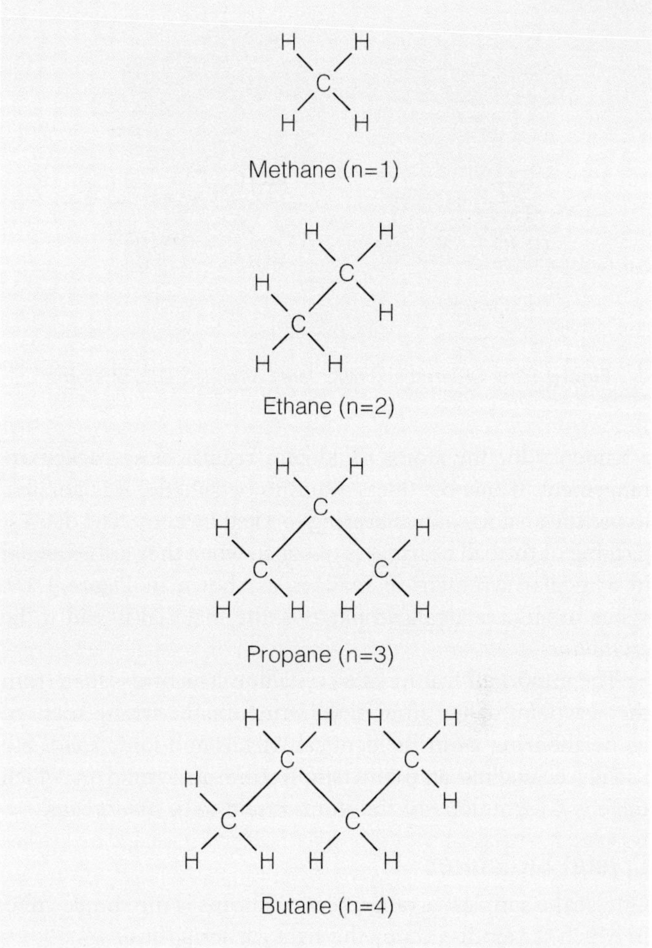

Figure 1.2.8 The first four members of the alkane family, which are straight-chain hydrocarbons, following the general formula C_nH_{2n+2}.

of the hydrogen atoms from each of the two methane molecules and join the molecules together through a carbon–carbon bond, we get ethane. We can continue to repeat this process and obtain very large molecules indeed (Figure 1.2.8).

Once the number of –CH₂– groups becomes very large, there is very little change in the properties of these materials, which are known collectively as *polymethylene*. This name is derived from the word *poly*, meaning *many*, and the basic structural unit on which it is based, *methylene*. A material with this type of structure is known as a *polymer*, since it consists of many repeat units called *mers*. How polymers can form a variety of solid structures will be discussed in detail in Chapter 1.5.

THE STRUCTURAL ARRANGEMENT OF ATOMS IN SOLIDS

Whereas the forces of attraction hold atoms close together, the mutual repulsion of the nuclei means that an equilibrium spacing is attained at which these forces balance. This interatomic spacing is presented as a_0 in Figure 1.2.1.

An external force is needed to move the atoms closer together or further apart. This interatomic spacing is the configuration of minimum energy, and in order to achieve this, there is

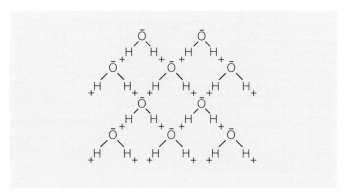

Figure 1.2.7 Hydrogen bond formation in ice.

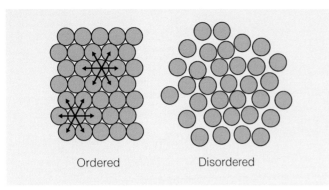

Figure 1.2.9 Ordered and disordered arrangements of atoms.

a tendency for the atoms to adopt a regular close-packed arrangement. If one considers atoms to be spheres, it is possible to use the analogy of ball bearings packed in a box. The densest packing of the ball bearings is obtained when they are arranged in a regular symmetrical manner, as shown in Figure 1.2.9. When atoms are arranged like this, the material is said to be *crystalline*.

The important feature of a crystalline structure is that, from the viewpoint of any atom in the structure, the arrangement of its neighboring atoms is identical. Metals and ionic solids are usually crystalline at room temperature. Any solid in which there is no symmetry of the atoms is said to be *amorphous*.

Crystal Structures

One of the simplest arrangements of atoms is the simple cube, in which the atoms occupy the eight corner positions.

Using the model of spheres for atoms again, this arrangement is shown in Figure 1.2.10a. Each sphere touches its nearest neighbor, such that the length of the side of the cube is equal to the diameter of the atom. If we consider a simple cube,

containing only a portion of the atoms within it, as shown in Figure 1.2.10b, we get what is known as the *structural cell*. By stacking these structural cells one on top of the other, a whole three-dimensional solid can be built up.

The atoms do not occupy all of the space of the structural unit. The fraction of space occupied by the atoms is called the *packing factor* and is easily calculated.

If we assume that each side of the cube is of length $2a$, then the volume of the structural cell is $8a^3$. Correspondingly, the radius of each sphere must be a, and its volume will be given by $4/3\pi a^3$. Each sphere actually only contributes 1/8 of its volume to the structural cell, but since there are eight such segments, the spheres within the cube occupy a total volume of $4/3\pi a^3$. Thus the packing factor for a simple cube is given by:

$$\text{packing factor} = \text{volume of atoms inside the cube}/ \text{volume of cube}$$
$$= 4/3\pi a^3/(2a)^3$$
$$= \pi/6 = 0.54$$

This indicates that nearly 50% of the space is unfilled.

It is, in fact, possible for other smaller atoms to occupy this free space without causing too much disruption to the crystalline structure, and this is something that we will return to later when discussing alloys. Given the large amount of free space in this simple structure, it is perhaps not surprising that there are other atomic arrangements where the packing factor is higher.

Two such arrangements that commonly occur in metals are the body-centered cubic (BCC) and the face-centered cubic (FCC) configurations, which are shown in Figure 1.2.11. The packing factors for these two structures are 0.68 and 0.74 for the BCC and FCC structures, respectively. With these larger packing factors, it is of course more difficult for smaller atoms to occupy the free space without upsetting the structure.

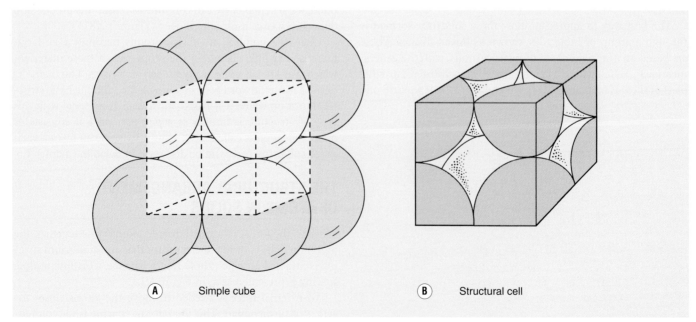

Ⓐ   Simple cube   Ⓑ   Structural cell

Figure 1.2.10 The simple cubic structure (a) and its structural cell (b).

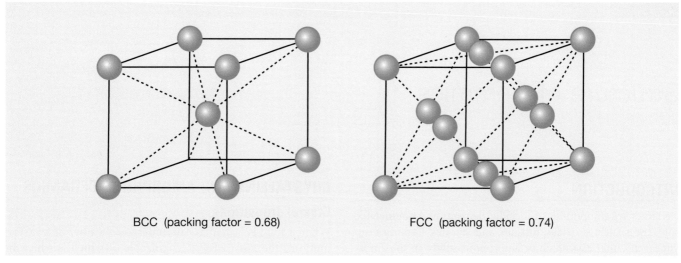

BCC (packing factor = 0.68)   FCC (packing factor = 0.74)

Figure 1.2.11 Atomic arrangements for body-centered cubic (BCC) and face-centered cubic (FCC) structures.

SUMMARY

In a sense, it is not surprising to find that there are three main groups of solids based on the three types of primary bonding, namely:

- ceramics – based on the ionic bond, which can exist in crystalline and amorphous forms, the latter being *glasses*
- metals – based on the metallic bond
- molecular solids – based on the covalent and secondary bonds, and including an important group of materials known as polymers.

There is one other important group of materials that have not yet been mentioned. These are the *composites*, which are based on a combination of two or more of the above solids.

There are many examples of composite materials, both natural and synthetic. Bone and dentine are natural composites, whose main constituents are collagen (a polymer) and apatite (a ceramic). Synthetic composites include fiber-reinforced polymers and polymers containing ceramic particles. A dental example of the latter is the composite restorative materials discussed in Chapter 2.2.

Structure of Ceramics

INTRODUCTION

Ceramics are compounds of metallic elements and nonmetallic substances such as oxides, nitrides, and silicates. Ceramics can appear as either crystalline or amorphous solids; in the amorphous state such materials are called glasses, and with an intermediate class, the 'glass ceramics', combining both amorphous and crystalline phases. This latter group presents particularly useful properties for dental materials: through careful processing and the inclusion of nucleating agents, one can attain a glassy material that contains crystalline inclusions, which has various favorable effects on properties such as a very low coefficient of thermal expansion.

In ceramics the negatively charged ions (*anions*) are often significantly different in size from the positively charged ions (*cations*). An example already considered is that of sodium chloride, which has a face-centered cubic structure.

The chlorine ions take up positions at the lattice points of the face-centered cubic (FCC) arrangement, with the sodium ions adopting positions between the chlorine ions, in what are called *interstitial positions*. The sodium ions are able to do this because they are considerably smaller than the chlorine ions and fit into the free space left between them. The exact lattice structure is shown in Figure 1.3.1. Another example of this type of structure is zinc oxide, which is widely used in dentistry. There are many other applications of ceramics in dentistry; they are used as fillers for composite resins, in glass–ionomer cements, and in investments and porcelains.

CERAMIC RAW MATERIALS

Silica (SiO_2) forms the basis of many ceramics. Although it has a simple chemical formula, it is a versatile material and can exist in many different forms.

Silica occurs as a crystalline material in the forms of quartz, cristobalite, and tridymite or as a glass, as in the example of fused silica. This ability of a compound such as silica to exist in different forms with distinctly different characteristics is known as *polymorphism*.

Silica is used as the basis for the formation of many complex ceramic formulations, particularly in combination with aluminum oxide, with which it forms alumino-silicate glasses as used in glass–ionomer cements. Similarly, feldspathic glasses are used in ceramic restorations and are compounds containing oxides of aluminum and silicon in combination with potassium, sodium, or calcium (e.g. $NaAlSi_3O_8$).

CRYSTALLINE AND AMORPHOUS CERAMICS

Crystal Transitions

When a solid is heated, it can undergo a number of transformations, the most easily recognizable of which is when the solid melts. This change of a crystal from solid to liquid is known as the *crystal melting transition* and is accompanied by a change in the volume of the material. The volume change can be monitored to allow such transformations to be detected.

A simple means of representing this change is to plot the specific volume of the material (i.e. the volume of a unit mass of the material) against the temperature. A curve such as that shown in Figure 1.3.2 results, and at the melting point of the crystal, there is a discrete (i.e. at a specific temperature) discontinuity in the specific volume.

The specific volume is effectively the inverse of the density. This specific volume–temperature curve shows that one effect of the melting of the crystal is an increase in the volume. This is not surprising when one thinks that this transition is one from an ordered crystalline structure to that of a disordered liquid; the packing density of the atoms in the liquid will be considerably less than that in the crystalline solid.

The specific volume–temperature curve for crystalline silica is as shown in Figure 1.3.3. In this example there are a number of solid–solid transitions, as well as the usual transition from solid to liquid. Silica is in the form of quartz at room temperature, which changes into tridymite at 870°C. A further transformation takes place at 1471°C, where tridymite changes to crystobalite and the crystobalite finally melts at 1713°C. Thus it is possible to detect both solid–solid and solid–liquid transitions in crystalline silica.

Glass Transitions

When an amorphous solid such as a glass is heated, it does not show a discrete solid–liquid transition as the material is not crystalline. Instead, what happens is that, at some point, there is an increase in the rate of change of the specific volume, as shown in Figure 1.3.4. The temperature at which this change in the slope of the specific volume occurs is known as the *glass transition temperature*, T_g. This is generally (although not always) the case for molecular solids as well.

A consequence of this is that there is no *sudden* increase in the volume (and hence the unoccupied volume). Instead, there is a *gradual* increase in the volume, with the rate of increase becoming more rapid above the glass transition temperature.

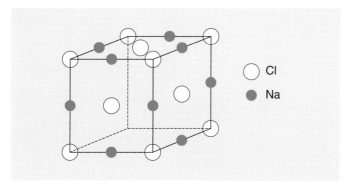

Figure 1.3.1 Face-centered cubic structure of sodium chloride.

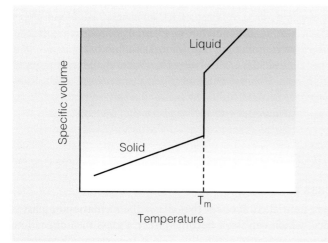

Figure 1.3.2 Transition from a solid to a liquid, where T_m is the melting temperature.

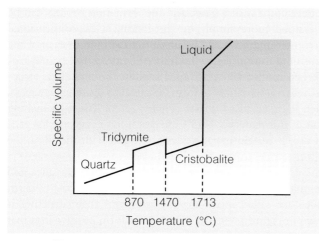

Figure 1.3.3 Solid–solid transitions for silica (SiO_2).

The converse of this is that a liquid, which cools without forming a crystalline structure, will contain a large amount of unoccupied volume. Solids, which are formed by moving through a glass transition rather than a crystal melting transition, will be amorphous and are referred to as *glasses*. Glasses

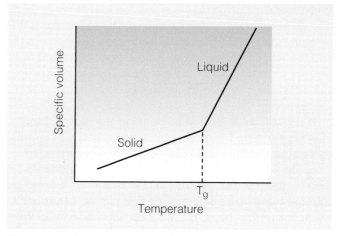

Figure 1.3.4 The variation of specific volume with temperature for an amorphous solid.

are an important group of materials and warrant some special attention.

THE FORMATION OF A GLASS

Given their regular shapes, atoms tend to form ordered structures. Small molecules such as methane are able to form crystal structures easily, and even some of the higher-order linear alkanes can form crystalline structures if the conditions are right. Once we arrive at larger, more complex molecules, however, regular arrangements become more difficult to achieve. Thus large irregular molecules have a high probability of forming a glass on solidification.

For crystal growth to occur, *nuclei of crystallization* must be present. These are usually in the form of impurities, such as dust particles, that are virtually impossible to exclude. Thus, if there is any chance that the material can take up an ordered crystalline arrangement, it will usually do so.

Silica can form either glasses or crystalline solids, and their specific volume–temperature curves are shown in Figure 1.3.5.

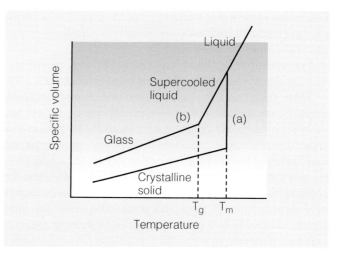

Figure 1.3.5 Cooling curves for a material that can form a crystalline solid (*a*) or a glass (*b*).

When crystallization occurs on cooling (curve a), there is a sharp, discrete reduction in the specific volume. This contraction is due to 'configurational contraction', as there is a large increase in the packing fraction when changing from a disordered liquid to an ordered crystalline solid. Once this sharp contraction has been completed, the material continues to contract by normal thermal contraction.

If crystallization did not occur, the material would follow curve b; the liquid continues to contract, partly by normal thermal contraction and partly by configurational contraction. The liquid takes up a less open structure, but there is no discrete jump in the specific volume. Below T_m, it forms an unstable *supercooled* liquid. This contraction continues as the temperature drops, until T_g, the glass transition temperature, is reached, whereupon the rate of contraction slows down markedly. At this point, the configurational contraction has stopped and only normal thermal contraction is taking place.

What happens at the glass transition temperature is that the supercooled liquid has become so viscous that configurational changes can no longer take place, and the liquid structure has been frozen in. The temperature at which this occurs is not a sharply defined point but is a range of temperatures of some 50°C, represented by the bend in the curve.

Once the supercooled liquid has cooled to below its glass transition temperature, it is now described as a *glass*. It is interesting to note that the viscosity at which this occurs is roughly the same for all glasses, about 10^{12} Pa s, although the temperature at which this happens can vary from −89°C for glycerine to over 1500°C for pure silica glass. The distinction between a supercooled liquid and a glass is that the latter has a viscosity greater than 10^{12} Pa s.

The term *transformation temperature* is somewhat of a misnomer, since no transformation actually occurs at this temperature. The configurational changes are still taking place at temperatures below T_g; it is just that the rate of change is now so small, because of the high viscosity, that to all intents and purposes, it has stopped. The glass transition temperature, that is, the temperature at which a glass that is being cooled effectively ceases to undergo configurational changes, is sometimes referred to as the *fictive temperature* of the glass. It is the temperature below which there is no spontaneous tendency for the glass to become more dense.

The question is: 'What happens at T_m that determines whether the crystal- or glass-forming route is followed?'

When silica melts, it produces an extremely viscous liquid, which means that the molecules can only move past one another very slowly. This is not conducive to the formation of a crystalline solid, since crystallization requires a substantial and rapid rearrangement of the molecules. Any crystal nuclei present will therefore tend to grow very slowly, especially given the complex structure of crystalline silica, which is similar to that of diamond. Thus, if the liquid is cooled quickly, the solid formed is likely to be a glass. The process of forming a glass is called *vitrification*.

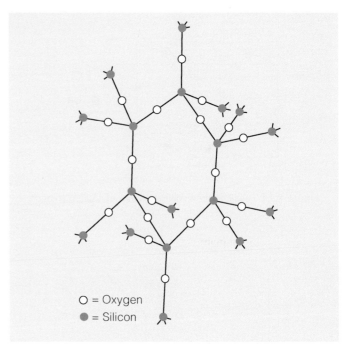

O = Oxygen
● = Silicon

Figure 1.3.6 Crystalline structure of cristobalite.

Glass Formers

The essential component that allows the formation of glass is silica, which can itself become either a glass or a crystalline solid on cooling. Cristobalite, one of the crystalline forms of silica, has a tetrahedron as its basic unit, with an oxygen atom at each corner and a silicon atom in the center, as shown in Figure 1.3.6.

This is a rather complex structure to use when visualizing the development of a glass, and the formation process can be understood more simply by considering a two-dimensional representation, in which one bond is missing from each of the atoms in the silica (Figure 1.3.7).

When molten silica is cooled rapidly, the crystalline structure does not have time to form, so the silica solidifies as a glass, which is called fused quartz (Figure 1.3.8). The high melting point of this material, 1713°C, makes it too expensive for general use. If certain metal oxides are mixed with the silica, the melting temperature is greatly reduced.

As an example, a composition of three-quarters silica and one-quarter sodium oxide will melt at only 1339°C. Such glasses are called *mixed oxide glasses*, and their structure is shown in Figure 1.3.9. The metal atoms form positive ions that disrupt the oxygen tetrahedra such that not all of the oxygen atoms are shared. The silica plays the role of a *glass former* and the metal oxide acts as a *glass modifier*.

Oxides of titanium, zinc, lead, and aluminum can all take part in the formation of the glassy network and produce stiff network structures. Soda (Na_2O) and lime (CaO) considerably lower the viscosity, and thus the glass transition

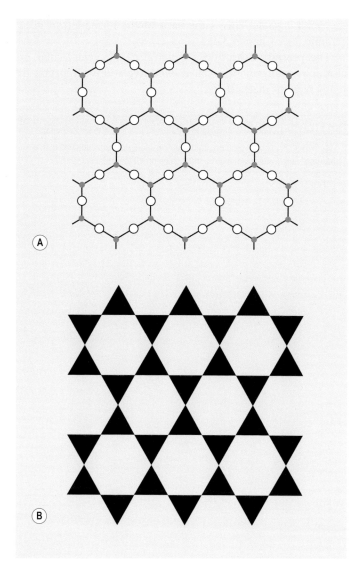

Figure 1.3.7 Two-dimensional representation of crystalline silica: (a) position of atoms, (b) oxygen triangles.

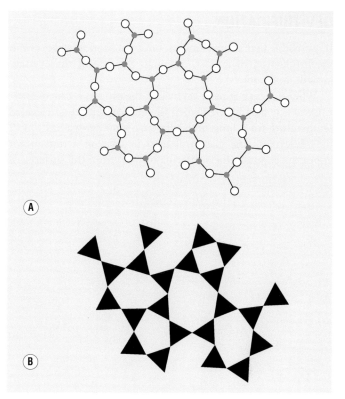

Figure 1.3.8 Two-dimensional representation of a pure silica glass: (a) position of atoms, (b) oxygen triangles.

temperature, by causing extensive disruption of the network. This eases the production of the glass. Boric oxide (B_2O_3) is also capable of acting as a glass former, producing boron glasses.

Although it is possible to make glasses from mixtures of crystalline silica and metal oxides, this is an expensive approach. It is much cheaper to use naturally occurring minerals with the required glassy structure, because nature has already carried out the vitrification process.

At one time, only naturally occurring feldspars were used by manufacturers, and these were modified with other metallic oxides to produce fillers and dental porcelains with the required properties. Nowadays, many glasses are produced synthetically, as this allows greater control over the composition and properties.

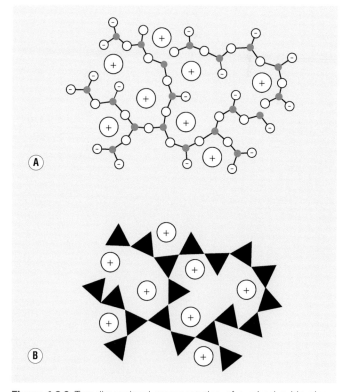

Figure 1.3.9 Two-dimensional representation of a mixed oxide glass: (a) position of atoms, (b) oxygen triangles.

DEVITRIFICATION

It is possible that a small amount of crystallization will occur in the production of a glass, although the rate of the crystals' growth is very low.

When a glass begins to crystallize, the process is called *devitrification*. It may happen when the glass is kept at an elevated temperature for a long time, allowing some reorganization of the molecules. The glass will tend to take on a translucent appearance, due to the scattering of light from the surfaces of the small crystals. This is the basis of the formation of glass ceramics (see Chapter 3.4).

The process of heating a material to allow molecular or atomic rearrangement is called *annealing* and is important in many types of materials.

CLINICAL SIGNIFICANCE

Ceramics tend to be extremely stable in the biological environment and are therefore perceived as among the most biocompatible of biomaterials.

Structure of Metals and Alloys

MICROSTRUCTURE OF METALS

Metals consist of aggregates of atoms regularly arranged in a crystalline structure. Whereas so far we have considered the formation of single crystals, metals do not often solidify (from what is known as the *melt*) as a single crystal, but instead are usually formed of a multitude of small crystals.

This happens because there are usually many *nuclei of crystallization* scattered throughout the molten metal. Such nuclei may form when four atoms lose sufficient thermal energy and become able to form a unit cell. These unit cells will grow as more metal atoms reach a low enough energy to join on, and hence crystal formation occurs. This process is known as homogeneous nucleation. It requires highly specialized equipment to grow a single crystal of metal from the entire melt.

More commonly, solidification is initiated by the presence of impurities in the melt. As the temperature drops below the melting point, metal atoms will deposit on these impurities and crystals begin to form. This process is known as heterogeneous nucleation. The crystals (or *grains*, as they are called) will continue to grow until all of the metal has solidified. During their growth, they will begin to impinge on one another, giving rise to boundaries between the crystals where the atoms are irregularly arranged. This boundary is called the *grain boundary* and is essentially a defect in the crystal structure of the metal.

The process of solidification of a metal is shown schematically in Figure 1.4.1. A fine grain size is usually desirable in a metal because it raises the yield stress, but the reason for this will not be considered now. One way in which to promote a finer grain size is rapid solidification, as used in the casting of dental gold alloys into an investment mold that is held at a temperature well below the melting temperature of the alloy. Alternatively, the presence of many nucleating sites will give rise to a fine grain size. This method is also employed in dental gold alloys by the addition of iridium. The iridium provides many sites for nucleation and acts as a grain-refining ingredient.

It is very useful to be able to study the detailed structure of metals, in terms of the sizes of the crystals, their shape, and their composition, because this information can tell us a lot about the properties of the metal and how it was made. Some idea of the structure can be obtained by examining the metal surface under a light-reflecting optical microscope.

Light is reflected from a polished metal surface, but the fraction of the incident light that is reflected from any region will depend on surface irregularities, as irregularities will cause the light to be scattered.

The action of chemicals on a polished surface (known as *etching*) can also reduce the amount of light reflected. A suitably chosen chemical will preferentially attack certain regions of the metal surface. These areas tend to be under high local stress, such as at the grain boundaries, where there is imperfect packing of the atoms. In effect, a groove is produced that scatters the incident light and therefore shows up as a dark line.

This effect is shown schematically in Figure 1.4.2 for a metal that has a very uniform grain structure. All the grains are of roughly the same size and shape; such a grain structure is described as *equiaxed*. An example of the grain structure for a hypoeutectoid stainless steel, revealed by etching, is shown in Figure 1.4.3. Many other shapes and sizes of grains are possible, and these properties often depend on the methods employed during solidification. For example, if molten metal is poured into a mold with a square or circular cross-section that is held at a temperature well below the melting temperature of the metal, the grains could look something like that depicted in Figure 1.4.4. Crystal growth will have proceeded from the walls of the mold toward the center.

Many metals are readily deformed, especially in their elemental (i.e. pure) form. This allows them to be shaped by hammering, rolling, pressing, or drawing through a die. A large casting, known as an ingot, can thus be turned into any desired shape, be it a wing-panel for a car, the shell of a boat, or a wire.

When deformed in this way, the metal is said to be *wrought*. If we were to examine the microstructure of a wire under the optical microscope, it would be seen to have a structure similar to that shown in Figure 1.4.5. The grains have been elongated in the direction of the drawing and have taken on a laminar structure. Thus, by looking at the microstructure of the metal, we can gain a lot of information.

ALLOYS

Elemental metals are not generally of much use because of the severe limitations in their properties. Most metals in common use are a mixture of two or more metallic elements, sometimes with non-metallic elements included. They are usually produced by the fusion of the elements above their melting temperatures. Such a mixture of two or more metals or metalloids is called an *alloy*. Two elements would constitute a *binary alloy* and a mixture of three is called a *ternary alloy*.

An alloy will often consist of a number of distinct solid *phases*, where a *phase* is defined as a structurally homogeneous part of the system that is separated from other parts by a definite

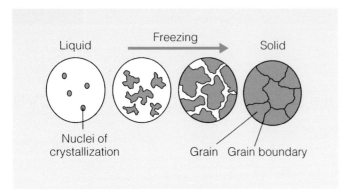

Figure 1.4.1 Solidification of a metal.

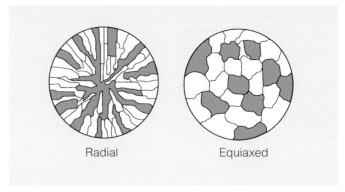

Figure 1.4.4 Grain structures arising from different conditions at solidification.

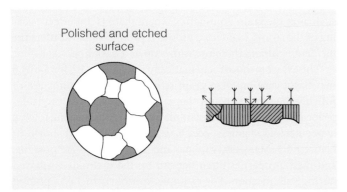

Figure 1.4.2 Reflection of incident light from an etched metal surface.

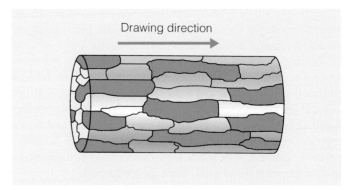

Figure 1.4.5 Elongated grains of a metal drawn into a wire.

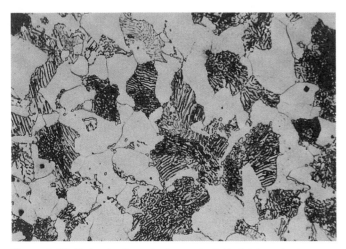

Figure 1.4.3 Grain structures for hypoeutectoid stainless steel.

physical boundary. Each phase will have its own distinct structure and associated properties.

The commonly cited phases are the gas, liquid, and solid phases, as these are markedly different from one another. A substance can exhibit several phases.

For example, water would be considered a single-phase structure, whereas a mixture of water and oil would consist of two phases. Sand would be considered a single-phase system, even though it is made up of lots of individual particles, since each particle of sand is identical.

A phase may have more than one component – as does saline, for instance, which is an aqueous solution of sodium chloride. Similarly, phases in metals can consist of a mixture of metals. Copper can contain up to 40% zinc without destroying its FCC structure. Such a *solid solution,* as it is called, will satisfy some special conditions (see below).

SOLID PHASES

When two different elements are mixed together, the resultant material can be a single-phase alloy or a multi-phase alloy. Which of these is formed depends on the solubility of one element in the other, and this is governed by the crystalline nature of the elements and their relative sizes.

There are essentially three different phases that can form an alloy: a pure metal, a solid solution, or an intermetallic compound. Of these, the solid solution and the intermetallic compound require further description.

Solid Solutions

A solid solution is a mixture of elements at the atomic level and is analogous to a mixture of liquids that are soluble in one another. There are two types of solid solutions: substitutional and interstitial.

Substitutional Solid Solution

If the solute atom can substitute directly for the solvent atom at the normal lattice sites of the crystal, a substitutional solid

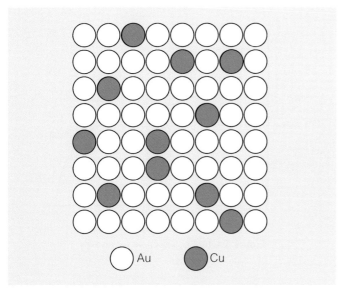

Figure 1.4.6 Substitutional solid solution.

TABLE 1.4.1	**Properties of Gold and Copper**		
Element	Atomic Diameter (Å)	Crystal Structure	Valence
Au	2.882	FCC	1 or 3
Cu	2.556	FCC	1 or 2

solution of the two elements will be formed. This will only be possible if:

- the atoms have a similar valency
- the atoms have the same crystal structure (e.g. FCC)
- the atomic sizes are within 15% of each other.

A dentally relevant example of such a system is a mixture of gold and copper (Figure 1.4.6).

Adding any amount of copper will always give a solid solution. Thus a *substitutional solid solution* can be made to range from 100% gold to 100% copper. This is because these two metals (Table 1.4.1) meet the above conditions.

Other metals that readily form solid solutions with gold are platinum (2.775 Å), palladium (2.750 Å), and silver (2.888 Å), all of which have an FCC crystal structure.

Interstitial Solid Solution

As the name implies, an interstitial solid solution is achieved when the solute atoms are able to take up the space in between the solvent atoms. For this to occur, the solute atom must, of course, be much smaller than the solvent atom. In practice, the diameter of the solute atom must be less than 60% of the diameter of the solvent atom. This is illustrated for the example of a type of steel that contains a small amount of carbon in iron (Figure 1.4.7).

The interstitial space is usually very limited, and some distortion of the lattice will occur to accommodate the extra atoms. Other elements that readily form interstitial solid solutions are hydrogen, nitrogen, and boron.

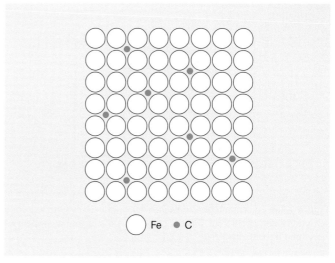

Figure 1.4.7 Interstitial solid solution.

Intermetallic Compounds

An intermetallic compound is formed when two or more metals combine, forming a specific composition or stoichiometric ratio. Some intermetallic compounds include zones of phases of different stoichiometric ratios. This has consequences for their physical properties: the phase structure tends to make the intermetallic compound more brittle, less ductile, than solid solutions. A dental example of an intermetallic compound is dental amalgam; the alloy may contain regions of an Ag–Sn phase (Ag_3Sn), a Ag–Hg phase (Ag_2Hg_3), and a Cu–Sn phase (Cu_6Sn_5). Amalgam is a more brittle alloy than many others used in dentistry, and this gives rise to a phenomenon known as ditching.

PHASE DIAGRAMS

Alloys can consist of a wide number of different phases, depending on the composition and temperature, and a means of representing this graphically has been developed, in what is known as a *phase diagram*.

Such a diagram indicates the phases (including the liquid phase) that are present at any given temperature, for any given composition of the alloy.

Solid Solutions

The simplest phase diagrams to understand are the binary phase diagrams.

An example of a phase diagram for such a simple system is shown in Figure 1.4.8. This phase diagram is for copper and nickel; the vertical axis represents the temperature and the horizontal axis the composition. Copper and nickel are so close in characteristics that they readily substitute for one another in the crystal lattice and form an example of a substitutional solid solution. Hence, throughout the compositional range from pure copper to pure nickel, only a single phase occurs.

Whereas one might expect the melting temperature of such an alloy to fall somewhere between that of pure copper and that

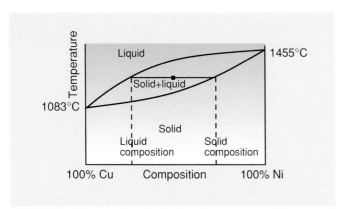

Figure 1.4.8 Equilibrium phase diagram for the Cu–Ni system, where a 50Cu:50Ni composition at 1300°C produces a mixture of a copper-rich liquid and a nickel-rich solid.

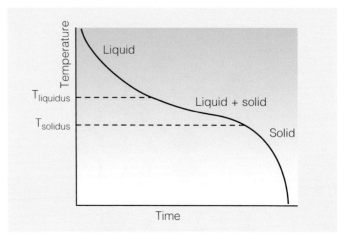

Figure 1.4.10 Cooling curve for an alloy.

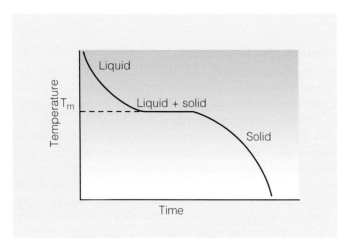

Figure 1.4.9 Cooling curve for a pure metal.

of pure nickel, it is not immediately obvious why there should be a region where there is a mixture of liquid and solid. The line that defines the transition from pure liquid to a mixture of liquid and solid is called the *liquidus,* and the line that separates the mixture of solid and liquid from the solid is known as the *solidus.*

When a pure metal solidifies, the transformation from a liquid to solid takes place at a well-defined discrete temperature; this is the characteristic melting temperature of the metal. If a temperature–time curve were constructed for such a metal as it cooled, it would look like that in Figure 1.4.9.

The plateau spans the period during which the metal is solidifying, and the liquidus and solidus are effectively one and the same point. The reason for this plateau is the release of energy (in the form of heat) during the solidification process, which maintains the metal at a constant temperature. This energy is called the *latent heat of fusion.*

When two metals are mixed to form an alloy, the cooling curve looks quite different (Figure 1.4.10), as the alloy solidifies over a range of temperatures. The liquidus and solidus are now separate points on the cooling curve.

The reason for the extended temperature range, covering the transition from liquid to solid for an alloy of copper and nickel, is that the copper and nickel atoms are not identical. As a consequence, in the region between the melting temperatures of the two metals, a copper-rich liquid and a nickel-rich solid are the most stable compounds.

For instance, for a 50:50 composition at 1300°C, solid nickel cannot contain more than 37 w% copper. Any copper atoms above the 37 w% level will therefore appear in the liquid phase, mixed with the remaining nickel. Such a mixture of solid and liquid provides a lower free energy than a single phase alone.

In effect, the solidus and liquidus represent the limits of solubility, and it is these that form the basis of the phase diagram. By creating a series of the cooling curves shown in Figures 1.4.9 and 1.4.10 for a range of compositions, it is possible to build up the phase diagram as shown schematically in Figure 1.4.11.

As the temperature of the 50:50 composition is reduced, the solubility of copper in nickel increases, until, at approximately 1220°C, all of the available copper can be dissolved in the nickel, and a single solid phase is the most stable configuration.

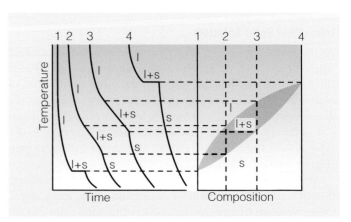

Figure 1.4.11 Construction of a phase diagram.

Partial Solid Solubility

More usually, the components of materials are not sufficiently soluble to form a complete series of solid solutions. Examples of this are copper and silver, which are sufficiently different in atomic size that their atoms are only partially soluble in one another.

The phase diagram for this system is shown in Figure 1.4.12. For a wide range of compositions, the material will consist of two solid phases, one being silver rich and one being copper rich; by convention, these are called the α- and the β-phase, respectively. The α-phase consists of predominantly silver, with a small amount of copper dissolved in it, whereas the β-phase consists of copper, with a small amount of silver dissolved in it.

At low concentrations of copper in silver, all of the copper is able to dissolve in the silver, and only a single phase exists. The maximum solubility of copper in silver is 8.8 w%, and this occurs at a temperature of approximately 780°C.

At lower temperatures, the solubility of copper in silver decreases, and the excess copper separates out as the second, β-phase.

Similar behavior occurs at the other end of the compositional range, where the limited solubility of silver in copper also gives rise to the formation of a two-phase structure.

An interesting and important feature of the phase diagram of the Ag–Cu system is the depression of the temperature of the liquidus at a composition of 72Ag:28Cu. At a temperature of 780°C, this composition of the alloy can exist as three phases: α, β, and liquid. This is called the *eutectic point*, and the temperature at the intersection of the three phases is the *eutectic temperature*. The composition is called the *eutectic composition* of the alloy.

If a eutectic liquid is cooled, it changes directly into two solid phases, without an interposing state as a liquid–solid mixture, something that occurs at all other compositions. This feature of some alloy systems can be utilized to form low-melting-temperature materials, such as alloys used as soldering materials.

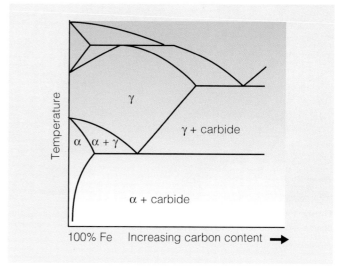

Figure 1.4.13 Equilibrium phase diagram for the Fe–C system.

In the same way that a eutectic involves the formation of two solid phases from a single liquid phase, such a transformation can also occur in solids.

The phase diagram of the Fe–C system, shown partially in Figure 1.4.13, is an example of this. For a composition of 0.8C:99.2Fe, the solid solution, γ, transforms to a solid solution of carbon in iron, α, and carbide (Fe_3C) at a temperature of 723°C. This is called a *eutectoid reaction* and differs only from the eutectic in that all three phases are solids.

Such transformations as described (and it should be noted that there are others) are extremely important in determining the microstructure and, consequently, the properties of the alloy.

NON-EQUILIBRIUM CONDITIONS

It must be stressed that the phase diagrams described above are what are known as *equilibrium phase diagrams*. The material would have to be held at a set temperature for a considerable time to achieve the phase structure shown in such diagrams. In practice, the solidification and cooling rates of alloys do not allow the formation of an equilibrium phase structure.

Above, it was noted that, for a composition of 50Cu:50Ni at 1300°C, a liquid phase rich in copper and a solid phase consisting of 63Ni:37Cu coexist. On rapid cooling, it is not possible for these liquid and solid phases to readjust their compositions, and some of the nickel-rich solid will be retained. As the material continues to cool, a composition richer in nickel will solidify, leaving the remaining liquid, and the subsequently formed solid, richer in copper. The overall effect of this is that the solid will consist of a multitude of crystals with a wide range of compositions, all in the same phase. This formation of a solid with a non-uniform composition is known as *compositional segregation*.

In systems with multiple phases the phase with the highest melting temperature will always be the first to solidify, followed by the phases with lower melting temperatures. As the first phase solidifies, it tends to form a lattice structure known as *dendrites* (Figure 1.4.14).

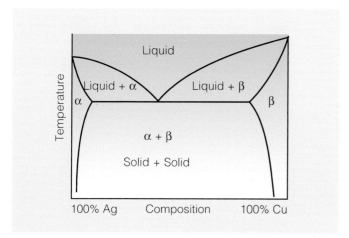

Figure 1.4.12 Equilibrium phase diagram for the Ag–Cu system.

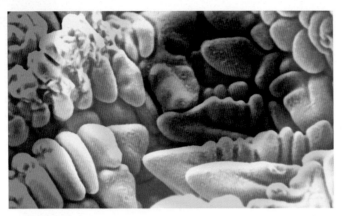

Figure 1.4.14 Scanning electron microscope (SEM) micrograph of the coarse dendritic structure for a Co–Cr alloy.

Compositional segregation can be eliminated, or reduced, by reheating the alloy to a temperature just below the solidus and holding it at that temperature for some time. This allows the atoms time to diffuse through the system and attain their equilibrium condition.

The process of heat-treating an alloy is known as *annealing*, and if the intention is to achieve a homogeneous composition, it is described as a *homogenization anneal*.

CLINICAL SIGNIFICANCE

In order to obtain the best mechanical properties, alloys rather than pure metals are used in dentistry. While alloys used in dentistry share many properties, such as high thermal conductivity and typically good mechanical properties, the intermetallic compounds – the main example being amalgam – exhibit a degree of brittleness not seen in other alloys.

Structure of Polymers

INTRODUCTION

Plastics and rubbers, as they are generally called in everyday life, have the common property of being *polymers*. Polymers are long-chain molecules, consisting of many repeating units, as discussed already in Chapter 1.2. Polymers are not a recent invention; they are, in fact, older than human beings themselves and in one form or another are the basic constituents of every kind of living matter, whether plant or animal. Examples of naturally occurring polymers are agar, cellulose, DNA, proteins, natural rubber, collagen, and silk. Examples of synthetic polymers in everyday use are PVC (polyvinyl chloride), polyethylene, spandex, and polystyrene.

Originally, the synthetic polymers tended to be regarded as substitutes for existing natural polymers, such as rubber and silk. Nowadays, such a wide variety of polymers can be produced that they have entered into every walk of life, satisfying needs that did not previously exist. Pertinent examples are medical applications, such as dialysis and oxygenator membranes, and dental applications such as filling materials.

The starting material for the production of a polymer is the *monomer*. In a material such as polyethylene the repeating unit is a CH_2 group, with many of these units joined together to form a long chain (Figure 1.5.1a). The monomer from which this polymer is derived is ethylene (Figure 1.5.1b).

A polymer with a similar structure to polyethylene is polypropylene. It is formed by joining molecules of propylene (Figure 1.5.2a). Propylene differs from ethylene in having a methyl group (CH_3) that replaces one of the hydrogen atoms, forming the polymer polypropylene (Figure 1.5.2b).

Polypropylene is slightly more complex than polyethylene, in that the arrangement of the methyl groups can vary so that they:
- are all on one side (*isotactic*)
- alternate from side to side (*syndiotactic*)
- are switched from side to side in a random manner (*atactic*).

A number of polymers based on vinyl monomers are presented in Table 1.5.1.

It should be noted that the chemical routes by which these different polymers are made are quite different, and that it is not a simple matter of modification to form one from the other. Each polymer has its own characteristic repeating unit, or 'fingerprint', and this unit is the basis for the widely differing properties of the polymers.

The most common polymers are those made from the organic compounds of carbon, but polymers can also be made from inorganic compounds, based on silica (SiO_2).

Silicon, being four-valent like carbon, provides the opportunity to form the backbone for the polymer, together with oxygen. An example of a silicone polymer is polydimethylsiloxane (Figure 1.5.3).

When a polymer is formed from a single species of monomer, it is called a *homopolymer*; when different species are included, it is called a *copolymer* or *heteropolymer*.

MECHANISMS OF POLYMERIZATION

The monomers shown in Table 1.5.1 all have a double bond in common, which is opened up to allow the monomer to bond to a neighboring monomer. This process of preparing polymers from monomers is called *polymerization*. There are two ways in which this may be achieved: *addition polymerization* and *condensation polymerization*.

Addition polymerization

Addition polymerization is defined as occurring when a reaction between two molecules (either the same to form a *homopolymer*, or dissimilar to form a *copolymer*) produces a larger molecule without the elimination of a smaller molecule (such as water).

This type of reaction takes place for vinyl compounds, which are reactive inorganic compounds containing carbon–carbon double bonds (see Table 1.5.1). The process of addition polymerization involves four stages to produce these polymers:
- activation
- initiation
- propagation
- termination.

Activation

The polymerization of a vinyl compound requires the presence of *free radicals* (•). These are very reactive chemical species that have an odd (unpaired) electron. The process of producing free radicals is described as *activation*. Activation occurs, for instance, in the decomposition of a peroxide.

The peroxide commonly used in dental materials is benzoyl peroxide. Under appropriate conditions, a molecule of benzoyl peroxide can yield two free radicals:

$$C_6H_5COO - OOCH_5C_6 \rightarrow 2(C_6H_5COO\cdot)$$

This in turn can decompose to form other free radicals:

$$C_6H_5COO\cdot \rightarrow C_6H_5\cdot + CO_2$$

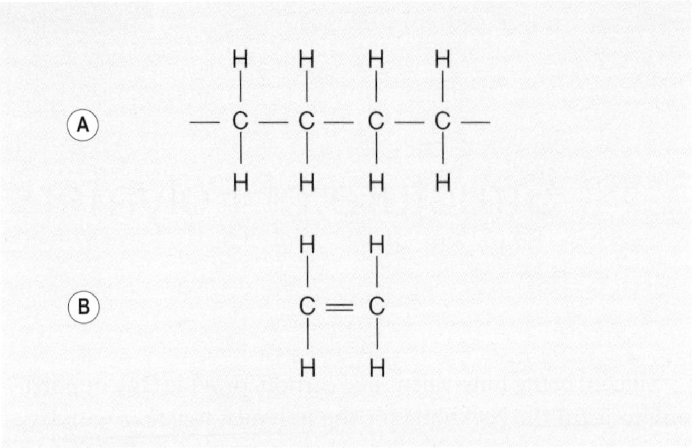

Figure 1.5.1 Polyethylene (a) is derived from ethylene (b).

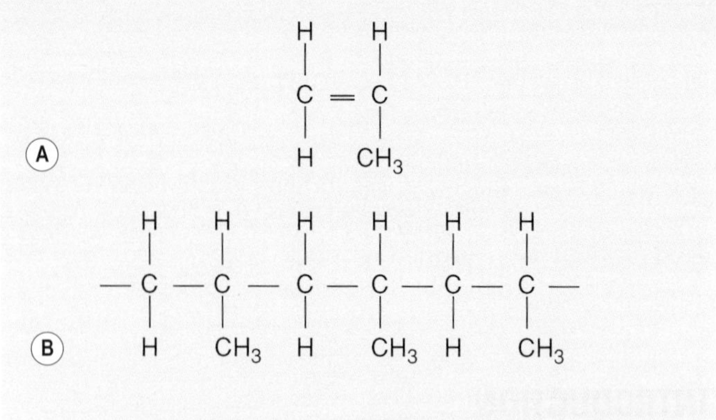

Figure 1.5.2 Propylene (a) polymerizes to give polypropylene (b).

TABLE 1.5.1 Some Monomers and Their Polymers

Name	Monomer	Polymer
Polyvinyl chloride (PVC)	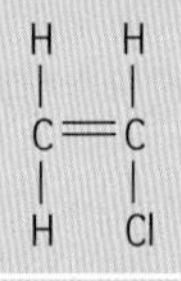 CH$_2$=CHCl	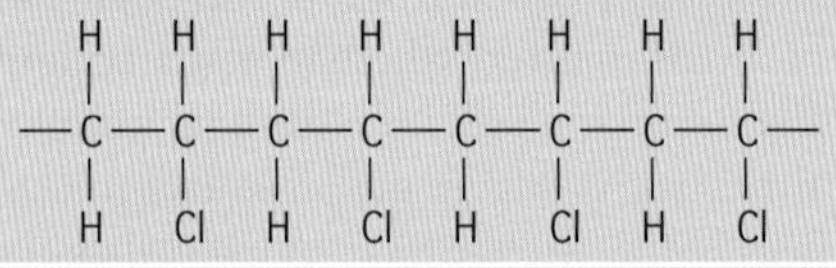 —CH$_2$—CHCl—CH$_2$—CHCl—CH$_2$—CHCl—CH$_2$—CHCl—
Polytetrafluoroethylene (PTFE)	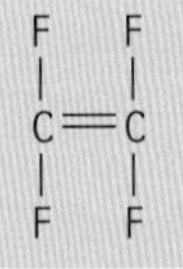 CF$_2$=CF$_2$	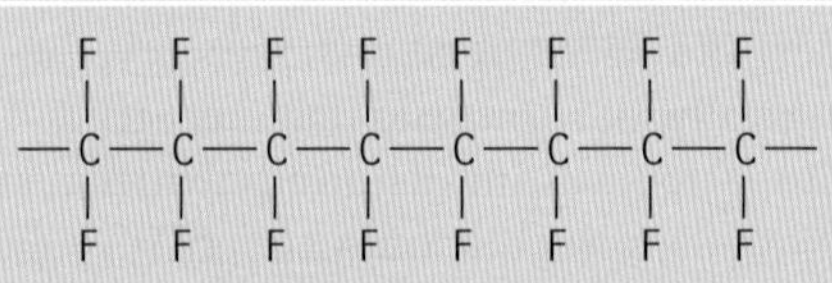 —CF$_2$—CF$_2$—CF$_2$—CF$_2$—CF$_2$—CF$_2$—CF$_2$—CF$_2$—
Polypropylene isotactic	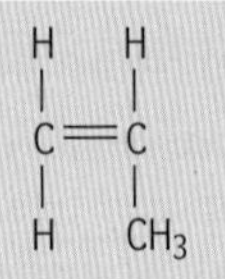 CH$_2$=CH(CH$_3$)	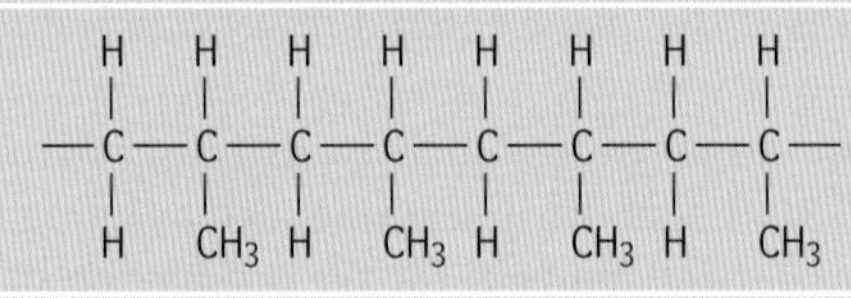 —CH$_2$—CH(CH$_3$)—CH$_2$—CH(CH$_3$)—CH$_2$—CH(CH$_3$)—CH$_2$—CH(CH$_3$)—
Polyacrylic acid	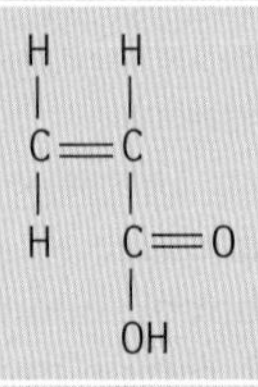 CH$_2$=CH(COOH)	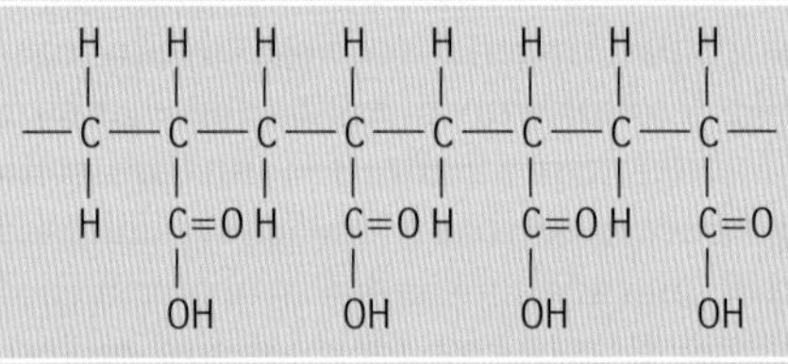 —CH$_2$—CH(COOH)—CH$_2$—CH(COOH)—CH$_2$—CH(COOH)—CH$_2$—CH(COOH)—
Polymethylmethacrylate	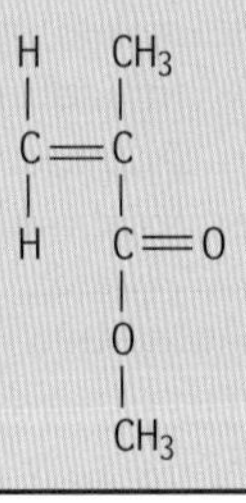 CH$_2$=C(CH$_3$)(COOCH$_3$)	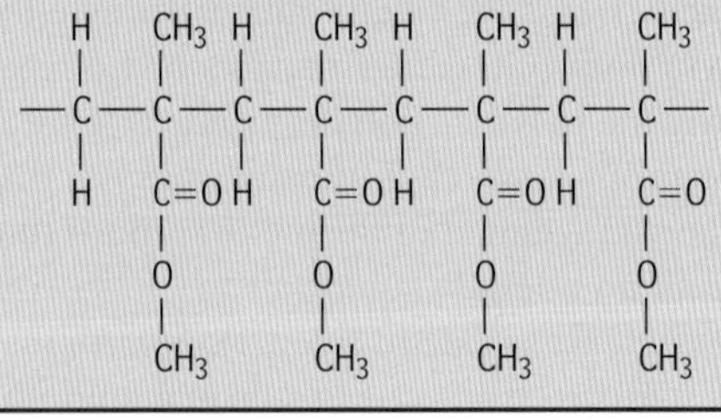 —CH$_2$—C(CH$_3$)(COOCH$_3$)—CH$_2$—C(CH$_3$)(COOCH$_3$)—CH$_2$—C(CH$_3$)(COOCH$_3$)—CH$_2$—C(CH$_3$)(COOCH$_3$)—

Such chemical species, known as *initiators,* are able to initiate vinyl polymerization, as described later, and are designated as R•.

Before initiation occurs, however, the benzoyl peroxide needs to be activated. This activation is achieved by the decomposition of the peroxide, due to the use of an *activator,* such as:

- *Heat.* When heated above 65°C, the benzoyl peroxide decomposes, as shown above. This is the method used in the production of acrylic resin denture bases (see Chapter 3.2).

- *Chemical compounds.* The benzoyl peroxide can also be activated when brought into contact with a tertiary amine such as *n,n*-dimethyl-*p*-toluidine (Figure 1.5.4). This method is employed in cold-cured acrylic resins, used, for example, in denture repairs, temporary restorations, orthodontic appliances, and special trays (see Chapter 3.2). The same method is also used in chemically cured composite restorative materials, which consist of a base paste containing the tertiary amine activator and a catalyst paste containing the benzoyl peroxide initiator (see Chapter 2.2).

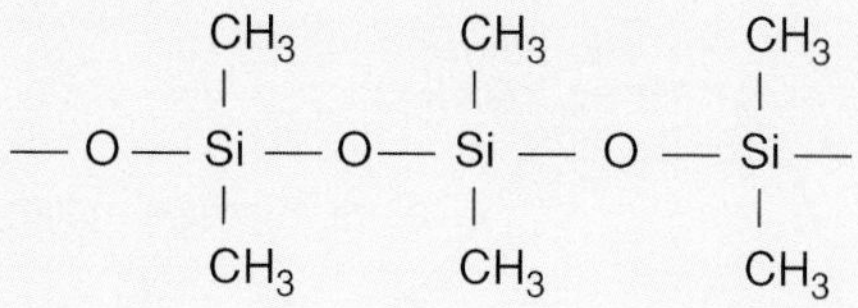

Figure 1.5.3 The structure of polydimethylsiloxane.

- *Light.* Yet another method for the creation of free radicals is employed by light-activated composites; these rely on light, usually in the visible part of the electromagnetic spectrum, as the activator of the polymerization reaction. In these instances, initiators other than benzoyl peroxide are employed, a common example being camphorquinone. Some materials employ more than one form of polymerization activator to allow, for instance, curing in the presence *and* absence of light.

Other forms of free radical production include the use of ultraviolet light in conjunction with a benzoin methyl ether, and visible light with an α-diketone and an amine (see Chapter 2.2).

Initiation

The free radicals can react with a monomer such as ethylene and *initiate* the polymerization process as follows:

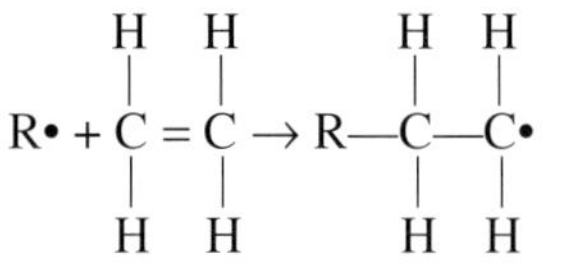

Propagation

The free radical is transferred to the monomer, which can, in turn, react with another monomer.

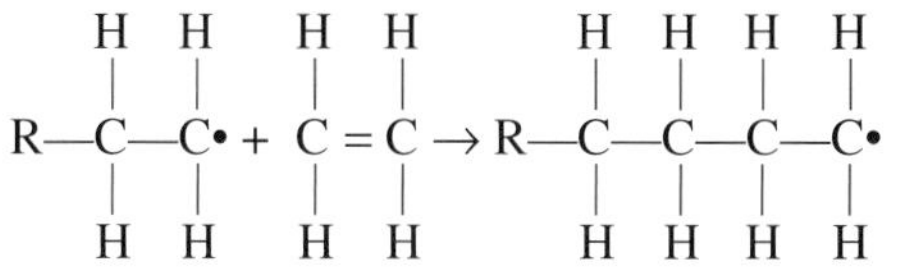

Repeating this process again and again generates the polymer chain until the growing chains collide or all of the free radicals have reacted.

Termination

Free radicals can react to form a stable molecule.

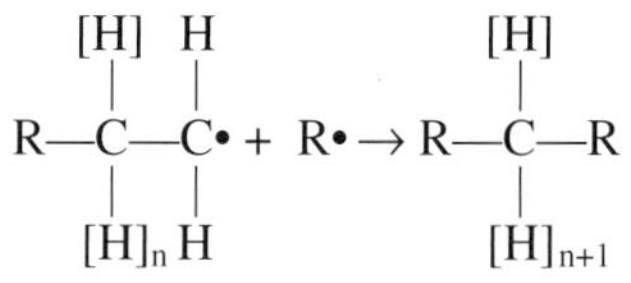

Since *n* will vary from polymer chain to polymer chain, a wide range of long-chain molecules are produced. In most situations, there will also be some unreacted monomer and some *oligomers,* which consist of just a few repeating units.

Condensation Polymerization

Condensation polymerization occurs when two molecules (not usually the same) react to form a larger molecule with the elimination of a smaller molecule (often, but not always, water).

In this case, monomer units with a carbon–carbon double bond are not necessary, as shown in the following example of a silicone, which is an inorganic polymer formed by the condensation of silanols.

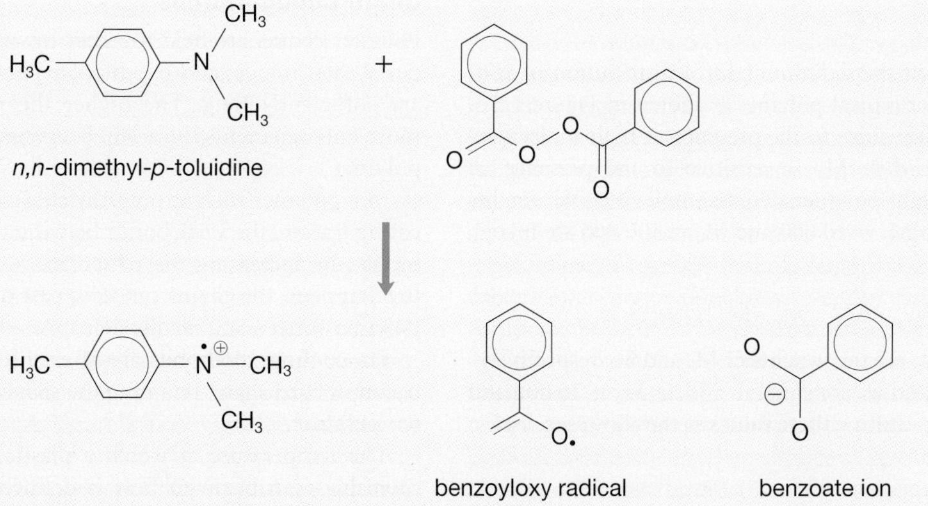

n,n-dimethyl-p-toluidine

benzoyloxy radical   benzoate ion

Figure 1.5.4 Benzoyl peroxide activated by a tertiary amine.

$$HO—\underset{\underset{R}{|}}{\overset{\overset{R}{|}}{Si}}—OH + HO—\underset{\underset{R}{|}}{\overset{\overset{R}{|}}{Si}}—OH \rightarrow$$

$$HO—\underset{\underset{R}{|}}{\overset{\overset{R}{|}}{Si}}—O—\underset{\underset{R}{|}}{\overset{\overset{R}{|}}{Si}}—OH + H_2O$$

In this case R is an organic group, such as a methyl (CH_3), and the by-product is water.

POLYMERIC STRUCTURES

Molecular Weight

The molecular weight of a polymer is equal to the number of repeating units (i.e. the *degree of polymerization*) multiplied by the molecular weight of the repeating unit. In both addition and condensation polymerization the length of the chain is determined by purely random events; not all of the chains will be of the same length and, in general, many different chain lengths will be present. Thus, the molecular weight can only be represented by an average value.

There are a number of ways in which the molecular weight can be determined for a polymer. Two main ones are the *number average molecular weight*, M_n, and the *weight average molecular weight*, M_w.

Number Average Molecular Weight (M_n)

M_n is obtained by counting the number of molecules in a given weight of sample. The general expression would be given by:

$$M_n = \Sigma n_i M_i / \Sigma n_i$$

Weight Average Molecular Weight (M_w)

M_w is obtained by measurement of the weight of the molecules in the total sample weight, given by the general expression:

$$M_w = \Sigma w_i M_i / w_i$$

The difference in the definitions for a distribution of molecular weights in a typical polymer is shown in Figure 1.5.5. M_w is particularly sensitive to the presence of high-molecular-weight polymers, while M_n is sensitive to the presence of low-molecular-weight polymers. For example, if equal weights of two polymers of $M_a = 10\,000$ and $M_b = 100\,000$ are mixed, M_w is given by:

$$M_w = (W_a \times M_a + w_b \times M_b)/(w_a + w_b)$$

where w_a and w_b are the weights of M_a and M_b respectively.

In this case w_a and w_b are equal to $\frac{1}{2}W$, as $M_a = 10\,000$ and $M_b = 100\,000$. Substituting these values in the above expression gives:

$$M_w = (\tfrac{1}{2}W \times 10\,000 + \tfrac{1}{2}W \times 100\,000)/W$$
$$= 55\,000$$

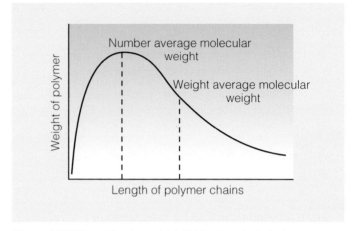

Figure 1.5.5 The molecular weight distribution of a typical polymer.

The number average molecular weight is given by:

$$M_n = (n_a \times M_a + m_b \times M_b)/(n_a + m_b)$$

where n_a and m_b are the number of molecules of molecular weight M_a and M_b, respectively. In this case $n_a = 10$ and $m_b = 1$, such that:

$$M_n = (10 \times 10\,000 + 1 \times 100\,000)/11$$
$$= 18\,200$$

The molecular weight of a polymer is of great value in explaining the variations in the physical properties of different polymers. For example, the tensile strength and the elongation required to break the polymer increase steeply for some polymers in the molecular weight range of 50\,000–200\,000.

However, improving the physical properties by increasing the molecular weight is accompanied by a rapid increase in the viscosity of the melt, and this raises the glass transition temperature, making it more difficult for the polymer to be processed.

Chain Configurations

Polymer chains are held together by weak secondary (or van der Waals) bonds, and by entanglement of the chains if they are sufficiently long. The higher the molecular weight, the more entanglements there will be, giving a stiffer and stronger polymer.

In a polymer such as polyethylene, which has a linear chain configuration, the weak bonds between the chains can easily be broken by increasing the temperature of the polymer. When this happens, the chains can flow past one another so that the polymer softens and readily deforms.

On cooling, the bonds are re-established, and the polymer becomes hard again, retaining the shape it was in at the higher temperature.

The temperature at which a plastic softens such that the molecules can begin to flow is defined as its *glass transition temperature*. These temperatures are similar to those for glasses, except that the temperatures involved are much lower in the case of plastics.

A polymer that can be softened and subsequently shaped by heating it above its glass transition temperature is known as a *thermoplastic polymer*. Examples of such thermoplastic polymers are polystyrene, polymethyl methacrylate, and polyethylene.

For some versions of polyethylene such as low-density polyethylene the chains are not linear but are branched (Figure 1.5.6). These branches give the polymer a three-dimensional network structure, which prevents the chains from moving past each other easily, even when heated. Thus the polymer will retain its properties up to reasonably high temperatures, until chemical breakdown of the polymer structure occurs.

Polymers that decompose on heating without showing a glass transition are known as *thermosetting polymers*.

Crystallinity in Polymers

In a polymer the molecules usually twist and turn, coil up, and criss-cross in a random fashion. Sometimes, however, there will be zones where the molecules are able to lie more or less parallel to each other, as shown in Figure 1.5.7. When this happens, the polymer exhibits a limited degree of crystallinity.

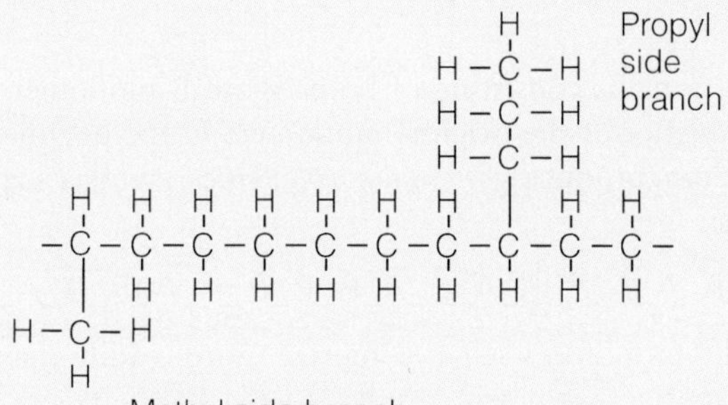

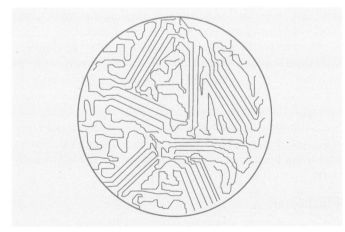

Figure 1.5.6 Branched polyethylene.

Figure 1.5.7 Partial crystallinity in a polymer.

The relative proportions of crystalline and non-crystalline regions in a polymer will depend on the chemical composition, the molecular configuration, and the method of processing. These polymers are not wholly crystalline solids but are composed of a large number of small crystalline regions in close proximity to one another, in an amorphous matrix.

Polyethylene is able to crystallize because of the regularity and simplicity of its polymer chain. As polymer molecules become more complex (whether due to branching or large side groups that restrict the motion of the chain), it becomes more difficult for them to attain crystalline regions.

Cross-Linking

When polymer chains are joined together by chemical bonds, the polymer is said to be *cross-linked*. As noted above, cross-linking has a profound effect on the properties of a polymer; it can make the difference between a thermoplastic polymer and a thermosetting polymer. More importantly, it can convert a liquid polymer into a solid polymer, a process used in the setting of many impression materials.

Silicone polymers have a glass transition temperature below room temperature and therefore are liquids at and above this temperature. When these polymers are cross-linked, the chains are no longer able to slide past each other, and a solid material is obtained. Extensive cross-linking in polymers results in hard, brittle materials, whereas more sparse cross-linking can produce a solid that is flexible: it can be deformed and distorted when handled but spring back to its prior shape when released. This is an important property of many impression materials: the solid material retains the form of the teeth and gums but is sufficiently flexible to be removed from the mouth without tearing or pulling the teeth away with it!

If the polymer consists of particularly long and flexible molecular chains, there may be cross-linking at several points along their lengths. The molecules can take up a highly coiled configuration when relaxed and can stretch over long distances (by uncoiling) when stress is applied. When the stress is removed, the chains will again take up their coiled configuration, governed by the cross-links. The amount of extension and the stress that can be borne by such a polymer depends on the lengths of the chains, the degree of cross-linking, and the strength of the bonds.

Materials that show the ability to stretch by large amounts, even to many times their original length, are known as *elastomers*. The characteristic features of an elastomer are that:

• the material is soft and has a low elastic modulus
• very high strains (>100%) are possible
• the strains are reversible
• the material is above its glass transition temperature.

The various polymer chain configurations for polymers are shown in Figure 1.5.8.

COMPOSITION OF REAL POLYMERS

Polymers are very rarely used in their pure form, for the same reasons that pure metals are rarely used in comparison to alloys;

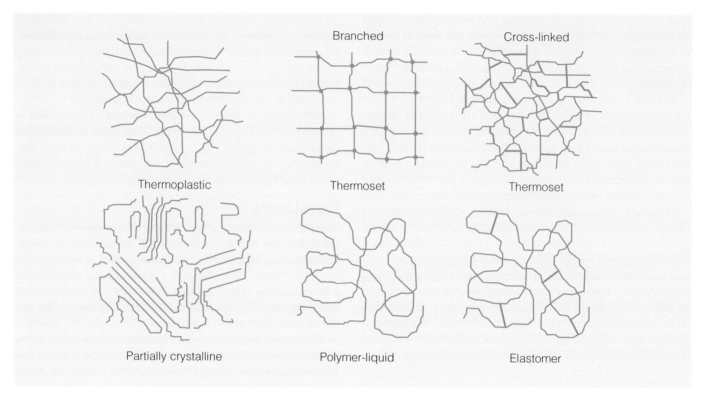

Figure 1.5.8 Polymer chain arrangements.

that is, the properties that can be attained are rather limited and unlikely to be ideally suited to a given application. Instead, modifications are carried out in order to improve the properties of the polymers.

One such modification that has already been considered is the cross-linking of polymer chains, to form thermosetting polymers from thermoplastic polymers. As thermosetting polymers cannot be softened and reshaped, the shape of the object has to be created before cross-linking, and this places serious constraints on the means of processing. However, various other processing options are available, such as blending, and the use of copolymers and composites.

Blending

Blending is a process commonly used in the processing of thermoplastic polymers and involves mixing two or more polymers prior to molding. The properties of the blended polymer will usually lie somewhere between those of the constituent polymers.

As the polymers have to be miscible (i.e. able to mix freely with one another), they tend to be of a similar chemical composition. This places a limit on the changes in properties that are possible by the blending process.

Copolymers

An alternative to blending is the mixing of two polymer-producing systems during the polymerization process; this is *copolymerization.*

For example, if monomer A and monomer B are mixed prior to polymerization, they will *copolymerize* to form polymer chains consisting of both A and B monomer units. The sequence of the original monomers in the polymer may be random, producing a *random copolymer*, giving a sequence such as:

_A_A_A_A_B_B_A_B_A_B_B_B_A_A_B_B_A_B_

If the monomers self-polymerize more readily than they copolymerize, what will result is a *block copolymer,* where segments of each homopolymer are linked:

_A_A_A_B_B_B_B_A_A_A_B_B_B

Such systems can produce polymers with properties that are quite different from the homopolymers. For example, one polymer may be quite rigid, while the other is very flexible. Producing a block copolymer would allow one to control the degree of flexibility of the final material by controlling the length of the blocks and the relative amounts of each polymer.

An example of a block copolymer is ABS (acrylonitrile butadiene styrene), which is formed from a mixture of three polymers. The acrylonitrile and styrene copolymerize to form a glassy block copolymer, while the butadiene forms spherical rubbery regions bonded to the rigid polymer matrix. Although this material has a lower stiffness and creep resistance than polystyrene, it is much tougher, to the extent that it has been considered for the manufacture of car body parts.

Plasticizers

If a low-molecular-weight substance is added to a polymer, it has the effect of lowering the glass transition temperature and the elastic modulus of the material. These plasticizers reduce the forces of attraction between the polymer chains, so the chains become more flexible and begin to flow past one another at a lower temperature, which accounts for the reduction in T_g.

If enough plasticizer is added, a brittle polymer can be transformed into a soft, flexible, and tough polymer.

Plasticizers are usually added to polymers to improve their flow (and hence their processability) and to reduce the brittleness of the product. An example is PVC, which is a very rigid polymer in its pure form but can be formed into flexible tubing after the addition of plasticizer.

The basic requirement to be met by a plasticizer is that it must be compatible with the polymer and have a permanent effect. Compatibility means that the plasticizer must be miscible in the polymer, and this implies the need for a similarity in the molecular forces active in the polymer and plasticizer.

For a plasticizer to be permanent and not easily leached out of the material, it must have a low vapor pressure and a low diffusion rate through the polymer.

A dental example of the use of a plasticizer is when dibutyl phthalate is mixed with polymethyl or polyethyl methacrylate for the production of soft liners for dentures (see Chapter 3.2).

Composites

A composite may be defined as a combination of materials in which the individual components retain their physical identity. More importantly, a composite material is a multi-phase material that exhibits properties of the constituent phases in such a way as to produce a material with a different, and more useful, combination of properties than could be realized by any of the component phases.

In two-component composites it is usual to refer to the *matrix* and the *filler*, the former being the component that binds the filler together. Enamel and dentine are excellent examples of composite structures, being made up of an organic matrix (collagen, proteins, water) and an inorganic filler (hydroxyapatite).

A wide variety of different composite structures can be created, as indicated in the simple classification scheme shown in Figure 1.5.9. In particulate composites the matrix may be a thermoplastic or a thermosetting polymer. The filler particles may be present simply to reduce the cost or may be used to perform a specific role, such as to impart color to an otherwise clear or colorless polymer. Their most crucial function, however, is when they are used to improve the mechanical

properties of the polymer. For instance, the inclusion of glass in a polymer increases the stiffness and sometimes increases the strength. The flow properties of elastomeric impression materials are to a large extent controlled by the amount of filler that is included.

The shape and distribution of the filler play an important role in the way the properties are modified. Besides particulate fillers, it is also possible to incorporate fibers or whiskers. The incorporation of fibers in a polymer matrix can have a profound effect on the properties of the resultant composite. Significant improvements in strength and stiffness, while retaining a low weight, can be achieved by the judicious use of fiber reinforcement. Whiskers are very thin crystals that have extremely large length-to-diameter ratios, as is the case with the example of a fluorcanasite structure shown in Figure 1.5.10. Typical tensile strength values for whiskers and fibers are provided in Table 1.5.2. The fibers may be short or long and can be distributed in a number of different ways in the resin matrix, depending on the sorts of properties required (Figure 1.5.11). An example of a structural composite is a material composed of sheets of material stacked one on top of the other, where each sheet may have fibers aligned in a certain direction. This can produce materials that have high strength properties in a multitude of directions (Figure 1.5.12).

In dentistry particulate fillers are most common, and a wide range of particle sizes are used, from the nanoscale up to tens of micrometers. Examples of uses of composite materials with

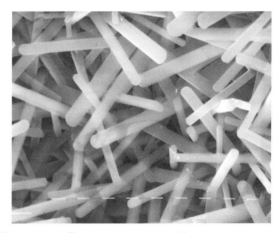

Figure 1.5.10 Fluorcanasite crystals with a large aspect ratio.

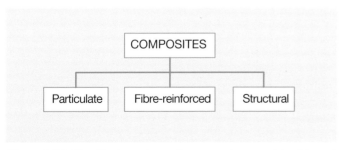

Figure 1.5.9 Classification scheme for composite materials. Adapted from Callister WD, Materials Science and Engineering: An Introduction. John Wiley & Sons Inc, New York, USA 1994.

TABLE 1.5.2 **Tensile Strength of Fibers and Whiskers**		
Material	**Type**	**Tensile Strength (MPa)**
Graphite	Whisker	20 000
Silicon carbide	Whisker	20 000
Aluminum oxide	Whisker	14 000–28 000
E-glass	Fiber	3500
Carbon	Fiber	1500–5500
Aramid (Kevlar 49)	Fiber	3500

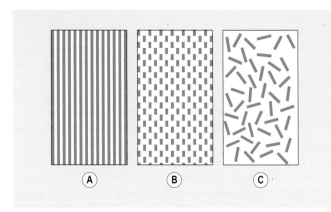

Figure 1.5.11 Schematic representation of fiber-reinforced structures: (a) continuous fibers, (b) short aligned fibers, and (c) randomly distributed short fibers.

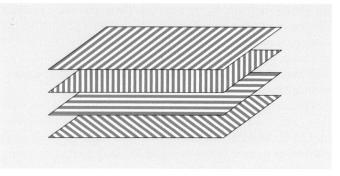

Figure 1.5.12 Laminate structure with sheets of fiber-reinforced resin placed on top of each other in different directions.

particulate fillers are impression materials (Chapter 2.7), resin-based composite restorative materials (see Chapter 2.2), and fiber-reinforced resin bridges and endodontic posts (see Chapter 2.6).

CLINICAL SIGNIFICANCE

Polymers are highly versatile materials in that they can be solid or liquid, and brittle or flexible at body temperature, depending on their composition and configuration. Many polymers are used in dentistry, most commonly copolymer composites that comprise more than one monomer species as well as inorganic fillers.

Mechanical Properties

INTRODUCTION

When one stretches a steel wire or an elastic band, the responses of the materials are quite different. The steel wire will hardly appear to change; although it will become longer, this change is normally so small that it is difficult to perceive. On the other hand, the elastic band will stretch quite readily and can easily double or triple in length. Obviously, different materials respond quite differently to the application of a load, and in order to select the right material for the job, we need to understand how that material will respond to the loads it encounters in day-to-day life.

We could make a component - a filling, denture, or impression, for instance and investigate its response to external loading. However, the data collected would be applicable only to that component and only to that specific three-dimensional shape. This approach would not allow us to predict the behavior of a differently shaped component that was made from the same material.

How are we to compare the performances of materials in different applications? We need some objective standard of comparison that is independent of the size and shape of the material. Once we have such a standard, it should be possible to compare the properties of different materials and to predict the behavior of objects made from them.

The bases for such an objective standard are the quantities called *stress* and *strain*. The description of the mechanical properties of materials is based on these, so we shall now consider them in some detail.

STRESS AND STRAIN

The simplest approach to understanding stress and strain is to consider a rod of material that is held under tension by being subjected to a *tensile force*, or *load*. As shown in Figure 1.6.1, the rod will extend.

Naturally, one would expect the rod to fail (i.e. to snap or to deform irreversibly) under a high enough load. The load at which failure occurs is a measure of the strength of the rod, but it is particular to a rod of those specific dimensions and specific material. The load that the rod could bear without failing would be increased if the diameter of the rod were greater and would decrease if the diameter were smaller.

The amount of extension of the rod at the time of failure depends on the starting length of the rod, such that the longer the starting length, the greater the extension. Thus force and extension do not represent the ideal means of defining the mechanical properties of a material.

The way to overcome the dependence on the dimensions of the rod is to introduce the parameters of stress, σ, and strain, e, for the material under test.

The definitions for these parameters are:
- Stress is the force per unit cross-sectional area that is acting on a material.
- Strain is the fractional change in the dimensions caused by the force.

Thus, if a rod is subjected to a tensile force, F, along its length, the stress, σ, is given by:

$$\sigma = F/A$$

where A is the cross-sectional area of the rod. The units used to measure stress are Newtons per meter squared ($N{\cdot}m^{-2}$ = Pascal = Pa).

At the same time as when the force is applied, the rod's length changes from its original length, L_0, to the extended length, L_1. The strain that results, e, is given by:

$$e = L_1 - L_0/L_0$$

This parameter is dimensionless, as it involves the calculation of length divided by a length.

In practice, we can measure the load–extension curve for a material and then convert this to a stress–strain curve. Once we have this information, it is possible to predict the load–extension curve for a rod of any cross-sectional area and length. We can also compare the response of different materials to the same tensile force.

Stress and strain are not material properties in themselves but allow the definition of a number of mechanical properties of a material that could not be defined otherwise. In the example described above the stress was generated by a load applied in an axial direction (i.e. along the rod), but in practice, a load could be applied in any direction, and in most situations there will be more than one load involved. These loads give rise to complex stress patterns in the structure.

The three principal types of stress are tensile stress, compressive stress, and shear stress, and these are shown schematically in Figure 1.6.2.

Definitions of Some Mechanical Properties

A typical stress–strain curve for a metal such as a brass alloy is shown in Figure 1.6.3. It can be used to identify several of a material's properties.

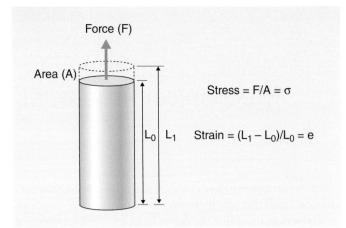

Figure 1.6.1 Rod of material being pulled in a uniaxial direction.

Stress = F/A = σ

Strain = $(L_1 - L_0)/L_0 = e$

CLINICAL SIGNIFICANCE

When a load is applied to a tooth, or a dental material, the load is transmitted through the material, giving rise to *stresses* and *strains*. Although the compressive force is easiest to visualize, owing to biting and chewing, the complex three-dimensional shape of teeth and restorations and the uneven distribution of load owing to point contacts means that compressive, tensile, and shear forces are all encountered by the material. If these stresses and strains exceed the maximum value the material can withstand, *fracture* is the most likely outcome. Repeated stresses and strains below this maximum can also cause gradual deterioration of the material, known as *fatigue*.

Elastic Limit and Plastic Flow

An important feature of the mechanical behavior of materials is the relationship between the stress and the strain. Immediately noticeable in Figure 1.6.3 is the fact that this brass alloy does not show a linear relationship between stress and strain along the full length of the curve.

The region where the stress–strain curve is linear is known as the *linear elastic region* and represents the range where *elastic deformation* occurs. In this region the removal of the stress from the material results in the material returning to its original shape.

Where the curve begins to deviate from its linear path, the material will have exceeded its *elastic limit* and will begin to deform permanently; removal of the stress from the material does not result in the return of the material to its original shape. This is known as *plastic flow* and is represented by the *region of plastic deformation* on the graph.

Young's Modulus

When a material is stressed, it is usually found that the stress is initially proportional to the strain, so their ratio is constant. In other words, the material deforms linearly and elastically. This can be represented by the expression:

$$\sigma/e = E$$

which allows us to define another property of the material: namely, *Young's modulus*, denoted by E. Young's modulus is the

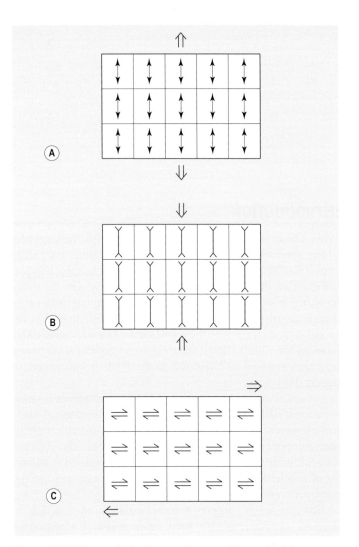

Figure 1.6.2 Three principal types of stress: (a) tensile; (b) compressive; (c) shear.

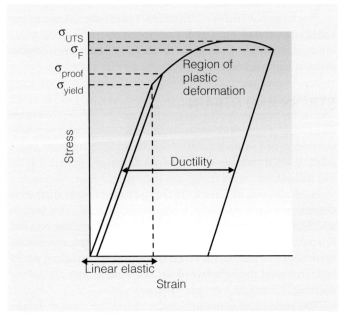

Figure 1.6.3 Stress–strain curve for a ductile metal. UTS, Ultimate tensile strength.

constant that relates the stress and the strain in the linear elastic region and is a measure of the stiffness of the material.

Note that the stiffness of a rod is dependent on its shape and dimensions *and* on the Young's modulus of the material from which it is constructed. Once we know the Young's modulus of a material, it is possible to determine the stiffness of any structure made from that material.

Since Young's modulus is obtained by dividing the stress by the strain, the units are the same as those of stress ($N \cdot m^{-2}$). The value of Young's modulus is often very large for real materials. To make the values more manageable, it is usual to express the value of Young's modulus in Gigapascals (GPa), where 1 Pascal is 1 $N \cdot m^{-2}$, and 1 Gigapascal is 10^9 $N \cdot m^{-2}$.

The Young's modulus is often described as simply the *elastic modulus*, or the *modulus of elasticity*.

Fracture Strength

It is now possible to define the *fracture strength* of the material, σ_f, since this is simply the stress required to break it.

Yield Stress and Proof Stress

The stress at which plastic deformation begins is defined as the *yield stress*, σ_y. In practice, this point is often difficult to detect since there is a gradual transition rather than a rapid change in the slope of the stress–strain curve.

The quantity known as *proof stress* is used as a measure of the onset of yielding of the material and is defined as the stress required to produce a certain amount of plastic strain, usually 0.2%.

CLINICAL SIGNIFICANCE

If, at any point in a metal restoration, such as a three-unit bridge, the tensile stress exceeds the yield stress, the restoration will deform permanently.

Ultimate Tensile Strength

In the tensile response depicted in Figure 1.6.3 there is a maximum stress that the specimen can withstand. This maximum stress is defined as the *ultimate tensile strength* of the material, σ_{UTS}, and is often different from the fracture strength, which, as noted above, is the stress at the point of fracture.

Ductility

The amount of plastic strain produced in the specimen at fracture is called the *ductility* of the material.

Ductility is measured by drawing a line from the point of fracture, which is parallel to the elastic region of the stress–strain curve. Where this line meets the strain axis is the measure of the ductility of the material and is frequently presented in terms of percentage elongation. A ductile material is one that displays substantial and plastic – permanent – elongation prior to fracture.

Metals and alloys used for wires are common examples. The converse is a brittle material: a material that displays little or virtually no plastic deformation.

Resilience and Toughness

When a wire is bent and then released, it will spring back to its original shape as long as the stress does not exceed the elastic limit.

TABLE 1.6.1 Fracture Toughness Data for a Variety of Materials

Material	K_{1c} (MPa m$^{1/2}$)
Ductile metals	100–350
High-strength steels	50–154
Aluminum alloys	23–45
Wood	11–13
Nylon	3
Porcelain	1

This is because the energy stored in the wire is recoverable when the stress is released. The amount of energy, which can be absorbed and subsequently released, is an indication of the potential springiness of the material.

The *resilience* is the amount of energy a material can absorb without undergoing any permanent deformation. It is measured from the stress–strain curve as the area under the linear elastic portion of the curve and is given by:

$$R = \frac{1}{2} \times \frac{\sigma_y^2}{E}$$

where R is the modulus of resilience, σ_y is the proportional limit, and E is the elastic modulus. The units are those of energy per unit volume, $J \cdot m^{-3}$ (1 Joule = 1 $N \cdot m$).

The total amount of energy that a material can absorb before it fractures is a measure of the *toughness* of the material and is indicated by the total area under the stress–strain curve. It is also expressed in terms of $J \cdot m^{-3}$.

Fracture Toughness

There are occasions when materials fail suddenly and unexpectedly. This is often as a result of fast fracture and arises when a crack in the material becomes unstable and grows at a very rapid rate. This mode of failure is usually associated with materials that have brittle behavioral characteristics, such as glasses and ceramics, although it can also happen for many metals that are not ductile, such as dental amalgam, solders, and welds, and for hard, brittle resins. The fracture toughness of a material is a measure of the ability of materials to resist propagation of a preformed crack. The method used to measure the fracture toughness of a material is to introduce a crack of known size and shape and then measure the stress required for this crack to grow and calculate a parameter known as K_{1c}. Typical values for the fracture toughness of a range of materials are presented in Table 1.6.1.

MECHANICAL TESTS

Tensile Test

The *tensile test* is a relatively simple test to understand and interpret, and is possibly also the most useful. In this test a sample of the material is stretched in a uniaxial direction in a tensile tester, as shown in Figure 1.6.4. The test is carried out at a constant strain rate (i.e. a constant rate of extension), and the load

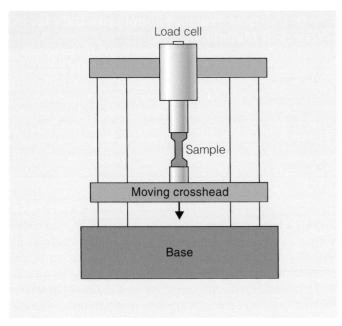

Figure 1.6.4 An arrangement for measuring tensile strength.

is measured from a load cell. The elongation corresponding to the applied load is measured simultaneously and can be done in a number of ways, possibly involving measurement of the separation of the moving crosshead, or by attaching strain gauges to the material if the strains are very low. The stress and corresponding strain can then be calculated according to the definitions already described.

A stress–strain curve can be constructed, from which many properties can be determined. Some typical examples of stress–strain curves for a range of materials are shown in Figure 1.6.5.

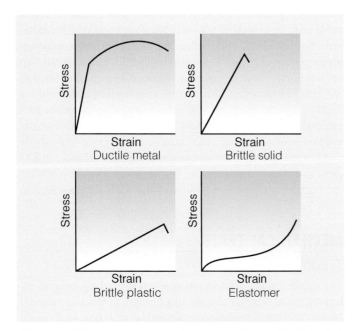

Figure 1.6.5 Stress–strain curves for a range of materials. Note that the stress and strain scales are not meant to be comparable.

An example of a ductile metal is mild steel, which shows a region of linear elastic behavior, a well-defined yield point, and a considerable degree of ductility. In contrast, a hard brittle solid, such as plaster of Paris, shows only a linear elastic region and then fractures without any evidence of plastic deformation.

Many plastics, such as polymethyl methacrylate, are also brittle, although they are less stiff than plaster of Paris. The elastomer, of which silicone impression materials are examples, shows a very different behavior when compared to the other materials. First, it does not appear to have a linear elastic region, and the region of elastic recovery is very large. The percentage elongation is much higher than that observed with either steel or plaster of Paris, and it is elastic in nature, since the elastomer will recover its original dimensions once the stress has been removed. The elastomer also has a significantly lower tensile strength.

Necking

During elastic deformation, there is a slight increase in the volume of the material because the atoms which make up the solid are being pulled apart. However, no such change in volume occurs during plastic deformation. During such deformation, an increase in the length of the material must result in a decrease in the cross-sectional area. This tends to occur in a localized region of the material, as shown in Figure 1.6.6, and is known as *necking*. This phenomenon occurs most readily in highly ductile materials.

The results of tensile tests can be very useful when designing structures, because a knowledge of the elastic deformation characteristics of the material is required in order to predict the behavior of the structure when it is placed under load.

The yield stress determines the maximum stress that the material can safely withstand, and, consequently, the maximum load the structure can withstand, although it is prudent to include some safety factor. The elastic modulus will allow the determination of the stiffness of the structure. For example, a combination of these properties would allow one to determine the resilience or springiness of a metal wire.

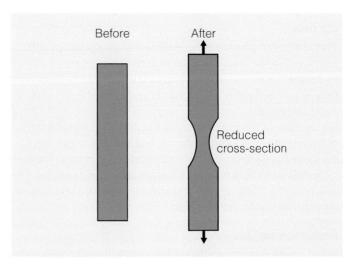

Figure 1.6.6 Necking, exhibited by a ductile material.

If fabrication techniques such as rolling, wire drawing, or pressing are involved in the manufacture of a product, then it is necessary to know how much plastic deformation the material can withstand. If the material shows high ductility, then it can be shaped, but if it shows no ductility, then shaping by the application of loads will not be possible.

Compression Test

For brittle materials in particular, the tensile test is difficult to carry out, and the results usually show a high degree of scatter. An alternative is a *compression test*, which is more easily performed on brittle materials and has results that show a lower degree of scatter. Another reason why such tests are done on brittle materials is that these materials are only used under conditions of compressive loading.

The configuration for a compression test is shown in Figure 1.6.7. As the sample is constrained by friction at points of contact with the platens of the tester, there is an increase in the cross-sectional area, with the material taking up a barrel shape. This 'barreling' effect gives rise to a very complex stress pattern in the material (also shown in Figure 1.6.7) that cannot be analyzed easily. This makes the interpretation of compression tests very difficult.

A compromise test is the measurement of *diametral tensile strength*, in which a disc of the material is subjected to a compressive load. The load applied to the disc results in a tensile stress in a direction perpendicular to the applied load, shown schematically in Figure 1.6.8. The tensile stress, σ, is calculated as follows:

$$\sigma = 2P\pi/DT$$

where P is the load, D is the diameter of the disc, and T is the thickness of the disc. It is a commonly used test for brittle dental materials, because it is simple and provides more reproducible results than a conventional tensile test.

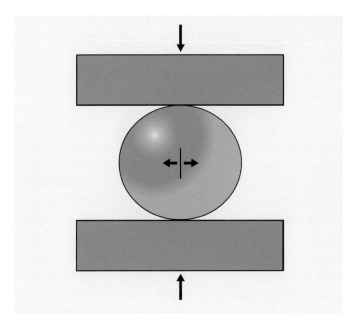

Figure 1.6.8 An arrangement for measuring diametral tensile strength.

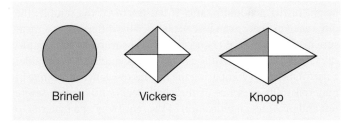

Figure 1.6.9 Surface indenters from different hardness testers.

Hardness Test

The *hardness test* measures the resistance of a material to an indenter or cutting tool. It provides an indication of the resistance of the material to scratching or abrasion. There is also a reasonable correlation between the hardness of a material and its ultimate tensile strength.

The test involves the use of an indenter, which can be in the shape of a ball (Brinell), a pyramid (Vickers or Knoop), or a cone (Rockwell), which of course must be harder than the material being tested. The indenter is pushed into the surface of the material for a given period, leaving behind an impression of the indenter (Figure 1.6.9).

The size of this impression will depend on the hardness of the material. The sizes can be measured, and an empirical hardness number calculated. The choice of hardness tester, to some extent, depends on the nature of the material being tested.

Impact Test

The *impact test* is designed to test the resistance of a material to the sudden application of a load. A standard notched bar is subjected to an impulse load provided by a heavy pendulum. The arrangement for the test is shown in Figure 1.6.10.

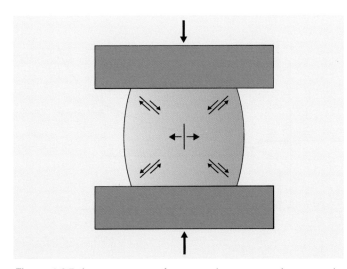

Figure 1.6.7 An arrangement for measuring compressive strength, showing where tensile and shear stresses develop.

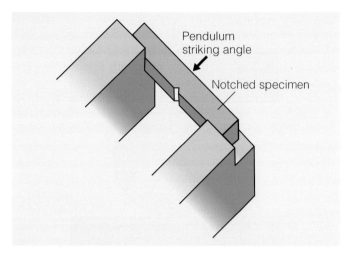

Figure 1.6.10 Specimen arrangement for a Charpy impact test. The pendulum has a hammer head, which is released from a fixed height.

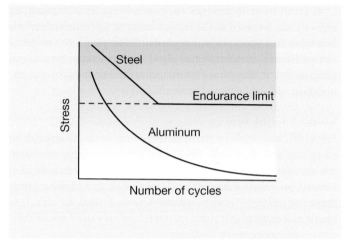

Figure 1.6.11 S–N curves for steel and aluminum.

The pendulum is released from a known height and then strikes and breaks the sample, which is placed across parallel supports. Some of the energy of the pendulum is used up in breaking the sample. From a knowledge of the initial and final height of the pendulum, after it has fractured the sample, the difference in energy can be calculated. This difference is a measure of the amount of energy that was absorbed by the sample, causing it to fracture. Although the test is empirical, it provides a useful means of comparing the impact resistance of a range of materials. The presence of the notch makes this a very severe test and provides an indication of the sensitivity of a material to notches in its structure.

Fatigue Test

In many practical situations materials are subjected to fluctuating stresses rather than the static loads that are considered above. The gradual accumulation of minute amounts of plastic strain produced by each cycle of a fluctuating stress is known as fatigue and a clinical situation where such failures may occur is for Ni-Ti files used in endodontics.

Fatigue can lead to failure at stresses well below the yield stress of the material. The test for fatigue strength involves subjecting samples of the material to cyclic loading for a range of loads. The number of cycles required to cause failure is counted in each case.

The stress is plotted as a function of the logarithm of the corresponding number of cycles required to cause failure. This gives an S–N curve, as shown in Figure 1.6.11.

Two forms of behavior can be observed. For some materials, as the number of cycles of loading is increased, the allowable stress decreases. In other materials, however, there is what is known as an *endurance limit*, which corresponds to a level of stress below which the material can be subjected for an indefinite number of cycles without fracturing.

The fatigue strength is very dependent on the surface characteristics of the material. Improvements in surface finish or surface compressive stresses, which may be induced mechanically or chemically, tend to raise the level of the S–N curve.

The testing environment will also have a profound effect on the S–N curve, with corrosive environments, particularly, lowering the fatigue strength.

CLINICAL SIGNIFICANCE

Whereas a material may be strong enough to withstand the loads placed on it when initially put into use, this does not mean it will always be able to withstand those loads. Fatigue can cause very small changes in the material that accumulate over time leading eventually to failure, even when the individual loads result in stresses well below the yield stress.

Creep Test

Under the influence of a constant stress, materials can deform permanently if the load is applied for a long time, even though the stress on the material may well be below its elastic limit. This time-dependent deformation of materials is known as *creep* and will eventually lead to fracture of the material.

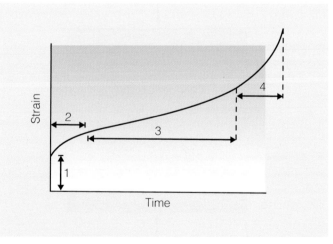

Figure 1.6.12 Creep curve, showing the four stages of creep for long-duration and high-temperature creep conditions.

It is particularly important when a material is used at a temperature above about half of its melting temperature or softening point, for example, some amalgam phases and many plastics. At temperatures 40–50% less than the absolute melting point, creep is negligible.

A typical creep curve is shown in Figure 1.6.12. Four stages of elongation can be identified:

- initial elongation due to the application of the load
- transient or primary creep, which tends to be a large effect
- steady state (secondary) creep
- tertiary creep.

We will not consider the mechanisms that give rise to creep.

CLINICAL SIGNIFICANCE

A wide variety of mechanical properties of materials can be measured. This allows comparisons to be made between dental materials, although their clinical meaning can be a matter of some considerable debate.

Physical Properties

INTRODUCTION

The uses to which many dental materials are put are not conducive to mass production, as each patient is different from the last, and the material has to be specially molded each time. Although there are a few exceptions to this such as preformed metal and ceramic crowns, as a rule, most materials used by the dentist, dental therapist, and dental technician require some form of processing before they are hardened.

This processing often involves mixing components of materials with each other to produce a dough or liquid that can then be placed and shaped to suit the patient's needs. The successful use of dental materials therefore requires some understanding of the way in which materials flow when they are mixed, poured, or molded. The study of the flow of materials is known as *rheology*.

When a patient consumes something hot or cold - a cup of tea, an ice cream - the temperature in the mouth can range from 5°C to 60°C. This can result in temperature differences within the tooth that can be quite pronounced and can differ greatly from the norm of around 37°C. When a filling, crown, bridge, or denture is placed, account must be taken of the *thermal properties* of the dental materials and the effect of differential temperature on the materials themselves and the surrounding hard and soft tissues.

The restoration of the human dentition was once primarily concerned with function, but nowadays aesthetic properties are as, or even more, important in the eyes of many patients. Patients often desire a restoration that is indistinguishable, to the untrained eye at least, from the natural teeth. Consequently, the *optical properties* of the materials that are selected and used by the dental professional have become of great importance.

RHEOLOGICAL PROPERTIES

Rheology is the study of the flow of materials. For liquids, flow is measured by the viscosity, whereas for solids, one considers creep and viscoelasticity. Creep has already been described in the previous section and only the viscosity and the viscoelasticity will be considered here.

Viscosity

When a substance flows under the influence of an external force (e.g. gravity), the molecules or atoms come into contact with different neighbors. Thus bonds must be broken and remade, and this gives rise to a resistance to flow, known as *viscosity*.

For a liquid such as water, the forces binding the molecules together are weak and easily overcome, so the water flows quite readily and has a low viscosity. For some fluids, the intermolecular attractions are much stronger. This is usually associated with large molecules, such as in the case of golden syrup or honey. The molecules may even become tangled up in one another, giving rise to very high viscosities. This is what happens with high-molecular-weight polymers.

When we stir a liquid, we are effectively applying a shear stress, and the degree of vigor with which we stir it can be quantified by the shear rate. Such a situation is shown in Figure 1.7.1. The shear stress and the shear rate are defined by:

$$\text{Shear stress} = \eta_s = F/A$$

$$\text{Shear rate} = \dot{e} = V/d$$

Several methods are available for measuring the shear stress over a range of shear rates for a fluid, and the information collected can be plotted as a *shear stress–shear rate curve*. This relationship is linear for many fluids, and a typical curve for such a fluid is shown in Figure 1.7.2. The slope of the curve is equal to the viscosity, so the exact scientific definition of viscosity, η, is given by:

$$\eta = \text{shear stress/shear rate}$$

The units of viscosity are Pascal seconds (Pa.s).

The viscous properties of substances that have a linear relationship between shear stress and shear rate are given entirely by this single value of viscosity and are said to be 'Newtonian' in behavior.

However, not all materials behave in this simple fashion, and some of the different forms of behavior are shown in Figure 1.7.3.

Liquids with *plastic* behavior will not flow until a threshold shear stress has been reached. The fluid will then flow in a Newtonian fashion.

Dilatant liquids show an increase in viscosity as the shear rate goes up. This means that the faster one tries to mix the fluid, the more difficult the liquid becomes to mix. It is not possible to define the flow characteristics of such a liquid by a single viscosity.

For some liquids, an increase in shear rate does not lead to a corresponding proportional increase in shear stress. This means that the liquid becomes easier to mix at higher shear rates than would be the case for a Newtonian or dilatant liquid. This behavior is described as *pseudoplastic* and leads to the feature of some liquids that is commonly known as *shear thinning*. A dental example of this type of behavior is in some flowable composite materials, where shear thinning makes it possible to easily dispense the composite through a fine syringe – high

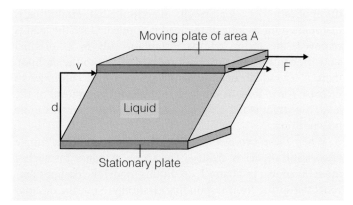

Figure 1.7.1 Shearing of a liquid between two rigid plates that are separated by a distance, d. The upper plate is moving at a velocity, v, relative to the stationary plate, and a force, F, is needed to overcome the resistance from the liquid.

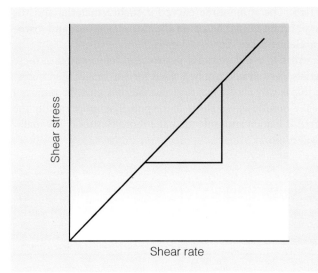

Figure 1.7.2 Shear stress versus shear rate for a Newtonian liquid.

shear – to aid placement, but once in position and being manipulated – low shear – the material is more viscous, that is, not so runny that it proves too difficult to handle.

Thixotropy

So far, it has been assumed that the viscosity can be determined from a knowledge of the shear stress and shear rate at any one instant in time. For some substances, the viscosity will change at a particular shear rate, and if one plotted the shear stress against the shear rate for such a liquid, one would typically find the response shown in Figure 1.7.4.

In this case the viscosity for an increasing shear rate is different from the viscosity for a decreasing shear rate, which is an example of *hysteresis*. In such cases the viscosity of the fluid is dependent on the previous deformations to which the fluid has been subjected.

This type of behavior occurs when there is some molecular rearrangement caused by the mixing, and a lack of time for the molecules to return to their normal arrangement before mixing again. The effect of this is that the longer the fluid is mixed at a given shear rate, the lower the shear stress and hence the viscosity will be. If the fluid were left for long enough, it would recover and the whole process could be repeated. A material which exhibits this type of behavior is described as *thixotropic*. A domestic example of a thixotropic fluid is non-drip paint, and some impression materials have been found to display thixotropic behavior. Thixotropy can be thought of as similar to pseudoplasticity, but with a time lag. In both cases stress causes the viscosity to reduce, and the removal of stress causes the viscosity to return to its earlier value. The difference is that with pseudoplasticity, the changes in viscosity are near-instantaneous, whereas with thixotropic materials, there is a time delay – time has to elapse after the removal of the stress, before the viscosity changes, since the behavior is due to the rearrangement of the polymer chains. Sadly, this distinction is often overlooked and many publications describe dental materials as thixotropic when in fact pseudoplastic would be a more accurate description.

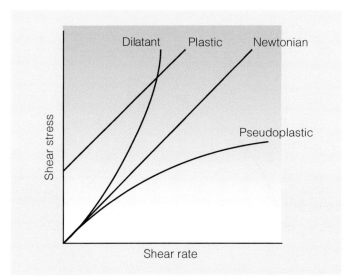

Figure 1.7.3 Rheological behavior of different liquids.

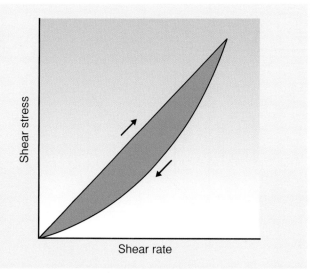

Figure 1.7.4 Thixotropic behavior.

CLINICAL SIGNIFICANCE

The rheological properties of a material are important, as these have a major influence on the handling characteristics of the material. Some rheological properties such as pseudoplasticity are exploited in dental materials for the convenience of the practitioner.

Viscoelasticity

A wide range of materials show behavior that is intermediate between that of a viscous liquid and that of an elastic solid. For an elastic solid, it has been assumed that the relationship between stress and strain is independent of any dynamic factors such as loading rate or strain rate. However, if given sufficient time to do so, some solids show a capacity to rearrange their molecules under the influence of an applied load, and this is reflected in a change in the strain. When the load is then released, the material does not immediately return to its original state. This means that the behavior of the material is dependent on such factors as the duration and the amount of load applied.

A simple and effective way of visualizing this problem is through the use of models based on a spring and a dashpot, which combine to give a system rather like a shock absorber. The spring represents the elastic element, and the dashpot represents the viscous element. The variation of the strain with time for these models is shown in Figure 1.7.5. For the spring, the application of a load results in an immediate strain that is maintained for as long as the load is applied. Once the load is removed, the spring returns instantaneously to its original state. In contrast, on the application of a load to the dashpot, there is a gradual increase in the strain, which continues to increase for as long as the load is applied. On removal of the load, the strain is not relieved, and the dashpot remains in its new position.

When these two elements are placed in parallel, a simple viscoelastic model is created. The strain response for such a model is shown in Figure 1.7.6. In this model the dashpot prevents the spring from responding elastically. Now, the dashpot gradually lets the spring approach its desired strained state. On removal of the load, the dashpot prevents the spring from contracting to its unstrained state, which it can now only achieve after some time.

A dental example of a group of materials that show viscoelastic behavior would be that of the elastomeric impression materials. The strain–time curve for such a material and the corresponding model based on the elastic, viscous, and viscoelastic elements are shown in Figure 1.7.7.

In order to avoid excessive permanent deformation of these materials, they should not be loaded for any longer than necessary; this is why elastic impression materials must be removed from the mouth with a short sharp pull. The more rapidly the material is loaded and unloaded, the more elastically the material will respond.

CLINICAL SIGNIFICANCE

Some materials have properties between that of a solid and a liquid, which makes them susceptible to distortion and has implications for how they should be handled in the clinic and laboratory.

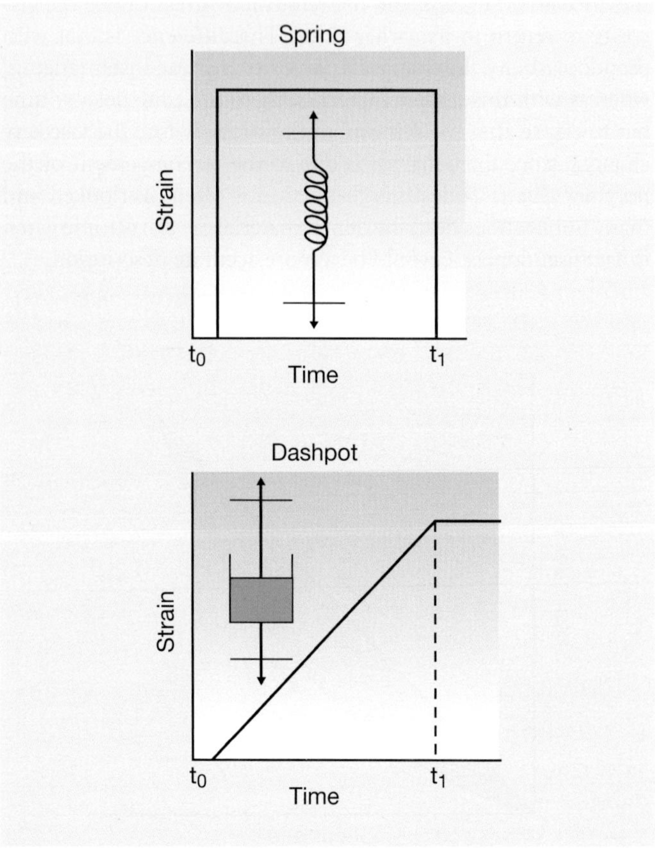

Figure 1.7.5 Elastic and viscous response for a spring and dashpot model.

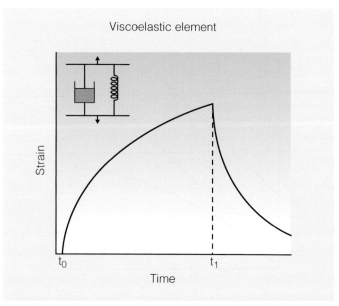

Figure 1.7.6 Viscoelastic behavior of a spring and dashpot in parallel.

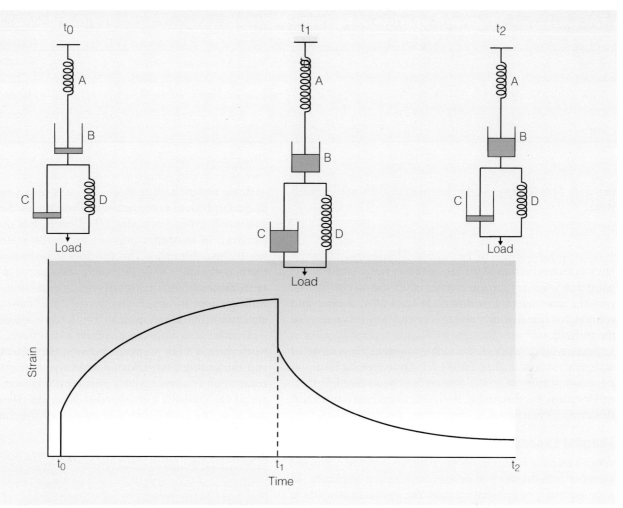

Figure 1.7.7 Viscoelastic model corresponding closely to the rheological behavior of a fully set elastomeric impression material. The load is applied at time t_0, and spring A extends instantaneously while spring D is prevented from doing so by dashpot C. With time, dashpots C and B allow further strain to develop. At time t_1, the load is removed, and spring A contracts immediately. Spring D is prevented from doing so by dashpot C. Eventually, at time t_2, spring D has returned to its original length. Some permanent strain remains, since dashpot B will not return to its original state.

THERMAL PROPERTIES

Materials can feel warm or cold to the touch; a metal or ceramic surface may feel cold while a fabric surface feels neutral or warm, even if they are in the same room with a steady ambient temperature. This response of a material to a source of heat, in this case the fingertips, is dependent on the ease with which heat is transferred through and absorbed within the material. A material that readily conducts heat is a *thermal conductor* and a material that resists the conduction of heat is a *thermal insulator*.

Thermal Conductivity

One factor which determines the ease with which heat is transferred through a material is its thermal conductivity. The thermal conductivity (K) is defined as the rate of heat flow per unit temperature gradient; its units are $cal \cdot cm^{-1} \cdot s^{-1} \cdot {}^{\circ}C^{-1}$.

Specific Heat

For some materials, the initial 'cold feeling' can rapidly disappear as the material heats up due to the transfer of heat energy from the heat source to the material. How rapidly the temperature increases depends on the specific heat of the material, which is defined as the heat energy required to raise the temperature of a unit volume by one degree Centigrade. Thus its units are $cal \cdot g^{-1} \cdot {}^{\circ}C^{-1}$ and the symbol used is C_p.

Thermal Diffusivity

The transfer of heat from a hot to a cold source is dependent on both the thermal conductivity and the specific heat, with the former regulating the rate at which the heat enters and passes through the material and the latter determining the rate at which the temperature will rise as heat enters the

TABLE 1.7.1   Physical Properties of Relevant Materials

	ρ (g·cm^{-3})	C_p (cal·g^{-1}·°C^{-1})	K (cal·cm^{-1}·s^{-1}·°C^{-1})	h (cm^2·s^{-1})
Enamel	2.9	0.18	0.0022	0.0042
Dentine	2.1	0.28	0.0015	0.0026
Silver	10.5	0.056	0.98	1.67
Silica	2.5	0.20	0.003	0.006
Water	1.0	1.00	0.0014	0.0014

material. This is presented by the thermal diffusivity, h, such that:

$$h = K/C_p\rho$$

where ρ is the density of the material. The thermal diffusivity gives a clear indication of the rate of rise of temperature at one point due to a heat source at another point and may be considered the most relevant in dental applications as it takes into account both the thermal conductivity and the heat capacity of the material.

Some typical values of the above properties for a range of materials are presented in Table 1.7.1. An interesting feature is the low diffusivity of water, showing it to be an excellent thermal insulator. For this reason, the Inuit can be quite warm when sheltering in their igloos.

Thermal Expansion

When a material is heated, the extra energy absorbed causes the atoms or molecules to vibrate with an increased amplitude. As a consequence, the material expands. The most common way of measuring this expansion is by taking a length of material, heating it to a certain temperature, and then measuring the resultant change in length. This change in length, when determined per unit length for a 1°C change in temperature, is called the linear coefficient of expansion, α. This change is so small that it is more usual to express it in terms of parts per million per degree Centigrade (ppm °C^{-1}). Some typical values for α are given in Table 1.7.2.

In an ideal restorative material the coefficient of expansion would be identical to that of the tooth tissues. If this is not the case, the thermal mismatch can give rise to marginal gap formation and the breakdown of adhesive bonds. Such effects will depend not only on the coefficient of expansion but also on the thermal diffusivity of the material.

TABLE 1.7.2   Coefficients of Thermal Expansion

Material	α (ppm °C^{-1})
Enamel	12
Dentine	14
Resin composite	20–55
Fissure sealant	80
Porcelain	12
Glass–ionomer cement	8

Some materials, such as silver, require only a small amount of heat energy to raise their temperature (low heat capacity) and readily expand or contract (high coefficient of thermal expansion). In contrast, composite restorative materials have a low thermal diffusivity. This provides some protection against thermal stimuli, as more heat energy is required to cause a rise in temperature and the corresponding expansion. However, if sufficient heat *is* supplied, the material *will* show a significant expansion/contraction mismatch with tooth tissues.

Fracture of castings can occur due to hot tearing on cooling, when there is a big mismatch between the refractory material and the casting alloy. Dimensional correction of the cooling contraction of alloys is vitally important if crowns and bridges are to fit. Similarly, metal-bonded porcelain relies on a close match of the coefficient of expansion of the metal and the porcelain.

CLINICAL SIGNIFICANCE

The thermal properties of a dental material can influence the sensation of hot and cold food and can cause fatigue and even mechanical failure (of the material or the adjacent, brittle, enamel) due to differential expansion and contraction.

OPTICAL PROPERTIES

In the real world every object we see is a result of the reflectance of light from that object reaching an extremely sensitive, if somewhat wavelength-limited, photodetector: namely, the eye (Figure 1.7.8). We therefore have a triplet, composed of the light source, the object, and the observer. Each of these will influence what we see. Hence, when we place an apple in front of three people and ask them to tell us the color of the apple, we may well receive three different answers. One will see it simply as red, another as crimson, and yet another as bright red. This is because our color sensitivity and past experience will be different.

There are three characteristics of the object that govern the nature of this reflected light, namely:
- *Color.* The color of an object that our eye detects will be a function of the light source providing the spectrum of light hitting a surface and how the object transforms this spectrum.
- *Translucency.* The amount of light reflected and the spectrum of light reflected from the object and detected by the eye will depend on the ability of the light to travel through

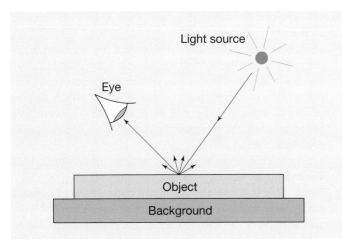

Figure 1.7.8 Perception of an object depends on the light source, the optical properties of the object, and the ability of the eye to discriminate the visible light spectrum landing on the retina.

the material, where it will change due to absorption and scattering properties of the material and the background against which it is held.

- *Surface texture.* Light can be reflected from a surface, as from a mirror, or scattered in all directions. In the first case the surface is an ideal reflecting polished surface, while in the second case it is a matte scattering surface.

Color

The perception of color is highly subjective, as it is a physiological response to a physical stimulus. For example, the choice of color of restorative material that we make in order to match a tooth tends to vary slightly from person to person. This happens because the eye is an ill-defined detector of light, followed by interpretation in the brain, of the energy scattered or transmitted by a material. This can present a challenge for those who suffer from color blindness, which basically means that their photodetector is deficient. The *perception* of color does not therefore lend itself to quantification, but this is not the case for the light itself.

Light is electromagnetic radiation that can be detected by the human eye. Newton (1666) was able to produce a spectrum of different-colored light by illuminating a glass prism, which split the light into a multi-colored band. This band of light was identical to the colors of the rainbow. He showed that white light is, in fact, the result of combining a broad spectrum of colored radiation. The spectrum of electromagnetic radiation is shown in Figure 1.7.9. From this, it can be seen that visible electromagnetic radiation occupies only a small part of the total spectrum and is in the range of 380–780 nanometers (1 nm = 10^{-9} m). This spectrum goes from violet (380–450 nm), through blue (450–490 nm), then green (490–560 nm), yellow (560–590 nm) and orange (590–630 nm), and finally to red (630–780 nm).

Light is focused on the retina and triggers nerve impulses that are transmitted to the brain. There are cone-shaped cells in the retina that are responsible for providing sensitivity to different-colored light and rod-shaped cells that are sensitive only to the brightness (i.e. the amount of light) that is focused on the retina. The response of the retina to light is indicated in Figure 1.7.10. It shows that the eye is most sensitive to light in the green–yellow

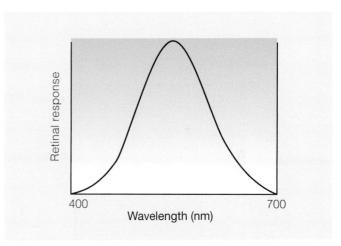

Figure 1.7.10 The relative response of the retina to visible electromagnetic radiation.

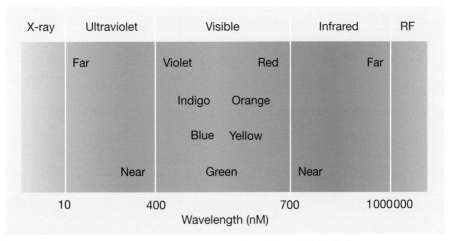

Figure 1.7.9 Spectrum of electromagnetic radiation. RF, Radio frequency.

range and is least sensitive at the extremes of the visible spectrum, that is, the reds and blues.

The cone-shaped cells have a threshold intensity. Exposure to excessive light of a given wavelength can cause these cells to switch off, resulting in eyestrain and a very different perception of color.

The actual light that we see is not of a single wavelength but is composed of a mixture of different wavelengths that combine to produce a distinctive color. The wavelength and intensity spectrum of the light we see depend on the source of the light. The light spectra for daylight and a tungsten filament lamp are quite different, as shown in Figure 1.7.11. Modern LED lighting is available with different colors such as 'warm' (longer wavelengths) and 'cool blue' (shorter wavelengths). The color of an object will appear different when it is viewed under light from different sources.

In order to allow us to convey color, for example, to a laboratory being asked to make a crown or a veneer, we need to have some mechanism for describing the color characteristics of the patient's teeth to which the restoration is to be matched. Various people have attempted to devise a method of quantifying color and expressing it numerically, with the aim of making color communication easy and accurate. In 1905 American artist A. H. Munsell came up with a method for describing

colors, which were classified according to their hue, chroma, and value:

- *Hue.* This represents the dominant color (i.e. wavelength) of the spectrum of light from the source. The possible colors are violet, indigo, blue, green, yellow, orange, and red. The three primary colors, from which all other colors can be produced, are red, green, and blue. This fact is used in TVs to create a full-color picture from only three distinctly colored light sources.
- *Chroma.* This is the *strength* of hue, in other words, how vivid the color is.
- *Value.* This is the brightness or darkness of the object and ranges from black to white for diffusive or reflective objects, and from black to clear for translucent objects.

Whereas hue and chroma are properties of the object, the value will depend on the incident light, the surface finish of the object, and the background if the material transmits light. For this reason, it is important that color matching should be carried out under an appropriate light source, with bright daylight or a 'daylight lamp' being preferable. The basis of the Munsell system is shown in Figure 1.7.12. This three-dimensional representation of color is not exactly practical, and initially this method of describing color involved a huge number of paper color tags, which was later updated to a numerical system. In this system any given color is expressed as a letter/number combination as visually evaluated using a Munsell Color Atlas. However, this system has its limitations in that the color stability of the atlas is such that it needs to be replaced periodically, and it has to be viewed under standardized lighting conditions.

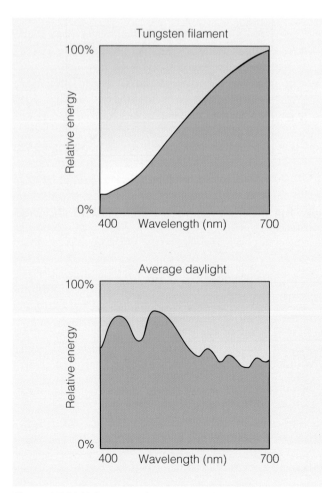

Figure 1.7.11 Light spectra for a tungsten filament lamp and daylight.

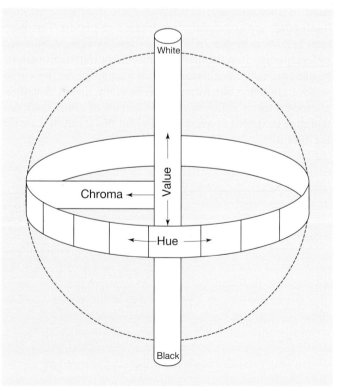

Figure 1.7.12 The three-dimensional Munsell color scheme for hue, chroma, and value.

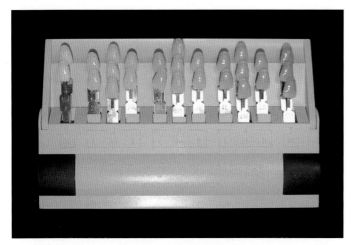

Figure 1.7.13 The VITA Linearguide 3D-MASTER tooth shade guide.

Besides, although it may be adequate for matching the color of a piece of cloth or a paint, which can be brought close to the atlas, it is not the most convenient method of assessing the color of a patient's teeth! Also, it has been shown that the range of tooth shades in humans only takes up something of the order of 2% of the Munsell color space. Hence, for dentistry, a simpler system based on a shade guide has been developed, of which the VITA Linearguide 3D-MASTER is one popular example (Figure 1.7.13). The VITA Linearguide 3D-MASTER tooth shade guide is structured on the principle of being able to make a decision in two steps and being able to do so quickly and accurately. A first selection is made with the VITA Valueguide by comparing the shade tabs with the patient's tooth. The Valueguide is numbered from 0 to 5. Once the appropriate value has been selected, the corresponding Chroma/Hueguide is selected and the closest match to the tooth in terms of chroma and hue is chosen. It is important that a shade guide is selected that corresponds with the restorative material being used. Ideally, the shade guide should be manufactured from the same material as that used to produce the restoration.

The fact that objects can change color under the influence of different light sources is known as *metamerism*. Metamerism occurs when two objects with different light-reflecting properties (spectral graphs) present an identical colored appearance in specific lighting and observation conditions and appear different when the lighting or observation conditions are changed. Most shoppers know that trying to match the color of two garments is best done under daylight rather than under the artificial lights of the shop. Ideally, a tooth shade should be determined in daylight conditions, or under a daylight-corrected lamp; under no circumstances should conventional lighting be used. The process should be completed in 5–7 seconds, as the eyes tire very quickly.

Another important feature of light is that some objects are able to absorb light of a wavelength near the ultraviolet range (300–400 nm) and then release it as light of a longer wavelength (400–450 nm). This is the property of *fluorescence*, and it occurs naturally in tooth enamel. This is the reason why teeth look so white under a fluorescent light and why sometimes crowns,

bridges, or fillings are more noticeable under a fluorescent light source than under daylight. If the materials used in the construction of the restoration do not have the property of fluorescence, then the restoration will look dark next to the fluorescing natural tooth under some lighting conditions.

CLINICAL SIGNIFICANCE

The color of an object is a human *perception*, which is a function of a triplet composed of the light source, the object, and the observer. Color selection of restorations should be done under carefully controlled lighting conditions to ensure a good match with the natural dentition.

Translucency

A *transparent* material such as window glass allows the passage of light in such a way that little distortion takes place, meaning that an object can be seen quite clearly through it. Selective absorption of certain wavelengths may take place, and this forms the basis for optical filters.

A *translucent* material allows some light to pass through it, absorbs some of the remainder, and scatters and reflects the rest from its surface or internal interfaces. An object viewed through such a material would have a distorted appearance.

An *opaque* material is one that does not transmit light but instead absorbs light and reflects or scatters it from the surface. The color of the object will depend on which wavelengths of light are reflected and which are absorbed. For example, red glass is red because it allows light with the wavelength of red light to pass through it but absorbs all other wavelengths. Consequently, it would appear opaque if the light source did not contain light with the wavelength of red light, since all the other wavelengths are absorbed.

A simple scale for the quantification of the degree of opacity is shown in Figure 1.7.14. In this system the opacity is presented by a contrast ratio between the daylight reflectance of a specimen

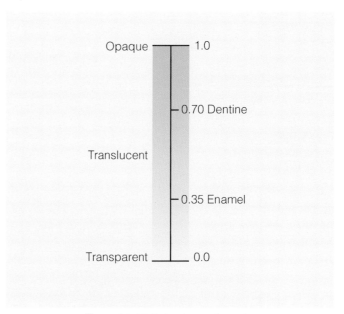

Figure 1.7.14 A simple opacity scale.

of standard thickness (normally 1 mm) when backed by a black standard, and the daylight apparent reflectance when backed by a white standard. The white standard has a reflectance of 70% relative to magnesium oxide ($C_{0.70}$). Restorative materials can be compared easily with enamel and dentine on this scale, to find their relative degrees of opacity.

Surface Texture

Whether a material has a shiny or a matte surface texture is a function of how smooth the surface is. Enamel has a shiny surface because it is extremely smooth and reflects a lot of the light falling on the surface. As a surface gets rougher, the light is scattered and it will begin to appear matte. This is an important consideration with regard to restorative materials, since the appearance of a restored tooth can be spoilt by the restoration having a matte surface finish, making it stand out from the rest of the tooth. The simplest way to assess this is visually, but it can also be assessed numerically using a device known as a profilometer. This device essentially consists of a stylus attached to a long lever arm, which is traced along the surface and records the up-and-down movement of the stylus, like an old-fashioned record player. An example of such a trace run across the surface of a composite resin restorative material is shown in Figure 1.7.15. It also allows the quantification of the surface roughness by calculating Ra, which is the arithmetic mean deviation of the profile; the higher this value, the rougher the surface.

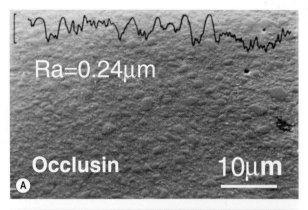

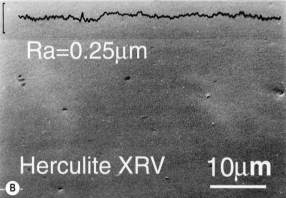

Figure 1.7.15 Surface profiles produced by a profilometer superimposed on scanning electron microscope views of a large particle hybrid composite resin (Occlusin, ICI) and a small particle composite resin (Herculite XRV, Kerr UK Ltd).

CLINICAL SIGNIFICANCE

The polishability of a restorative material is an important consideration in its selection, as it dictates how smooth the surface can be made, a factor in determining how well the material will blend in with the tooth tissues.

Chemical Properties

INTRODUCTION

The oral environment is an aggressive environment. Materials may dissolve in the water that is present in saliva or release soluble components, they may deteriorate due to the presence of dietary or intrinsic acids, they may discolor or break down due to absorption of substances from saliva, or they may tarnish and corrode.

All of these can adversely affect the chemical stability of the materials and in doing so cause changes to their mechanical and physical properties, thereby limiting their durability. The by-products released due to dissolution or corrosion may have an adverse effect on the biological environment, both locally and systemically.

Dental ceramics are mostly compounds of oxygen, such as silica (SiO_2) and alumina (Al_2O_3). These are chemically stable under most circumstances and immune from the oxidation process associated with electrochemical (or wet) corrosion. Degradation of ceramics generally involves a process of chemical dissolution. In contrast, metals are susceptible to wet corrosion. With the notable exception of some *noble metals*, such as gold and platinum, metals are usually found in nature as compounds (principally oxides or sulfides), from which the metal is extracted. Corrosion of metals is, in effect, the reversal of the reactions employed in the extraction process. Frequently, the corrosion product of a metal is very similar to the compound from which the metal was originally extracted. For instance, iron is extracted from naturally occurring iron oxide, and rust is simply hydrated iron oxide. Generally, polymers are not stable either, as many will burn once ignited, showing that the polymer oxidizes readily. However, polymer degradation is generally physicochemical in nature, such as swelling, dissolution, or covalent bond rupture. The latter may be due to heat or radiation and invariably results in a deterioration in mechanical properties such as strength and toughness.

CLINICAL SIGNIFICANCE

In general, it could be said that polymers tend to suffer from absorption and loss of soluble components, metals are prone to tarnish and corrosion, and ceramics may be subject to chemical dissolution.

DEGRADATION OF POLYMERS

Water Sorption and Soluble Fraction

Many polymers used in dentistry, such as those used in resin composites, dentures, and soft liners, are susceptible to absorption of solvents, particularly water, and the loss of soluble components. The solvent molecule forces the polymer chains apart, causing swelling. As the strength of the bond decreases, the polymer becomes softer, the glass transition temperature is reduced, and the strength may be lowered. Nylon is particularly susceptible to water sorption, and this is a significant contributing factor to limiting the life of a toothbrush. In the case of resin composites, water sorption is believed to be a contributory factor to the gradual discoloration of the restorations and the hydrolytic degradation of the resin–filler interface that sometimes occurs. Soft denture liners lose their flexibility due to the loss of water-soluble plasticizers, have an increased propensity to creep, and may even fracture under the osmotic pressure that can build up. Water sorption can have a significant effect on the properties of glass ionomer cements, as too much or too little water can lead to loss of translucency or surface crazing, respectively.

Generally, it is desirable for both the water sorption and soluble fraction of polymers to be as small as possible. This ensures that the polymer retains its characteristic properties and that no components are leached out which might adversely influence the biocompatibility of the material.

The simplest method of assessing the water sorption and soluble fraction of a polymer is to monitor the change in mass of a sample when immersed in water. The detailed analysis of the amount of water sorption by polymeric materials is complicated by the concurrent loss of water-soluble components such as residual monomers or plasticizers, as these two processes take place simultaneously, although at different rates. It is important in the characterization of these factors that the two processes are separated.

Both processes are controlled by the rates of diffusion of water and the water-soluble components through the material, such that the higher the rates of diffusion, the faster water will be absorbed and the faster the soluble fraction will be lost. It is important that any water that the sample has absorbed from the atmosphere has been removed prior to its immersion in water. To this end, samples must be stored in a desiccator until a constant mass is attained.

The kinetics of a sorption and desorption cycle are shown in Figure 1.8.1. The peak in the mass of the sample in the first cycle is a consequence of the different rates of diffusion of water *into* the sample and diffusion of the soluble fraction *out of* the sample. Water is usually absorbed more rapidly than the soluble components are removed, such that there is an initial rapid weight gain until the sample is nearing saturation. At this point,

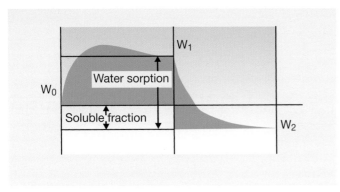

Figure 1.8.1 A schematic representation of the kinetics of water sorption and the dissolution of the soluble fraction.

the loss in mass due to the soluble fraction begins to show, as its release is aided by its dissolution into the absorbed water. The amount of water sorption and the soluble fraction can be calculated from the following:

$$\text{Weight \% water sorption} = (w_1 - w_2)/w_2 \times 100$$

$$\text{Weight \% soluble Fraction} = (w_0 - w_2)/w_2 \times 100$$

If the volume, V, at the end of the desorption cycle is calculated, and W_2 replaced by V, then the water sorption and soluble fraction can be expressed in terms of $\mu g\ mm^{-3}$, as recommended in the international standard (ISO/DIS 4049).

For most polymers, the amount of water sorption is approximately 30–50 $\mu g\ mm^{-3}$. For resin composites, the value will be lower, due to the presence of the glass fillers, but if this is taken into account, the amount of water sorption into the resin should be in the range given above for polymers. Higher values for water sorption have been recorded for some resin composites, which may be associated with the presence of porosity, free space formed due to the removal of the soluble fraction, hydrolytic breakdown of the resin–filler interface, or dissolution of the glass filler.

> ### CLINICAL SIGNIFICANCE
> Excessive water sorption can lead to discoloration and degradation of dental restorative materials.

Bond Rupture

The degradation of polymers by the breakdown of covalent bonds is known as *scission*. Many polymer properties are governed by the molecular weight of the polymer chains. If the polymer chains are broken by chain scission, reducing the molecular weight, this can result in a significant loss of mechanical properties. Bond rupture can be due to radiation, heat, or chemical attack.

Some forms of radiation, such as ultraviolet (UV) light, can penetrate the polymer and interact with the bonds holding the polymer together. One possibility is ionization, where the UV radiation removes an electron from a specific atom, converting this atom into an ion. The result is that the bond with that atom is broken and the polymer chain length is reduced. Another possible outcome is that a cross-link may be formed, and this can also be utilized to good effect to improve the mechanical properties. An example of this is the γ-radiation of polyethylene to introduce cross-links, which improves its resistance to softening and flow at high temperatures.

If a polymer is subjected to elevated temperatures, this can result in chain scission. This can arise simply due to localized overheating during polishing. The ability of a polymer to resist high temperatures depends on the bond energies between the various constituent parts of the polymer (see Chapter 1.2 for bond energies).

Another factor to consider is the chemical attack of polymers by solvents such as alcohol. The absorption of alcohols causes swelling of the polymer matrix, and the weaker polar interactions between the polymer chains can result in a softer material that is more susceptible to wear. However, there are situations in which the breakdown of the polymer can work to our advantage. An example of this is biodegradable polymers, such as soluble sutures and resorbable implants. In this case the degradation process converts the polymer to smaller products (carbon dioxide, water, salts etc.), which can be ingested by cells and transported away from the implant site.

TARNISH AND CORROSION OF METALS

Tarnish is a surface discoloration due to the formation of hard and soft deposits, for example, sulfides and chlorides. Tarnish does not cause a deterioration of the material itself, but can be unsightly, and is easily removed from the surface by polishing the metal. In contrast, corrosion is a chemical reaction between the material and its environment and is therefore a potentially much more serious problem.

The corrosion process for metals is driven by a decrease in the free energy as the metal reacts with a liquid or a gas. For metallic materials, the corrosion process is normally electrochemical, involving the loss of electrons (e^-) in what is called an oxidation reaction:

$$M \rightarrow M^{n+} + ne^-$$

with the metal becoming a positively charged ion. The site at which the oxidation takes place is called the *anode*. The electrons will transfer or become part of another chemical species in a reduction reaction. For example, in an acid solution containing dissolved oxygen, the reduction takes the form of:

$$O_2 + 4H^- + 4e^- \rightarrow 2H_2O$$

The site of the reduction reaction is known as the *cathode*. All metals are prone to corrosive attack when the environment is sufficiently aggressive. Corrosion is highly undesirable, as it weakens materials and may lead to fracture. Similarly, the corrosion products may react adversely with the biological environment. This latter factor is of major concern in the use of metals in dental applications, such as amalgams, crowns and bridges, rubber dam clamps, and orthodontic brackets and archwires.

Dry Corrosion

Other than gold and a few other noble metals, all metals will form a surface oxide coating when the surface comes into contact with the oxygen in the air (Figure 1.8.2). Sometimes this thin film of surface oxide can be seen, as is the case of titanium when it can be made to produce interference colors that are used to good effect in the production of jewelry.

Since the formation of the surface layer of oxide involves the addition of oxygen atoms to the surface, a material that oxidizes will gain weight. This process can be monitored; the three possible outcomes of such an experiment are shown in Figure 1.8.3. Which of these will actually happen depends on the stability of the oxide formed.

If the oxide is very stable, then the corrosion process is self-limiting and there comes a point where the metal ions take so long to diffuse through the thickening oxide layer (whereupon they come into contact with oxygen and react with it) that the oxidation virtually stops. In this case there is an initial rapid gain in mass that gradually tails off; this gives the parabolic mass-gain curve.

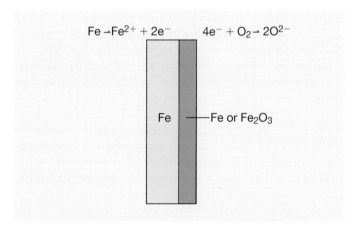

Figure 1.8.2 Oxide formation on the surface of a metal.

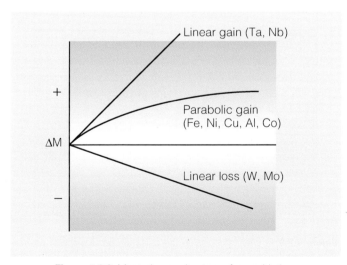

Figure 1.8.3 Mass change due to surface oxidation.

Some oxides are not very stable, and as they form on the metal surface, they tend to crack or to separate partially from the surface, exposing the underlying metal and allowing a new oxide coating to form. In this case there is a gradual build-up of the oxide, causing a continuous gain in mass.

The third possibility, mass loss, is less common and only occurs during the oxidation of certain metals at high temperatures. If the temperature is sufficiently high, the oxide evaporates as soon as it is formed, offering no barrier to further oxidation of the metal. Consequently, material, and thereby mass, is lost as the oxide layer evaporates.

These forms of oxidation are described as *dry corrosion*. Most metals are stable under such processes due to the protective first layer of the oxide coating itself. Hence surplus aircraft are stored in the desert, where it is hot but, more importantly, dry, and cars are less susceptible to rust in hot, dry climates. In the presence of an aqueous environment different conditions prevail and the material's response is much altered.

Wet Corrosion

Wet corrosion can take place in neutral, acid, or alkaline environments. When a metal is placed in an aqueous environment, metal ions and electrons are released into the water (Figure 1.8.4).

An oxidator, commonly oxygen dissolved in the water, withdraws electrons from the metal, in what is known as the *cathodic process*. This extraction of electrons produces a current called the *cathodic current*. This loss of electrons from the metal causes the metal to become positively charged, and positive ions are released into the water, producing an *anodic current*.

Metals do not all oxidize with the same ease and the relative reactivity of metals is presented in what is known as the galvanic series. This is shown in Table 1.8.1 for a series of metals when placed in seawater, where the alloys near the top of this ranking are the least reactive.

If the metal ions are removed from the surface evenly, the process is called *uniform* corrosion. Under suitable conditions, *localized* as opposed to *uniform* corrosion can take place, and this is generally far more dangerous. *Galvanic* and *crevice* corrosion are examples of such localized corrosion.

Galvanic Corrosion

Galvanic corrosion occurs when two dissimilar metals are brought together, resulting in the corrosion of one of the metals being significantly increased.

A classic example of this is the corrosion of zinc in acid. When zinc is in contact with platinum, as shown in Figure 1.8.5, the platinum reacts very quickly with the hydrogen ions that are supplied by the acid and releases electrons, producing hydrogen (this is an example of the cathodic process). This generates an electrical imbalance between the zinc and the platinum, such that electrons flow from the zinc to the platinum. This enhances the release of metal ions from the zinc (the anodic process), such that the zinc corrodes faster when it is in contact with the platinum.

To what degree dissimilar metals will be susceptible to this form of corrosion depends primarily on their relative rates of reaction. Platinum is a particularly effective oxidizer. Other

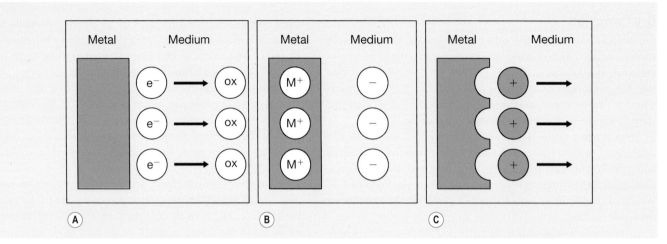

Figure 1.8.4 Oxidation of a metal in an aqueous environment. The oxidator withdraws electrons from the metal in what is known as the cathodic process (a). This causes the metal to become positively charged and the medium negatively charged (b). Due to the positive charge of the metal, metal ions are released, in what is known as the anodic process (c).

TABLE 1.8.1 **The Galvanic Series in Seawater**	
↑	Platinum Gold Titanium Silver
Increasingly inert	Stainless steel Copper Nickel
Increasingly active	Tin
↓	Lead Cast iron Aluminium Zinc

noble metals will not have quite the same effect, as they are not quite so effective at oxidation.

A combination of metals behaving in this way is described as a *galvanic cell* and can occur within alloys due to the presence of different phases with different rates of oxidation. An example is the galvanic cell set up between the γ_1 and γ_2 phases in dental amalgam, where the γ_2 phase corrodes significantly faster than the γ_1 phase.

Crevice Corrosion

When there is a sharp crack or fluid-filled space, as shown in Figure 1.8.6, this space is usually depleted of oxygen. The metal ions will still be released into the space and will form corrosion

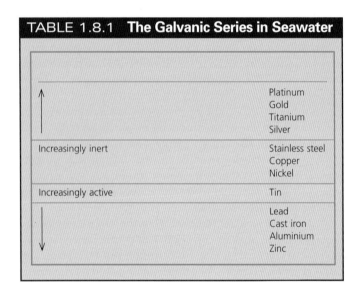

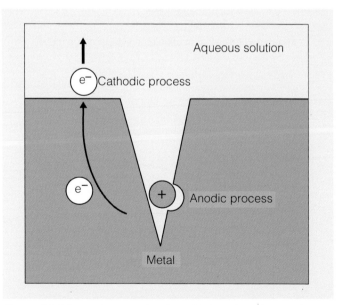

Figure 1.8.5 Galvanic corrosion of zinc in contact with platinum. The noble metal (platinum) is more easily oxidized than the base metal (zinc), such that the anodic process takes place at the zinc surface and zinc ions are released into the aqueous environment.

Figure 1.8.6 In crevice corrosion the oxidation takes place at the surface (cathodic process) and metal ions are released from within the crevice (anodic process).

products, whereas the electrons are unable to react because of the lack of oxygen. Thus the oxidation reaction must take place where there *is* oxygen, which will be at the main surface, such that the electrons will have to travel through the metal, making the base of the crevice anodic and the surface cathodic. Material is therefore lost from the base of the crevice. As the corrosion products are formed, they tend to build up in the crevice such that the supply of oxygen is further restricted. There is nothing to stop this reaction from continuing, which makes this form of corrosion highly insidious. The same process can take place when there is a break in the surface oxide coating, which is known as *pitting* corrosion.

The concentrated attack on one area of the metal is highly undesirable, as it causes the metal to weaken due to the formation and growth of cracks. The damage done is totally out of proportion to the amount of material destroyed by the corrosion process, as the surface cracks seriously reduce the net strength and structural integrity of the structure. Thus localized corrosion is far more dangerous than uniform corrosion.

CLINICAL SIGNIFICANCE

If the conditions are favorable, corrosion of metals can be a rapid and highly damaging process.

DEGRADATION OF CERAMICS

In contrast to metals, ceramics are in general very resistant to electrochemical corrosion but are still susceptible to chemical corrosion. For example, a glass made from only SiO_2 and Na_2O will rapidly dissolve in water, and CaO is added to reduce its susceptibility to dissolution. On the other hand, the dissolution capabilities of certain acids such as hydrofluoric acid are used

to great effect to create microscopically roughened surfaces and improve adhesion to resins by the preferential dissolution of certain phases in the ceramic.

Chemical corrosion can also have a profound effect on the strength of ceramics. The failure of ceramics is usually associated with a crack that has become so large that the component can no longer support the stresses applied. This can manifest itself as a sudden disintegration of the ceramic, such as the apparently inexplicable shattering of a drinking glass or car windscreen. These failures are frequently caused by the slow and undetectable growth of a crack until the crack becomes a critical size and progresses spontaneously and catastrophically. As far as the patient is concerned, the restoration failed suddenly and out of the blue, whereas in fact the failure process has been proceeding, unbeknownst to them, for quite some time. Chemical interaction between the ceramic and the environment at the crack tip can have a profound effect on the rate of crack growth. Water or water vapor at a crack tip can react with the Si–O–Si bond at the tip of the crack in a silica-based glass, forming hydroxides (Figure 1.8.7). This process is often referred to as *static fatigue*. When the environmental conditions are combined with high levels of stress in the ceramic, either by the application of an external load or built-in stress, the rate of growth of the crack will be much accelerated. Under such circumstances, the failure may be described as resulting from *stress corrosion cracking*.

CLINICAL SIGNIFICANCE

All materials are susceptible to attack from the oral environment, such that virtually all materials will degrade in the longer term. The extent and nature of the degradation will dictate whether the material can continue to fulfill its function or needs to be replaced or repaired.

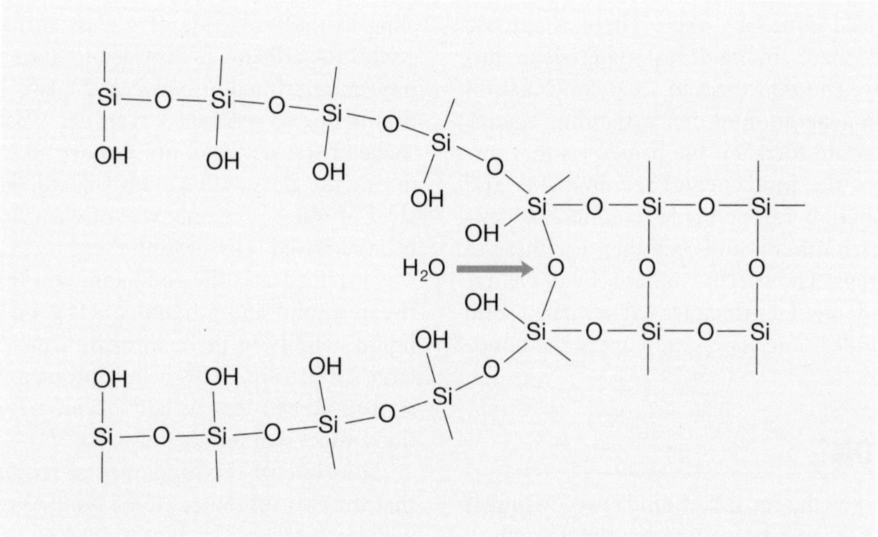

Figure 1.8.7 Crack growth in a ceramic due to local hydration at the tip of the crack.

1.9

Principles of Adhesion

INTRODUCTION

The acid-etch technique of bonding to enamel was introduced into dentistry over 50 years ago, and the application of adhesive products has developed very substantially since this time. New adhesive techniques and materials are introduced to the market at a pace that can be quite bewildering to the clinician; although, as we shall see, later, some of the 'new' products are not so new when you dig down to the science that underpins them.

Two examples of adhesive restorative procedures that moved forward our understanding of the requirements that need to be satisfied in order to obtain robust and resilient bonds are resin-bonded bridges and porcelain veneers. These procedures have been possible because of our improved knowledge and understanding of the surface characteristics of enamel and dentine, and how materials may be made to interact with them. The early adhesive techniques and products, although they have largely been superseded now, laid a foundation for the development of the contemporary materials and techniques that are used in enamel and dentine bonding today.

There are many materials that we wish to bond to enamel and dentine, and to each other. Consequently, numerous adhesive products have been developed to cope with the diversity of the applications; so much so that adhesion of dental materials is one of the greatest sources of confusion among students and experienced clinicians alike. There is intense competition for market share among dental materials manufacturers and as such we should expect to see a continuation of the trend for the *n*th generation of dental bonding agents. As such, the student should focus on the principles that underpin such products – the fundamental requirements and processes by which materials can be made to adhere to dentine and enamel and each other – and only then use these to relate to specific materials. The specific materials will change and evolve, but the fundamental principles will remain a solid foundation to use to understand, assess, and apply the bonding agents of the future.

WHAT IS ADHESION?

Adhesion can be defined as the force that binds two dissimilar materials together when they are brought into intimate contact. This is distinct from *cohesion,* which is the attraction between similar atoms or molecules within one substance.

Adhesion Between Solids

At an atomic level, surfaces are rough. This means that, when they are brought into contact, the only place where intimate contact is achieved is at the tips of the *asperities* (Figure 1.9.1). Very high pressures can be generated at these points, such that, in the absence of any contaminants, an effect called *local adhesion* or *cold welding* can result. If an attempt is then made to slide one surface over the other, a resistance known as *friction* is experienced.

Friction is caused by the need for the local adhesions to be sheared, or broken. In general, the local adhesions are so strong that the shearing process does not take place at the interface but actually within the solids themselves; this explains the general phenomenon of frictional wear.

While frictional forces due to local adhesion can be quite high, adhesion *normal* (i.e. perpendicular) to the surface is usually undetectable. This has been attributed to the build-up of elastic stresses in the normal direction, which are released when the load on the material is removed.

Only very soft metals, such as pure gold, can relieve these elastic stresses by flow and prevent rupture of the junction when a normal load is applied. A dental example of this is the use of cohesive gold.

Adhesion Between a Solid and a Liquid

It is a matter of common observation that a drop of water will cling to the underside of a glass surface. This effect demonstrates the adherence of water to glass that arises by virtue of molecular attraction between the two substances. The attraction is due to secondary (van der Waals) bonds. Even a hard shake of the glass will not remove all of the water and merely drying the glass with a cloth will still leave a very thin residual layer of water. The only way of ensuring that all the water has been removed is by heating the glass in an oven.

This illustrates the good adhesion that may be obtained between a solid and a liquid. Such good adhesion is due to the liquid's ability to make intimate contact with the solid over a large surface area. This is in contrast to the poor adhesion (described above) that usually occurs between two solids, where the contact is at points only.

Thus one of the fundamental requirements of adhesion is that the two substances to be bonded must be in close contact with each other. The importance of this statement cannot be overemphasized, as a strong bond can be created only in the case of intimate molecular contact. This may seem a simple

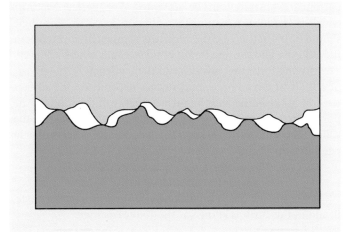

Figure 1.9.1 Point-to-point contact of two solid surfaces at a microscopic level

requirement, but it is not particularly easy to achieve intimate contact at the microscopic level, as noted for solids above.

Given that the distance between the interacting molecules must be less than 0.0007 μm (micrometers; 1 mm = 1000 μm) for adhesion to occur, one appreciates that adhesion is virtually impossible for two solid surfaces. This is a serious obstacle when there is a need for adhesion between two solids, and in order to overcome this, we use a third substance, usually in a fluid or semi-fluid state, to act as an intermediary.

The substance that binds the two materials is defined as the *adhesive*, and the surfaces of the materials are the *adherend* or *substrate*. The point at which the substrate meets the adhesive is described as the *interface* (Figure 1.9.2).

Naturally, what happens at the interface is crucially important to the success or failure of an adhesive bond. This applies equally to industrial and dental adhesives, so it is useful in the first instance to consider the general requirements of an adhesive and then to look more closely at the bonding mechanisms.

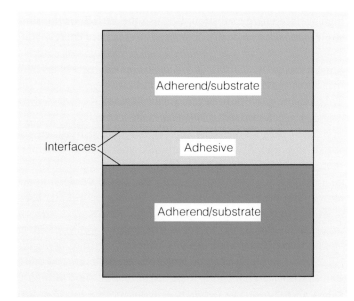

Figure 1.9.2 Terminology for the description of an adhesive joint

CRITERIA FOR ADHESION

When reading the instruction leaflet for a pack of superglue, one sees that one of the first requirements is invariably that the surfaces to be bonded are both clean and dry. This is important for a variety of reasons. A clean, dry surface ensures that the adhesive has the best possible chance of creating a proper bond with the solid material. The presence on the surface of anything that could be considered a contaminant will prevent the formation of a strong bond, since the contaminant itself is weakly bonded to the solid and will prevent the adhesion of the adhesive to the substrate.

The factors that govern the ability of the adhesive to make intimate contact with the substrate are:
- the *wettability* of the substrate by the adhesive
- the *viscosity* of the adhesive
- the *morphology* or *surface roughness* of the substrate.

Wettability

In order for the adhesive to create a bond between two materials, it must make intimate contact with the surfaces of the substrates such that no air voids (which would weaken the overall bond) are formed. The ability of an adhesive to contact a substrate depends on the *wettability* of the adhesive on that particular substrate. *Good wetting* is the ability to cover the substrate completely so that the maximum benefit is obtained from whichever adhesive mechanism is activated.

The ability or inability of fluids to wet a surface is frequently encountered in everyday life. An example of a surface that is extremely difficult to wet with water is PTFE (polytetrafluoroethylene or Teflon®), as used in non-stick saucepans. When water is placed on a PTFE surface, it forms globules that will not spread in an even layer across the surface. This is an example of poor wettability. This and the other possible responses are depicted in Figure 1.9.3.

The interaction between the substrate and the adhesive is governed by a driving force that tends to spread the adhesive over the substrate, and resistance to spreading that depends on the viscosity of the adhesive, the surface irregularities, and the presence of contaminants. The driving force is provided by the surface energies of the adhesive and the substrate.

Surface Energy

In the bulk of a solid or a liquid the molecules are subjected to attractive forces in all directions, such that the molecule is in dynamic equilibrium with its surrounding molecules. At the surface, however, this delicate balance is destroyed, resulting in a net inward attraction directed toward the large number of molecules in the mass of the material. It is this inward force that

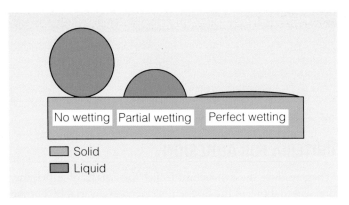

Figure 1.9.3 The possible wetting characteristics for liquids on a solid surface

gives rise to the *surface energy* of a material. In liquids the surface energy is known as the *surface tension*.

One of the effects of surface tension is the tendency for liquids to take up a spherical shape in preference to any other. This arises because a sphere has the minimum surface area (and hence the minimum surface energy) for a given volume of liquid, allowing the total energy stored in the liquid to be a minimum.

Whereas the surface tension of a liquid is a real surface stress, in the case of a solid work is done in stretching and not in forming the surface. The measurement of the surface energy of a solid is not achieved as readily as it is with liquids. An approach that has now gained wide acceptance is one pioneered by Zisman, who introduced the concept of the *critical surface energy*.

Contact Angle

When a solid and a liquid make contact, the angle between the liquid surface and the solid surface is known as the *contact angle* and is dependent on the surface tension of the liquid and the surface energy of the solid (Figure 1.9.4).

By measuring the contact angle between the solid and the liquid, a useful measure of the wettability of the liquid on a particular substrate can be obtained. For perfect wetting, which is the ideal situation for adhesion to occur, this angle should be 0°. In this case the surface is completely covered with the adhesive and the maximum bond strength can be achieved. The driving force that gives rise to the tendency, or otherwise, of a fluid to spread on a solid surface depends on the surface tension of the liquid and the surface energy of the solid. At the point where the surface of the liquid meets the surface of the solid, their surface tensions must balance, in order to be in equilibrium:

$$\gamma_{SV} = \gamma_{sl} + \gamma_{lv}\cos\theta$$

This relationship can be rearranged to give the contact angle, θ, and in this form is known as the *Young equation*:

$$\cos\theta = (\gamma_{SV} - \gamma_{sl})/\gamma_{lv}$$

where γ_{sl} is the surface energy at the solid–liquid interface, γ_{sv} is the surface energy at the solid–vapor interface, and γ_{lv} is the surface energy at the liquid–vapor interface.

Critical Surface Energy

If one measures the contact angle of a number of different liquids on the same substrate and plots the cosine of the contact angle against the known surface tension of the liquids, then a linear relationship results.

This relationship is shown in Figure 1.9.5; it shows the linear curve being extrapolated to the point where it crosses the line at which the cosine of the contact angle is equal to 1. This is the situation under which the contact angle will be 0°, representing the condition of perfect wetting.

The value of the surface tension at which the cosine of the contact equals 1 is defined as the *critical surface energy* of the solid. This critical surface energy is equal to the surface tension of a liquid that will *just* spread on the surface of the solid; such a liquid may be real or hypothetical. Any liquid that has a surface tension less than the critical surface energy of the solid will wet the surface of the solid effectively.

Thus a low surface energy liquid will readily spread over a high surface energy substrate because the surface of the substrate is replaced by a surface with a lower surface energy.

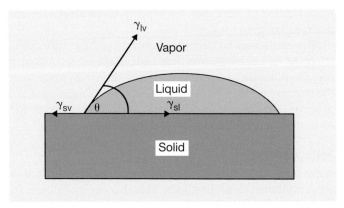

Figure 1.9.4 The contact angle θ between a liquid and a solid, where γ_{sv} is the surface tension between the solid and the vapor, γ_{sl} is the surface tension between the solid and the liquid, and γ_{lv} is that between the liquid and the vapor

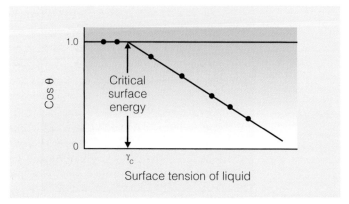

Figure 1.9.5 Zisman plot for the determination of the critical surface energy, γ_c, of a solid

TABLE 1.9.1 Typical Surface Energies	
Material	Surface Energy × 10⁻³ J m²
Perfluorolauric acid	6
Methyl chloride	16
Polytetrafluoroethylene (PTFE)	18
Polytrifluoroethylene	22
Ethyl alcohol	24
Polyvinyl chloride (PVC)	39
Water	73
Plate glass	200
Steel	230
Iron oxide	350
Alumina	560
Mercury	488

PTFE has a very low surface energy, making it difficult to find liquids with lower surface tensions that could wet it successfully. Another material with a similarly low surface energy is silicone rubber. Again, it is extremely difficult to make anything adhere to this material.

On the other hand, silicone polymers in their liquid form tend to adapt well to most surfaces due to their low surface energies. These polymers are used to great effect in impression materials.

Examples of the surface energy of some substances, expressed in units of $J \cdot m^{-2}$ ($N \cdot m^{-1}$) for convenience, are provided in Table 1.9.1. In the case of perfluorolauric acid, only condensed inert gases can spread on this surface.

CLINICAL SIGNIFICANCE

Before bonding to a surface, one must make sure it is scrupulously clean, or no adhesive bond will form. An adhesive must be compatible with the surface to be bonded. For example, hydrophobic resins will not stick to hydrophilic surfaces.

Viscosity

For an adhesive to be effective, it must be able not only to make intimate contact with the substrate but also to spread easily on it, yet not so easily that it is impossible to control. The driving force for the spreading of the liquid is provided by its wettability on the solid surface and is resisted by the liquid's viscosity. Too high a viscosity is undesirable, as it prevents the fluid from flowing readily over the surface of the solid and penetrating into narrow cracks and crevices.

In general, contact angles are directly proportional to the viscosity of the adhesive, but this can be a misleading statement if the adhesive is a solvent containing additives.

The use of low surface tension solvents with highly viscous solutes will give misleadingly low contact angles. Although a low contact angle is obtained, the resistance to flow offered by the high viscosity of the solute will continue to resist the spreading.

Similarly, a highly filled adhesive, such as a composite resin, can be difficult to spread, which may lead one to think it has a high surface tension and poor wettability. However, the substrate only experiences contact with the low-viscosity resin that may readily wet the surface if it has the correct surface tension. The spreading of the composite resin is merely resisted by its own stiffness and not by any reluctance on the part of the resin to wet the underlying surface.

The ability of a liquid to fill cracks and crevices can be quantified by what is described as the penetration coefficient (PC), which is a function of the surface tension (γ) of the liquid and its viscosity (η), according to the equation:

$$PC = \gamma Cos\theta/2\eta$$

The penetration coefficient is a measure of the ability of a liquid to penetrate into a capillary space, such as interproximal regions, gingival pockets, and pores. An example of the penetration coefficient for mouth rinses is shown in Figure 1.9.6.

Surface Roughness

The measurement of contact angles assumes that the surface of the substrate is perfectly smooth. In reality, the surface may be quite rough at a microscopic level. This roughness has the advantage of increasing the potential area for bonding but can also give rise to the entrapment of air. Such entrapment will significantly reduce the effective bonding area and result in a weak bond. Cracks and crevices constitute surface irregularities and the adhesive must be able to flow into these.

Adhesives with a high viscosity are particularly prone to causing entrapment of air because their stiffness may be such that they bridge the small cracks and crevices in the surface rather than flowing into them.

In the absence of air capillary action ensures that the adhesive penetrates the cracks and crevices. For this penetration to occur readily, a high surface tension adhesive is desirable, as this means that the capillary attraction is also high. This effect is demonstrated by the fact that the higher the surface tension of a liquid, the higher the liquid will climb up a capillary placed in it.

The driving force that causes capillary action must work against the pressure of the air that is trapped by the adhesive

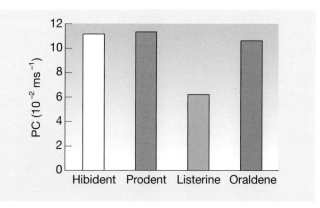

Figure 1.9.6 Penetration coefficients for mouth rinses. Adapted from Perdok et al. Physicochemical properties of commercially available mouthrinses. J Dent 1990; 18: 147.

and must also overcome the viscous resistance forces. However, the surface tension of the liquid must also be sufficiently low to wet the substrate perfectly. Hence the ideal adhesive would have a surface tension just below the surface energy of the solid. If this condition is satisfied, then the surface irregularities can be advantageous in improving the bond strength of the adhesive.

An irregular surface has a higher surface area than a smooth surface, so more chemical bonds can be created. If the irregularities are of a particular morphology, such that undercuts are present at the microscopic level, the bond can be enhanced by the process of micromechanical interlocking.

MECHANISMS OF ADHESION

First, let us assume that the initial criterion for adhesion is met, in that intimate contact at the molecular level between the adhesive and the substrate is achieved. Let us now look at what happens when the materials are in contact and see how they may interact. An adhesive bond can be mechanical, physical, or chemical and is more usually a combination of all of these.

Mechanical Adhesion

The simplest method of adhesion is that of the mechanical interlocking of components. This form of adhesion can result from the presence of surface irregularities, such as pits and fissures that give rise to microscopic undercuts.

A primary condition for this form of adhesion is that the adhesive can penetrate readily into the pits before it begins to set. This condition is determined by the wettability of the adhesive on the substrate, which in turn is governed by the relative surface energies and the resultant contact angle, the ideal situation being that of perfect wetting. To improve the level of contact, any air or vapor in the pits must be able to escape in front of the advancing liquid. If the adhesive is able to penetrate these spaces and subsequently to set solid, it remains locked in by the undercuts (Figure 1.9.7). The degree of penetration will depend both on the pressure used in the application of the adhesive and on the properties of the adhesive itself.

If the adhesive is to disengage from the substrate, then it must fracture in the process of debonding, as it cannot withdraw from the undercut. This is not unlike the concept of retention, used in the placement of restorations, except that it occurs at a microscopic level. However, one important difference is that good wettability is not a prerequisite for macro-retention,

whereas it is of paramount importance for micromechanical interlocking.

The general view is that undercuts frequently provide important mechanical characteristics but that they are not usually sufficient to act as the mechanism of adhesion in themselves. There are a number of additional adhesive mechanisms that are due to what can be described as physical and chemical causes. The term *true adhesion*, or *specific adhesion*, is commonly used to distinguish physical and chemical adhesion from mechanical adhesion. However, such terms should be discouraged, as these are inappropriate.

True adhesion implies that there is also false adhesion, but a material is either adhesive or not. Physical adhesion and chemical adhesion are distinguished from mechanical adhesion by virtue of the fact that they involve a molecular attraction between the adhesive and the substrate, whereas mechanical adhesion does not require such interaction at the interface.

Physical Adhesion

When two surfaces are in close proximity, secondary forces of attraction arise through dipole interactions between polar molecules (see Chapter 1.2). The attractive forces that are generated can be quite small, even if the molecules have a substantial permanent dipole moment or have a large polarizability.

The magnitude of the interaction energy is dependent on the relative alignment of the dipoles in the two surfaces but is usually less than 0.2 eV. This is considerably less than primary bonds, such as ionic or covalent bonds, which are typically 2.0–6.0 eV.

This type of bonding is rapid (because no activation energy is needed) and reversible (because the molecules remain chemically intact on the surface). This weak physical *adsorption* is easily overcome by thermal energy and is not suitable if a permanent bond is desired. Even so, the hydrogen bond in particular can be an important precursor to the formation of a strong chemical bond.

It follows that non-polar liquids will not readily bond to polar solids and vice versa because there is no interaction between the two substances at the molecular level, even if there is good adaptation. Non-polar liquid silicone polymers exhibit such behavior and will not form bonds to solids other than themselves; this bonding is only possible because the chemical reaction of cross-linking provides sites for bonding between the solid and the liquid.

Chemical Adhesion

If a molecule dissociates after adsorption onto the surface and the constituent components then bond themselves separately by covalent or ionic forces, a strong adhesive bond will result. This form of adhesion is known as *chemisorption* and can be either covalent or ionic in nature.

The sharing of electrons between the two atoms in the chemical bond distinguishes it from the physical interaction. Adhesives must be strongly attracted chemically to the surface of application in order for strong bonds to form and require the presence of reactive groups on both surfaces. This is particularly so for the formation of covalent bonds, such as occurs in

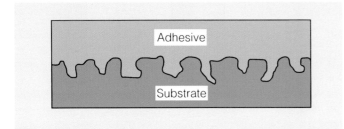

Figure 1.9.7 Microscopic mechanical interlocking between an adhesive and the substrate

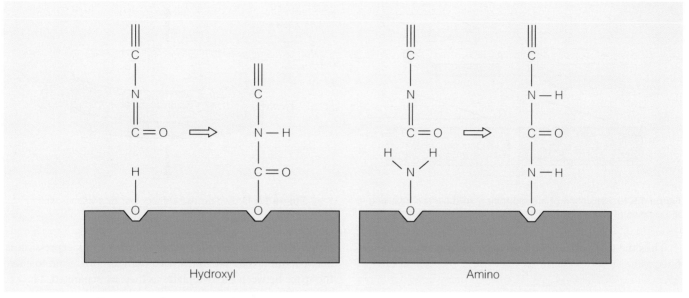

Figure 1.9.8 Covalent bond formation between an isocyanate and a hydroxyl and an amino group on the surface of the substrate

the bonding of reactive isocyanates to polymeric surfaces containing hydroxyl and amino groups (Figure 1.9.8).

In contrast, a metallic bond is readily created between a solid metal and a liquid metal, which forms the basis for soldering or brazing. The metallic bond is provided by free electrons and is chemically unspecific. However, the bond will only be possible if the metal surfaces are scrupulously clean. In practice, this means that fluxes need to be used to remove oxide films that would otherwise prevent the metal atoms from meeting.

The mechanical breaking of these chemical bonds becomes the only way of separating the adhesive and the substrate, and there is no reason why these bonds should be broken in preference to any other valence bond. This places a restriction on the strength that can be achieved. If the bond strength exceeds the tensile strength of the adhesive or the substrate, then a cohesive failure of the adhesive or substrate will occur before the bond fails.

Adhesion Through Molecular Entanglement

So far, it has been assumed that there is a distinct interface between the adhesive and the substrate. In effect, the adhesive is adsorbed onto the surface of the substrate and can be considered as being *surface active,* collecting on the surface but not dissolving in the medium below. In some instances, the adhesive, or a component of the adhesive, is able to penetrate the surface of the substrate and absorb *into* it rather than *onto* it. It should be stressed that the absorption of molecules is a *result* of good wetting and not the cause.

If the absorbing component is a long-chain molecule or forms a long-chain molecule within the penetrated layer, the resultant entanglement between the adhesive and the substrate is capable of producing very high bond strengths (Figure 1.9.9).

Thus adhesives must be strongly attracted chemically to the surfaces of application in order to form a strong bond.

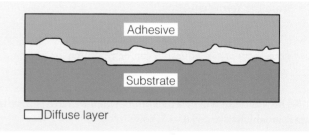

Diffuse layer

Figure 1.9.9 Diffuse interpenetrating layer arising from molecular entanglement between the adhesive and the substrate

CLINICAL SIGNIFICANCE

It is important to know what type of bond one is trying to achieve so that the bonding steps are understood. This way, there is less chance of making an error that can compromise the strength or longevity of the bond.

THE STRENGTH OF THE ADHESIVE BOND

A reasonably strong bond can result from the cumulative action of a number of bonding mechanisms that act in concert, such as a large area of intimate contact providing numerous sites for the creation of weak secondary bonds, and the presence of surface undercuts at the microscopic level.

Theoretical Strength

It is possible to determine roughly the theoretical strength of an adhesive joint between a liquid and a solid.

If we assume that we have the unit surface area of the solid in contact with the liquid, the energy required to separate these materials will be the difference between the energy of the surfaces when joined and the energies of the individual surfaces when separated (Figure 1.9.10).

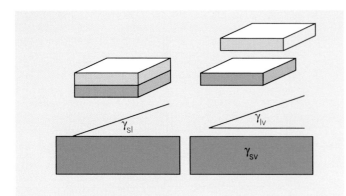

Figure 1.9.10 Separation of a liquid from a solid surface, resulting in the creation of two surfaces

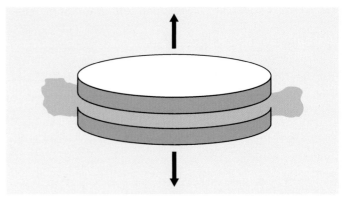

Figure 1.9.11 Two plates held together by a viscous liquid

Thus the work of adhesion per unit surface area can be defined as:

$$W_a = \gamma_{sv} + \gamma_{lv} - \gamma_{sl}$$

This is known as the *Dupré equation,* which states that the work of adhesion is the sum of the surface free energy of the solid and the liquid, less the interfacial energy between the solid and the liquid.

From the Young equation:

$$\gamma_{sv} - \gamma_{sl} = \gamma_{lv} \cos\theta$$

Thus the work of adhesion can be rewritten as:

$$W_a = \gamma_{lv}(1 + \cos\theta)$$

This adhesion will be a maximum when we have perfect wetting, in which case $\cos\theta = 1$, so:

$$W_a = 2\gamma_{lv}$$

For a hydrocarbon liquid, the surface tension is approximately 30 mJ·m^{-2}. If it is assumed that the attractive force falls to 0 at a distance of 3×10^{-10} m, then the force required to pull the liquid away from the solid surface is given by the work of adhesion divided by the distance, giving about 200 MPa. This value is, in fact, far in excess of anything found in the real situation. For example, two slides held together by an interposing liquid are difficult to separate by pulling apart but separation is readily achieved by shearing the two slides apart, as the liquid has no resistance to such a shearing action other than its viscosity.

Thus it is not enough for the fluid adhesive to wet the surface of the substrate and provide a chemical bond. It must also be able to resist tensile and shearing forces, which would cause failure within the adhesive. Increasing the viscosity would make shearing more difficult, and this is the basis on which adhesives, such as single-sided sticky tape, work.

When two plates that are held together by an interposing viscous substance are separated (Figure 1.9.11), the relationship between the force required to do so and the viscosity of the liquid is given by:

$$F = \frac{3}{2}\left(\pi\eta R^4 / h^3\right)(\delta h/\delta t)$$

where η is the viscosity, R is the radius of the plates, and h is the thickness of the adhesive.

We will not concern ourselves with how this expression is derived, but it is based on the need for additional fluid to enter the space between the two plates as they are separated. The expression shows that the force is dependent on the viscosity and the thickness of the adhesive layer. The higher the viscosity of the adhesive and the thinner the adhesive layer, the more force is required to separate the two plates. This expression also shows that the force depends on the rate of separation.

High rates of separation are resisted more strongly than low rates. The adhesive bond is not resistant to long-term low loads, as it would fail by viscous flow in this manner. The best resistance to shear would therefore be offered by a liquid that turns into a solid, as this greatly increases its shear strength.

Real Bond Strengths

The actual strengths of adhesive joints are found to be at least an order of magnitude smaller than those predicted from theoretical strength calculations. Another common observation is that bond failure does not often take place at the interface between the substrate and the adhesive but actually somewhere *within* the adhesive, which is essentially a cohesive failure.

Where the failure is genuinely adhesive in nature, it is most probably due to the inability of the adhesive to adapt to the substrate, such that no interaction at the molecular level is possible. Alternatively, contamination or the entrapment of air or other gases at the interface can prevent a good contact from being established. In this case again, the failure will be at the interface, occurring due to the nucleation and growth of cavities at weak spots along the joint. This highlights the importance of contaminant-free surfaces for bonding.

In practice, the strengths of many adhesive bonds are governed by the presence of stress concentrations in the adhesive or at the interface rather than being a function of the local forces of attraction at the interface. This is especially the case when the bonded structure is subjected to environmental attack or highly stressed loading conditions. In general, adhesives tend to have poorer mechanical properties (i.e. tensile strength and shear strength) than the substrates being bonded, such that surface and internal defects can play a major role in determining the bond strength of the adhesive joint.

For example, if the exposed surface of the adhesive contains numerous defects, then the probability of finding a defect of a critical size is increased as the exposed surface area of the adhesive is increased. For this reason, it is important that the thickness of the adhesive layer is kept to a minimum. The adhesive must be able to adopt a very thin film thickness, which imposes limits on the addition of fillers that might be incorporated to improve the strength.

There is another reason why the minimal application of adhesives is desirable, and that is because of the shrinkage associated with the setting process of the adhesive. When an adhesive shrinks on setting, the contraction may be away from the surface of the substrate such that debonding of the adhesive occurs immediately after placement. Even if the bond holds out during the initial contraction, the stresses generated may be sufficient to eventually cause breakdown of the bond. The thinner the layer of adhesive, the smaller the shrinkage will be. This is one reason why it is important that indirect restorations such as veneers, crowns, and bridges have as good a marginal fit as it is possible to achieve, if the restoration is to be bonded to the tooth structures. The setting shrinkage of resin-based restorative materials such as resin composites, which is a consequence of the polymerization process, can generate very high localized interfacial stresses and contribute to the failure of the bond.

CLINICAL SIGNIFICANCE

More often than not, a bond failure for a compatible adhesive system, such as acid-etched enamel and resin, is usually due to part of the procedure not having been followed properly since, when properly executed, the bond is extremely strong.

ADHESION PROMOTERS

There are many instances in which two materials need to be bonded to each other but will not do so under normal circumstances because they have no particular affinity for each other and consequently will not wet each other.

A dental example of this would be the desire to obtain a strong and durable bond between the glass filler particles used in a composite resin and the resin itself. To allow these two materials to bond by means other than the physical adsorption of one on to the other (which would be inadequate in itself), it is necessary to modify one or other of the two surfaces to achieve a bond. In this instance an intermediary substance is used that is able to bond to both of the materials in question and such a material is known as a *coupling agent*. Alternatively, it is possible to modify the characteristics of the surface of one of the two materials so that a bond can be created. These materials are known as *primers*.

Coupling Agents

The surface of glass, being ionic in nature, readily adsorbs water, forming a well-bonded surface layer that may be many molecules thick. The formation of this water layer cannot be avoided during the commercial processing of glass.

As a consequence of this, when glass is mixed with a resin to produce a composite, be it a fiber composite or a particulate composite, the resin will not wet the surface of the glass and the two are poorly bonded. This has the effect of producing a very weak composite because the glass is not able to take on a load-bearing role and acts merely as a space filler. Some method needs to be devised to dispose of the adsorbed water. One such approach is the use of *coupling agents*. An appropriate coupling agent, applied to the glass, will displace the water on the surface if the bond created between it and the glass is more stable than that between the water and the glass.

The function of the coupling agent is to displace the adsorbed water and provide a strong chemical link between the oxide groups on the glass surface and the polymer molecules of the resin. Silane coupling agents are extensively used for this purpose and have the general formula:

$$R - Si - X_3$$

where R represents an organo-functional group and the X units are hydrolyzable groups bonded to the silane. The latter are only present as an intermediate, since they are hydrolyzed to form a silanol as follows:

$$R - Si - X_3 + 3H_2O \rightarrow R - Si(OH)_3 + 3HX$$

These trihydroxy-silanols are able to compete with the water on the surface of the glass by forming hydrogen bonds with the hydroxyl groups on the glass surface.

When the silane-coated glass is now dried, the water is removed and a condensation reaction occurs between the silanol and the surface. The two stages involved are shown in Figure 1.9.12. Once this bond is formed, it is no longer susceptible to hydrolysis.

When the resin is now placed in contact with the silane-treated glass, the organo-functional group, R, reacts with the resin, and forms a strong bond to it. For this process to succeed, it is important that the organo-functional group is so chosen so as to be compatible with the particular resin system employed.

This approach produces a strong, water-resistant bond. Without the coupling agent, the bond would deteriorate rapidly

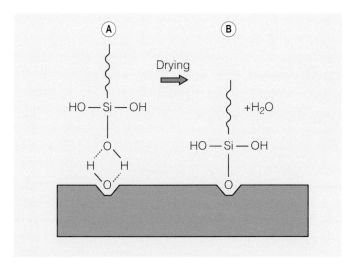

Figure 1.9.12 Hydrogen bond formation between a silane and a surface hydroxyl group (a), which, after drying, forms into a covalent bond with the release of water (b)

as water diffuses through the resin and re-adsorbs onto the glass surface, displacing the resin.

The bond, as depicted in Figure 1.9.12, will be very rigid, as the organo-functional groups are very short. Strains generated by shrinkage during setting, or possibly by differential thermal shrinkage, could be sufficient to cause the bond to fail. This problem can be overcome by making sure that the organo-functional groups consist of reasonably long molecules, providing the necessary degree of flexibility. In a sense the interface created by the use of coupling agents should be treated as two interfaces: namely, the glass–silanol interface and the resin–organo-functional group interface.

Two commonly used silane coupling agents are γ-methacryloxypropyltrimethoxysilane and γ-mercaptopropyltrimethoxysilane.

Primers

Primers, like the coupling agents, are another group of substances that seek to make the surface of the substrate more amenable to accepting a bond. Primers are usually applied in conjunction with an adhesive.

A typical example of a primer is one that is used to seal the surface of wood prior to applying the adhesive. If a primer were not applied, the adhesive would be soaked up by the porosity of the wood, such that none remained at the interface.

There are many dental examples of primers, such as phosphoric acid, which is used for preparing the enamel surface, and the wide variety of dentine conditioners, which are used in conjunction with dentine-bonding agents. Unfortunately, in the dental literature the distinction between primers and coupling agents is lost, and the two terms are used interchangeably.

SUMMARY

Adhesion is not a simple phenomenon, nor is it comprehensible with a single model. The formation of an adhesive bond depends on a multitude of factors and rarely involves a single adhesive mechanism.

CLINICAL SIGNIFICANCE

Adhesion has become one of the major cornerstones of dentistry. In operative dentistry it has created the opportunity to produce a marginal seal around restorations. In prosthetic dentistry it has provided the opportunity to explore new materials and techniques. There is no aspect of dentistry that has not been touched in some way by our improved understanding of the molecular interactions between materials at their interfaces.

Clinical Dental Materials

Dental Amalgam

INTRODUCTION

An amalgam is a particular variety of alloy, formed when mercury reacts with another metal or metals. Mercury is liquid at room temperature (solidifying at $-39°C$), and it reacts readily with metals such as silver, tin, and copper to produce alloys, which are soft and pliable for a short time, and set to become hard, rigid solids. From a dental perspective, the reaction is convenient in its speed, in that once the mercury and other metals are mixed together, the resulting material remains pliable for a few minutes, long enough for the clinician to manipulate it into the cavity and carve the final desired profile, but then becomes solid and strong soon afterward, allowing the patient to go about their day without undue inconvenience.

Dental amalgam had a fairly inauspicious beginning when it was first used as a restorative material, being made by mixing Spanish or Mexican silver coins with mercury early in the 19th century. In the early days dentistry was not regulated, and materials – and indeed practices and practitioners – varied enormously in their quality. The development of modern, reliable, and reproducible dental amalgams is due, in no small way, to one of the most famous dentists ever, G.V. Black, who recognized the need to determine the properties of dental amalgams with some accuracy if their performance was ever going to be predictable. By the beginning of the 20th century, because of his research work, amalgams could be produced with reasonably predictable handling characteristics.

Although the composition and presentation of amalgam has evolved over the intervening century, the pace of change in amalgam has been sluggish compared to the development and evolution of the other direct restorative materials of composite resins, glass ionomer cements, and the related materials. While these various materials have in some instances superseded amalgam, amalgam still has its place. Although amalgam use continues to decline for reasons we shall discuss later in this chapter, it is and will be used in many parts of the world for some time to come, and the clinician in dental education today can expect to encounter amalgam restorations in need of scrutiny, repair, or replacement, for many decades. It is important therefore to understand this material in full and not to consign it to the dustbin of history prematurely.

In this chapter we discuss modern amalgams, their composition and properties, and how these have developed over timescales of relevance to the modern practitioner (that is, to the extent that they might encounter 'old' amalgams still in patients' mouths today).

CLINICAL DENTAL AMALGAMS

Presentation

As outlined above, an amalgam is defined as an alloy that has mercury as one of its component metals. Dental amalgam is an alloy of mercury with silver, tin and copper. The material is supplied in a capsule with two compartments: one compartment containing the mercury and one containing all of the other metals, in the form of an alloy. Thus we refer to the mercury and the alloy that are brought together to make the dental amalgam. When the clinician selects a certain dental amalgam, they are effectively selecting the chemistry and presentation of the *alloy* with which the mercury will be mixed and react.

Strictly speaking, the material that is supplied by the manufacturer cannot be called a dental *amalgam*. An amalgam has mercury as one of its component metals. When supplied in its special capsule, the mercury is still separate from the other metals; at this stage, it is mercury and an alloy, not an amalgam. It only becomes an amalgam when the mercury and other metals come into contact and react with one another – *amalgam* is the material produced as a *consequence* of the reaction between the mercury and the alloy. However, this distinction is usually overlooked, and arguably it would make the marketing of the material somewhat confusing if the product had to be described as 'a capsule containing mercury and other metals that when they react together will form amalgam' rather than simply 'amalgam'. We will therefore follow this unscientific but convenient convention and refer to the material supplied by the manufacturer as a dental amalgam, as well as (correctly) the material that forms the filling in the patient's mouth.

Alloy Form

The alloy is used in the form of a powder, and the size and shape of the particles in this powder are critical to the handling characteristics and the final properties of the restoration. The alloy powder is available as either *lathe-cut* particles or *spherical* particles, as shown in Figure 2.1.1.

Lathe-Cut Alloy Particles

The lathe-cut particles are produced by machining a solid ingot of the alloy on a lathe. The chippings that are produced are graded, and only those in the right size range are used. The alloy is available as coarse-, medium-, or fine-grained powder, and each will handle slightly differently. The individual chippings will have become highly stressed during the machining, and this

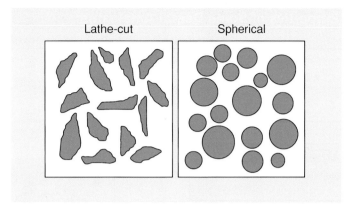

Figure 2.1.1 Schematic representation of the lathe-cut and spherical shapes of alloy particles used in amalgams

makes their surfaces very reactive to mercury. A consequence of this is that the setting reaction is far too rapid unless heat treatment (which relieves the internal stresses) is applied.

Spherical Alloy Particles

The production of the spherical particles is by a quite different route. The various ingredients of the alloy are melted together and then sprayed into an inert atmosphere, where the droplets solidify as small, spherical pellets of various sizes. This method of manufacture has the advantages that no further machining processes are required and that the composition of the alloy can be readily altered. What is important to the manufacturer is that the yield of particles of the correct size is as high as possible, since this minimizes the cost of production. The particles that are rejected because they are either too big or too small are simply recycled.

Admixed or Dispersed Phase Alloy Particles

Lathe-cut and spherical alloy particles each offer certain advantages, and a product evolved that contained a mixture of the two particle shapes, in an attempt to benefit from the favorable properties of both. These are usually known as admix(ed) or dispersed phase amalgams, and the majority of modern amalgams fall into this category.

Composition

The mercury in an amalgam forms around 40–50% of the total mass and needs to be very pure, as any contaminants interfere with the setting reaction; for this reason, the mercury is triple distilled. The remaining 50–60% of the material is made up of the alloy. Traditional dental amalgam, widely used from the 1960s onward, was made using an alloy consisting mainly of a mixture of silver and tin in roughly a 3:1 ratio (Table 2.1.1). Copper was sometimes added in small quantities (below about 6% by mass) to increase the strength and hardness of the amalgam, and small additional quantities of mercury (typically 1–2%) were also sometimes added to the alloy to provide a more rapid reaction, in what is referred to as *pre-amalgamation*. Zinc was present in some formulations as a result of the method of production of the alloy, but this led to undesirable traits such as delayed expansion owing to the formation of zinc oxide and

	% In Traditional Amalgam Alloy	**% In High Copper Amalgam Alloy**
Constituent		
Ag	67–74	60–70
Sn	25–28	18–30
Cu	0–6	12–30
Hg	0–3	0–3
Zn	0–2	0

TABLE 2.1.1 Composition of Traditional and High-Copper Dental Amalgam Alloys

Note that the alloy is mixed with roughly equal quantities of mercury, so the composition of the finished amalgam will be roughly half the values shown here, with the other half being mercury.

as a consequence is rarely, if ever, found in modern amalgams (Table 2.1.2).

This traditional formulation was used fairly successsfully for many years, but it did display one particular undesirable trait, which was a tendency to corrode. While a little corrosion is generally considered to be acceptable in relation to amalgam – amalgam corrosion products build up in the microscopic voids between the amalgam and the dental hard tissues and provide a seal, preventing the ingress of bacteria – too much corrosion is damaging. Furthermore, amalgam can be subject to different *forms* of corrosion, and some are more insidious and destructive than others. If the conditions for corrosion are right, the material can deteriorate quite rapidly, losing strength and integrity, becoming rough and dull, and more prone to fracture.

Fortunately, as the understanding of these corrosion processes developed, so did the understanding of how to limit or prevent them. It was found that by increasing the copper content from 0–6% in traditional amalgams in the range of 12–30%, the setting chemistry was adjusted in such a way as to reduce the corrosion and improve various other properties, which we shall come on to shortly. A typical composition of these high copper amalgams is given in Table 2.1.1. To understand the effects of changing the alloy composition, we need to look in some detail at the setting process of these materials and the resultant final structure of the traditional and high-copper amalgams.

TABLE 2.1.2	**Selected Properties of Some Dental Amalgams**					
Material	**Manufacturer**	**Type**	**% Cu Content**	**% Creep**	**Compressive Strength (MPa)**	
					1 hour	**24 hours**
GS 80	SDI	Admix	28.7	0.1	225	510
Dispersalloy	Dentsply	Admix	12	0.25	226	440
Tytin	Kerr	Spherical	12	0.1	260	472

CLINICAL SIGNIFICANCE

Modern dental amalgams are almost exclusively of the high-copper variety owing to their corrosion resistance.

SETTING REACTIONS OF AMALGAMS

Silver and tin are major constituents of the alloy of both traditional and high-copper amalgam and are mostly present as the intermetallic compound Ag_3Sn, known commonly as the γ *phase*. The phase diagram for the Ag–Sn system is shown in Figure 2.1.2 and shows that the Ag_3Sn phase is the third pure phase in the system, hence the Greek symbol γ (gamma). The setting reaction between the Ag_3Sn or γ phase and the mercury is initiated by a vigorous mixing of the two ingredients. This mixing causes the outer layer of the alloy particles to dissolve into the mercury, forming two new phases, which are solid at room temperature. The reaction is as follows:

$$Ag_3Sn \quad + Hg \quad \rightarrow Ag_3Sn \quad + Ag_2Hg_3 + Sn_7Hg$$
$$\gamma \quad + \text{mercury} \rightarrow \gamma \quad + \underbrace{\gamma_1 \quad + \gamma_2}$$

| powder | liquid | unreacted | amalgam | matrix |
| | | alloy | | |

As can be seen from the reaction, not all of the alloy particles dissolve in the mercury. On the contrary, a considerable amount remains, so the final structure is one of a core of γ held together

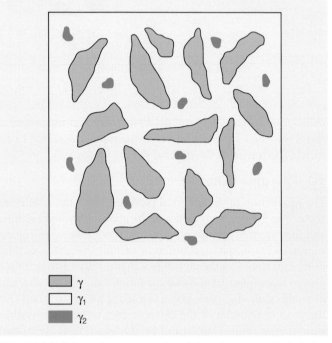

	γ
	γ_1
	γ_2

Figure 2.1.3 Schematic representation of the microstructure of a lathe-cut alloy-based amalgam

by a matrix of predominantly γ_1, which is interspersed with γ_2. The structure of the set material is shown in Figure 2.1.3. The γ_2-phase has various undesirable attributes, as we shall see in the next section.

The effect of the additional copper used in high-copper amalgams is to modify the setting reaction, creating a parallel reaction pathway as follows:

$$\gamma_2 + Ag\text{-}Cu \rightarrow Cu_6Sn_5 + \gamma_1$$

The outcome is that in high copper amalgams the γ_2 phase is very much reduced, or eliminated, and converted to more γ_1. The structure of this amalgam is shown in Figure 2.1.4. While the copper-tin phase that is produced alongside the γ_1 is still more corrosion-susceptible than the γ or γ_1, it is much less so than γ_2, and thus overall, the material is more resistant to corrosion.

The method of incorporating copper into the alloy powder is different for the different forms of alloy and this has implications for the properties. The copper in the lathe-cut alloy is present in the form of discrete areas of Cu_3Sn and remains mainly within the original alloy in its unreacted form. In the case of the

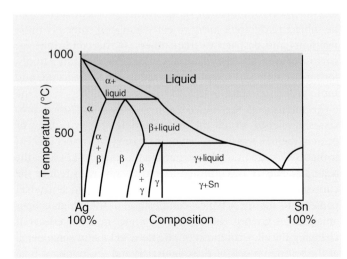

Figure 2.1.2 Phase diagram for the Ag–Sn system

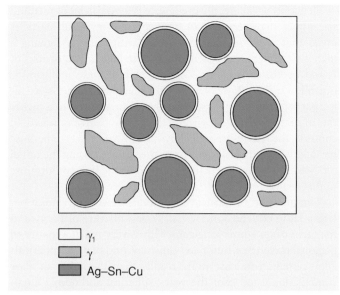

Figure 2.1.4 Schematic representation of the microstructure of a dispersed-phase amalgam. The halo around the spherical particles is a Cu–Sn phase

Phase	Tensile Strength (MPa)
γ	170
γ₁	30
γ₂	20
Amalgam	60

TABLE 2.1.3 Tensile Strengths of Phases of Amalgam

spherical particles the copper is uniformly distributed, and the alloy can be considered a ternary alloy of silver, tin, and copper. Hence, in the final structure of the spherical alloy amalgam, the copper is not present as a discrete phase but is widely distributed throughout the material. This is better suited to allowing the copper to react according to the equation shown below and is part of the reason that spherical or dispersed phase alloy powders are more popular than purely lathe-cut alloys.

$$Ag\text{-}Sn\text{-}Cu + Hg \rightarrow Ag\text{-}Sn\text{-}Cu + \gamma_1 + Cu_6Sn_5$$

PROPERTIES OF AMALGAM

Strength

The strength of an amalgam is extremely important, since the restoration has to be able to withstand the considerable loads generated during mastication, and any lack of strength is likely to lead to marginal ditching of the restoration or even gross fracture.

Most attention has been paid to the final compressive strength of the set material, and while this is important, it is arguably more important to consider the tensile strength of the material, as this is much lower than the compressive strength and more likely to be the cause of failure. Also important is the rate at which the final strength is acquired, since if this occurs slowly, the material may be vulnerable in the short term while the setting process is still ongoing.

The final strength of the amalgam is a function of the properties of the individual phases. It is not easy to determine the properties of the three main phases of an amalgam, but micro-hardness measurements suggest that the γ phase and the γ_1 phase have a similar hardness, while the γ_2 phase is considerably softer. The tensile strength of the γ_2 phase has also been measured to be only a fraction of that of the original γ phase, with

the γ_1 phase falling in between (Table 2.1.3). This means that the weak link within the amalgam structure is the γ_2 phase, and if its proportion in the final composition can be minimized, a stronger amalgam will result. This highlights how important it is that the γ_2 phase is eliminated from the amalgam by the presence of copper; otherwise, the net strength of the material will be considerably lower than would otherwise be the case. The amount of γ_1 formed is strongly dependent on the amount of mercury in the final composition. The higher the mercury content, the weaker the material will be, because larger amounts of the weaker (in tension) phase will be produced.

The final mercury content of the amalgam is dependent on the quality of the condensation technique, with a properly condensed amalgam having a mercury content of just less than 50%. Besides the condensation technique, the size and shape of the alloy particles will also affect the final mercury content. The initial ratio of alloy to mercury is lower in amalgam made with spherical alloy particles than with lathe-cut alloy particles because the material is more easily condensed.

The particle size is also important. For a given amount of alloy that is to be amalgamated with mercury, choosing smaller alloy particles results in more of the alloy surface being exposed to the mercury. This means that more of the alloy will dissolve in the mercury, producing more of the mercury-containing phases. Consequently, too small a particle size is contraindicated.

Whatever the form of the alloy used, the conscientious removal of excess mercury during the placement of a restoration is vitally important.

Flow and Creep

It has been postulated that the excessive flow of an amalgam resulting from repeated occlusal loading can cause flattening of contact points, overhanging margins, and protrusion of the restoration from the tooth surface at the margin. The latter has been implicated as a major source of marginal breakdown. Although flow is measured for amalgam in laboratory tests, the measurement is usually carried out over a short period very soon after mixing and is therefore of limited clinical relevance. A more appropriate measurement would be that of creep. This is the flow caused by loads acting over long periods. Creep is dependent on both the yield strength of the material and the temperature of the environment and only becomes a serious problem when the environmental temperature is greater than half the melting temperature of the material.

Since the amalgam phases have very low melting temperatures (about 80°C) and the restorations are subjected to repeated loadings, there is the possibility of creep occurring.

The phases most prone to creep will be the mercury-based γ_1 phase. Consequently, the lower the proportion of the mercury-rich phase present (as may be achieved by proper condensation), the less susceptible the amalgam will be to creep.

Corrosion

It is well recognized that amalgams corrode in the oral environment and, as explained above, a limited degree of corrosion is sometimes cited as an advantage in that corrosion products help to produce a good marginal seal! Nevertheless, other forms of corrosion are definitely undesirable. Crevice corrosion, caused by the formation of an oxidation cell in the marginal gap, can cause a rapid deterioration in the properties of the amalgam. The corrosion process is especially associated with the γ_2 phase. The γ_2 phase is considerably more electronegative than the γ and γ_1 phases. This means that, in the presence of an electrolytic solution, the γ_2 phase will act as the anode of the oxidation cell and will gradually dissolve. The reaction is as follows:

$$\text{tin-mercury phase} + \text{oral fluids} \rightarrow \text{tin salts} + \text{free mercury}$$
$$Sn_7Hg + \text{oxygen} \rightarrow \text{oxides \& chlorides} + Hg$$

Normally, the formation of oxides would help slow down the corrosion process by forming a protective surface coating. However, in the gap between the amalgam and the tooth tissues a surface oxide is not formed, as the reaction products from the corrosion process precipitate out. The process is also very insidious, since the production of free mercury allows further reaction with γ, and the formation of more γ_1 and γ_2. This process will severely weaken the amalgam structure and is often cited as a cause of marginal breakdown – another reason that the high-copper amalgams have overtaken their low-copper or copper-free competitors.

CLINICAL SIGNIFICANCE

Traditional dental amalgams suffered from a lack of strength and excessive creep and corrosion. High copper amalgams – used exclusively today – have reduced corrosion and creep and improved, more consistent strength owing to the reduction or elimination of the γ_2 phase.

SELECTION AND HANDLING OF DENTAL AMALGAMS

Even as amalgams become less prevalent in the marketplace, there are still various options available to the clinician and the choice that the individual makes is largely down to personal preference. There are also several steps in the placing of the amalgam and the choices made for each have implications for the success – or otherwise – of the final restoration. The following section sets out some of the choices that can be made, and their implications.

Particle Size and Shape

The alloy particles' size and shape need to be considered seriously because they not only determine the handling characteristics of the alloy but also affect the final composition.

Generally speaking, the preference is for particles of medium size rather than very fine or very coarse. Very small particles mean that more mercury will react with the alloy, giving a higher final mercury content, and hence higher proportions of γ_1 and γ_2. The early compressive strength of these amalgams is much lower than those of amalgams made with larger-sized alloy particles, and they have been shown to give rise to a higher rate of marginal breakdown, and their use is contraindicated. In contrast, the coarse-grained alloys are difficult to carve because particles are easily dislodged from the surface during the initial set. Medium to fine particles appear to be the best compromise in this respect.

The question of particle shape boils down to a choice between lathe-cut and spherical alloy or a mixture of the two in the form of an admix amalgam. This is very much a matter of personal preference, but many clinicians find that the spherical-alloy systems condense more readily than the lathe-cut alloy compositions, and over the years, spherical and admix amalgams have largely prevailed over the purely lathe-cut variety.

Proportioning and Trituration

In times gone by, it was possible for the dental practice to purchase amalgam as separate containers of mercury and alloy, and the dentist or nurse would measure out and mix these themselves. As mercury is highly volatile in its elemental form, it is perhaps not surprising that the practice of handling elemental mercury in a clinical setting has now ceased and amalgam is now provided only in sealed, pre-proportioned capsules, that are only opened once the mercury has been brought into contact with the alloy and the amalgamation reaction – which chemically binds the mercury to the other metals and prevents its release into the air – has commenced.

Trituration is the mixing of the mercury and alloy and is one of the most important of the variables under the control of the operator (as opposed to the manufacturer). Adequate trituration is essential to ensure a plastic mix and thorough amalgamation. The trituration time that is needed is dependent on the type of alloy being used. The spherical alloys tend to mix more readily and in general require a shorter trituration time than amalgams containing lathe-cut alloy particles, as spherical particles are more easily wetted than the irregular and high surface area lathe-cut particles. The trituration time is also a function of the amalgamator itself – different instruments vary in respect of the range of speeds they can attain and the 'throw' or distance of travel. It is important to familiarize yourself both with the specification of the particular brand of amalgam you are using *and* the amalgamator, to ensure that device time and speed are set to the correct values to ensure successful trituration.

The general recommendation is that it is better to err on the side of over-trituration than under-trituration. If the amalgam comes out looking crumbly or dry, which might give the appearance of having set already, in fact, the trituration time must be *increased* and not decreased, as is often thought; the extra trituration will provide a more plastic mix with a longer working time. However, if the trituration time is set too long, this will reduce the setting time because the material

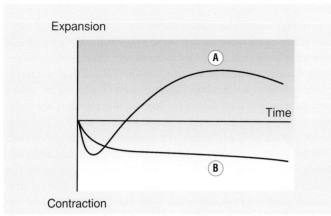

Figure 2.1.5 Dimensional change for a traditional hand-mixed amalgam (A) and a modern mechanically mixed amalgam (B)

heats up during the vigorous mixing action. Trituration times also affect the dimensional changes that occur when amalgams set. In short: ascertain the precise instructions for the specific amalgam and amalgamator, and follow these, for the best results.

Prior to the introduction of capsules and amalgamators, the traditional amalgams contained large alloy particles, which were hand-triturated; these formulations showed a slight expansion once fully set. The dimensional change with time is shown in Figure 2.1.5.

There is an initial contraction as the mercury diffuses into the alloy. This is followed by an expansion as the γ_1 phase forms, due to the γ_1 crystals impinging on one another and producing an outward pressure, which opposes the contraction. This occurs only if sufficient mercury is present to produce a plastic mix.

The near-universal adoption of high-speed mechanical amalgamators, reduced mercury:alloy ratios, small alloy particle sizes, and high condensation pressures reduces the amount of mercury in the mix and favors a contraction of the amalgam, such that modern amalgams show a small net contraction on setting.

Condensation

The term *condensation* when used in relation to amalgam refers to the process of firm taps or impacts applied to the amalgam *in situ* in the mouth that causes the material to adapt to the cavity and eliminates air voids. The most important demands on the condensation technique are that as much excess mercury is removed as is possible, that the final restoration will be nonporous and that optimum marginal adaptation is achieved so as to prevent postoperative sensitivity.

For the lathe-cut alloys, a final mercury content of 45% can be achieved. Although reductions below 50% mercury have little effect on the compressive strength after 24 hours, a much higher *early* compressive strength is achieved and the susceptibility to creep is much reduced. A high early strength reduces the likelihood of gross amalgam fracture during the first few hours after placement. This applies equally well to the spherical

alloy systems, except that in these cases the final mercury content should be approximately 40%.

The important components in condensation are the use of sufficient force, suitably sized condensers in relation to cavity size, multiple and rapid thrusts, and the placement of small increments. Although condensation pressures of 30–40 N are generally recommended, this does not mean that lower condensation pressures will result in a poorer result, as low condensation pressures can be compensated for by the placement of small increments. The placement of large increments will not only lead to the formation of large amounts of γ_1 and γ_2 but will also produce a high level of porosity.

The condensation of the spherical alloy amalgams requires a different approach from the lathe-cut systems. As the mix flows more readily under even light pressures, small loads need to be applied by larger condensers, if possible. However, close marginal adaptation appears to be more difficult with the spherical alloy amalgams, which is due to the coarser grain structure of the spherical alloys.

Carving and Polishing

The end result of carving and polishing an amalgam is a function of the size and shape of the alloy particles. In general, the spherical alloys produce a better initial surface finish than the lathe-cut alloys. Polishing improves the aesthetics and contributes to the removal of any high levels of residual mercury in the surface layer. A controversy has been going on for decades concerning whether it is necessary to burnish the amalgam restoration. Some have commented that the burnishing of amalgams may give rise to a mercury-rich surface layer, which would increase the possibility of corrosion or fracture. Others claim that the overall effect of burnishing is to increase surface hardness, reduce porosity, and decrease corrosion while also improving the marginal adaptation of the amalgam. Ultimately the data to support either position is weak and there is no clear consensus regarding the benefits of burnishing. This has been the case for many years and is unlikely to change; amalgam rarely attracts research efforts as there are newer and more 'exciting' materials to entice today's dental materials researchers.

An as-carved surface finish for an amalgam is decidedly rough, however, and some form of polishing is necessary, even if burnishing is not carried out. For many years, it was thought necessary to delay for 24 hours before polishing, and some clinicians still stick to this, but more recent data suggests this may not be necessary and immediate polishing is now often practiced.

PROPERTIES OF DENTAL AMALGAM

High Thermal Conductivity

As one would expect from a metallic material, the thermal conductivity of dental amalgams is high. Problems presented by this, such as pulpal sensitivity due to the hydrodynamic effect of pumping fluid through the marginal gap and up and down the dentinal tubules, are readily dealt with by suitable cavity preparation techniques, involving the use of varnishes or liners (see Chapter 2.4).

Galvanic Effects

When two metallic restorations consisting of metals with different degrees of electronegativity are placed in close proximity to one another in an electrically conducting medium (in the dental case, this medium is saliva), it is possible that a galvanic cell will be set up. This process can result in a metallic taste in the mouth and can accelerate the corrosive breakdown of the more electronegative metal. Consequently, although the problem rarely arises, the use of different metals in contact in the mouth is not recommended.

Lack of Adhesion

The need for the use of retentive cavity designs with dental amalgams imposes a severe constraint. Often it is necessary to remove large amounts of perfectly sound enamel or dentine to achieve a retentive cavity. This is undesirable, as amalgam can never be a substitute for healthy tooth tissues. New ideas in cavity preparation have been developed, with the aim of minimizing the loss of healthy tooth tissue, but these can never be as conservative as the approach of using adhesive restorative materials. In order to overcome this shortcoming of dental amalgams, bonding of amalgam to teeth can be carried out using resin cements. This has the benefits of reinforcing the tooth, aiding retention, and preserving tooth structure but of course the requirements of the resin cement such as the need for moisture exclusion and surface preparation add to the complexity and duration of the procedure, and one might well ask: Why not just place a composite restoration? This limits the uptake of this approach.

Lack of Strength and Toughness

As noted previously, dental amalgams are very brittle, low-tensile-strength restorative materials. The way to deal with this is to use the material in bulk, as this reduces the degree to which the restoration will bend and flex, which in turn reduces tensile stresses. Hence cavity preparations are designed such that thin sections of the amalgam filling are avoided. This means that boxes have to be cut deep and margin angles need to be as near to 90° as possible. The consequence of this is that dental amalgams inherently do not conserve tooth structure. In situations of small primary caries lesions, the use of dental amalgam may well be contraindicated as being too destructive of tooth tissue, and an alternative material, such as a composite resin, would be preferable.

Lifespan of Dental Amalgam Restorations

Hundreds of thousands of amalgams are placed each year; around half of these are replacements for existing restorations. The longevity of amalgam restorations has been the subject of a number of clinical studies, with some suggesting that half need replacement within 4–5 years.

On average, the survival time of amalgam restorations is broadly inversely proportional to their size: the smaller the restoration, the longer it is likely to survive. To compound this problem, every time an amalgam restoration is replaced, the cavity outline is increased by at least 0.5 mm, leading to a larger restoration. Data comparing the longevity of amalgam restorations with alternative materials such as composites is by its nature hard to obtain, as the pace of development of composites means that data relating to composites placed, say, 10 or 20 years ago, refers to composites that were *sold* 10 or 20 years ago and have now been superseded by more modern versions! However, what data is available that compares the longevity of amalgam and composite restorations that has been conducted in such a way as to ensure that we are comparing like-for-like (not comparing large amalgams with small composites, for instance, which would naturally benefit the smaller composites) indicates that for patients at low caries risk, the composite has a slightly better rate of survival, whereas for patients at high caries risk, the converse is true with slightly better survival of amalgam restorations. The differences *are* small, however, and it should be remembered that modern composites designed specifically as amalgam alternatives were not available at the time those restorations were placed.

Of all the disadvantages mentioned above, the lack of longevity and the destructive nature of the procedure are matters of the greatest concern. Ways of making amalgam restorations last longer will be considered in the next section.

IMPROVING THE LONGEVITY OF AMALGAM RESTORATIONS

The most common causes of ailing and failing amalgam restorations are associated with:

- tooth fracture
- recurrent caries
- gross amalgam fracture
- marginal breakdown.

The latter may arise from fracture of either the amalgam margins or the enamel margins. Of the factors cited, the most common reason for replacing an amalgam restoration (accounting for some 70% of replacements) is considered to be recurrent caries.

Some of the failures are unavoidable, being related to inadequacies in the properties of the amalgams, but others *can* be avoided by considering amalgam's limitations and by adopting appropriate techniques by avoiding faults in cavity design and poor clinical technique.

Tooth Fracture
Weakened Tooth Structure

The more tooth tissue that is removed, the weaker the tooth becomes. A dental amalgam acts as an effective space filler, but since it has no adhesive qualities, it does not help in strengthening the underlying tooth structure. Thus techniques involving the minimal removal of tooth tissue should always be employed.

By cutting enamel along the plane parallel to the prism direction, it is possible to keep outline form to a minimum. This practice also ensures that cavo-surface angles will be close to 90°, which is optimal for the amalgam, with acute cavo-surface angles encouraging marginal breakdown of the amalgam.

Resin adhesives allow bonding of the amalgam to the tooth tissues, which will provide additional support to both the restoration and the cusps and should help strengthen the restored tooth crown, although the design of the cavity should still be such that potential sites for fracture are avoided. With severely weakened cusps, alternative techniques, such as gold onlays or resin-bonded ceramics, might have to be considered.

Undermined Enamel

The principle of providing flat walls and floors to a cavity can give rise to undermined enamel, as shown in Figure 2.1.6 for a box in a proximal restoration. The unsupported enamel will break free and leave a gap, which can lead to recurrent caries.

Residual Caries

It is of paramount importance that any residual caries is removed. If not, the caries will spread and undermine the cusp, eventually causing it to fracture. The leakage of bacterial toxins will also cause pulpal inflammation.

Recurrent Caries

Contamination

Contamination of the cavity with blood or saliva will result in poor adaptation of the restoration to the cavity margins.

Poor Matrix Techniques

A poorly adapted matrix band can be the cause of proximal overhangs, or of poor contact points with the adjacent teeth. Overhangs are particularly prone to plaque accumulation and may initiate recurrent caries. If the overhang is subgingival, it may cause soft tissue irritation and can eventually lead to bone loss and pocketing. Overtightening of the matrix band can cause the fracture of tooth cusps that have been weakened by the removal of large amounts of tooth tissue.

Poor Condensation

As already noted, poor condensation results in porosity of the amalgam and the presence of excess mercury, both of which reduce the strength of the amalgam. Marginal adaptation will also be poor, increasing the potential for marginal leakage, recurrent caries, and corrosion. For good condensation, it is important that the amalgam is well mixed, and that the appropriate trituration time is selected. Under-trituration, in particular, should be avoided, as this will result in a dry amalgam mix that will not condense properly.

Gross Amalgam Fracture

Shallow Preparations

Dental amalgams have a fairly low tensile strength, certainly when compared to most alloys. When placed in thin sections and subjected to bending forces, they will break. Shallow preparations are only acceptable in very small restorations, where the surface area is small compared to the depth. For large mesial occlusal distal restorations, there must be sufficient depth to the cavity on the occlusal floor to provide enough bulk to resist the bending forces. This may require the removal of large amounts of sound tooth tissue.

Non-Retentive Proximal Boxes

A frequently observed failure of mesial occlusal, distal occlusal, or mesial occlusal distal restorations is the fracture of the proximal boxes from the occlusal section of the filling. To some extent, this is due to the low tensile strength of the amalgam restoration, as an occlusal load can force the amalgam to splay outward. However, sharp internal line angles aggravate the situation, which ultimately leads to the fracture and loss of the box. The risk of this happening can be reduced by cutting retention grooves in the lateral walls and gingival floor of the boxes. This technique ensures that the box is self-retentive and opposes the

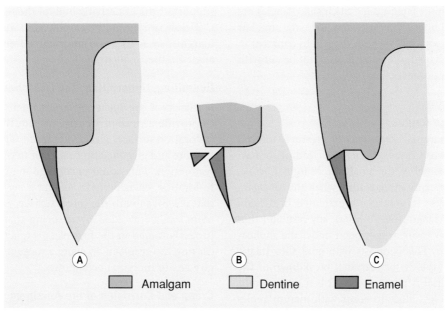

A   B   C

⬜ Amalgam   ⬜ Dentine   ⬛ Enamel

Figure 2.1.6 If the gingival floor of the proximal box is finished (A), then unsupported enamel will break away (B) and lead to recurrent caries. Beveling the enamel (C) prevents this from occurring but it is necessary to place a groove in the gingival floor of the dentine to resist the displacement of the restoration proximally

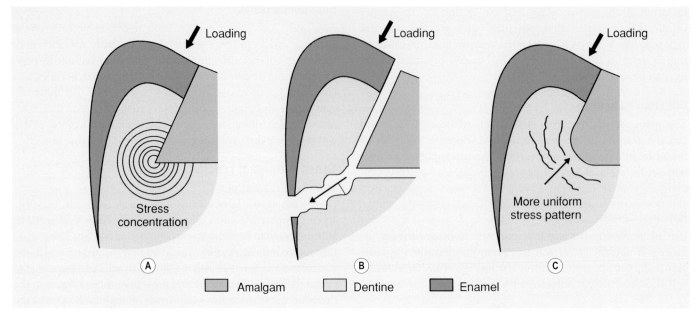

Figure 2.1.7 Sharp internal line angles (A) may lead to cusp fracture (B) under heavy occlusal loading. Tensile stresses are concentrated at the line angle and can be considerably reduced by creating rounded line angles (C)

splaying action from an occlusal load by resisting the displacement of the restoration in a proximal direction. An added advantage is that an occlusal lock is not required for retention of the restoration. Thus the additional preparation of occlusal fissures is not required when a primary lesion is confined to the proximal surface only; this type of preparation is generally described as a 'wedge' preparation.

Sharp Internal Line Angles

The presence of sharp internal line angles concentrates stress at these sites, which increases the risk of fracture of both the tooth and the filling, as shown in Figure 2.1.7. Such sharp angles are avoidable, and rounded internal surfaces should be the aim. For example, proximal boxes should be pear shaped, to conform to the extent of the underlying lesion, and should not be cut with sharp line angles in their corners.

Marginal Breakdown
Incorrect Cavo-Surface Angles

The primary cause of marginal breakdown of a restored tooth is the presence of an incorrect cavo-surface angle, leading to marginal fracture of the enamel or the amalgam. Marginal breakdown of the amalgam occurs more readily when the amalgam has an acute margin angle. As amalgam is extremely brittle and has a very low tensile strength (60–70 MPa), any resultant thin wedges will fracture very easily as they bend under the application of an external load. This contrasts with gold alloy inlays, which do not show symptoms of marginal breakdown of the alloy because this material is tough and ductile. Consequently, marginal breakdown is less likely to occur with margin angles greater than 70°, as this avoids thin wedges of the amalgam.

The practice of cutting perpendicular cavity walls on the occlusal aspect of the cavity is conducive to producing an acute

margin angle for the amalgam (Figure 2.1.8a). Changing the angle for the whole of the cavity wall is not possible, as this may cause the cavity outline to come close to the pulp horn or to perforate it (Figure 2.1.8b). An acceptable method of overcoming this problem is to confine the sharp angulation to the enamel only, as depicted in Figure 2.1.8c.

For occlusal cavities of minimal width, it is not necessary to prepare 90° cavo-surface angles in the enamel because the amalgam may be carved flat without interference with the opposing dentition. The amalgam margin angle will then be obtuse, which will give the margin added strength due to the support of the underlying bulk of the restorative material.

Great care should be employed in the preparation of cavity margins, so as to avoid undermined enamel or acute margin angles in the amalgam.

Overfilling, Underfilling, and Overcarving

If a cavity is overfilled and is not then carved back sufficiently to provide a smooth transition from the tooth surface to the restoration surface, a ledge will result. This ledge will eventually fracture and give the appearance of marginal breakdown of the restoration. This could encourage the clinician to replace the restoration when, perhaps, all that is needed is to trim it back so that it is flush with the tooth surface. Such unnecessary treatment can be avoided by ensuring that the surface has been properly carved in the first place. Equally, underfilling or overcarving can result in an acute amalgam margin angle that will give rise to marginal breakdown.

Creep and Corrosion of the Amalgam

The problems associated with amalgam as a filling material have already been covered in detail, both in terms of the limitations imposed by their mechanical and physical properties and their

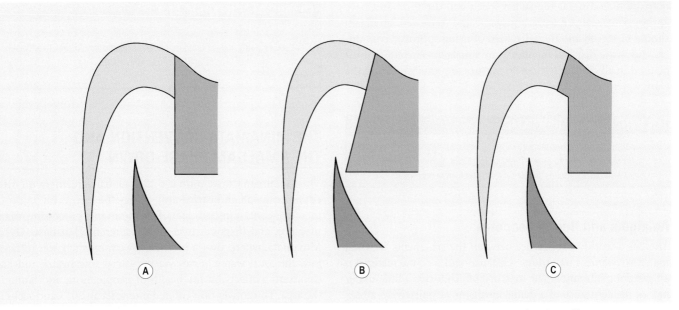

Figure 2.1.8 An obtuse cavo-surface angle (A) produces an acute margin angle in the restoration that will lead to marginal fracture and should be corrected. In (B) the cavo-surface angle is now closer to the ideal but may give rise to a pulpal exposure. An acceptable method is shown in (C), where adjustment is confined to the enamel without increasing the outline form

handling. Most short-term failures are avoidable if the above factors are addressed and if careful attention is paid to the detail of cavity preparation and the handling of the materials. In the longer term, amalgams will eventually fail. When such failures are specifically material related, they are usually associated with creep or corrosion that has caused marginal breakdown.

CLINICAL SIGNIFICANCE

Dental amalgams continue to be a restorative material of choice for certain clinical situations, but their days are numbered and there is an ever-increasing array of alternative materials. This notwithstanding, with careful attention to material selection and handling and an appreciation of its limitations, amalgam can provide the patient with restorations that will give satisfactory function for many years.

LIMITATIONS OF DENTAL AMALGAMS

Dental amalgam has long been an emotive subject, with many calling for their phasing out (on both rational and irrational grounds, as we shall see later in this chapter), and others campaigning vigorously for their continued use. As with any material, there are pros and cons. We have discussed some of amalgam's favorable characteristics – particularly its mechanical properties, ease of use, and long history of good service – and will now consider some of its limitations.

Poor Aesthetics

Being metallic restorations, amalgams are not the most visually attractive of options, although if they are polished regularly, they *can* look quite presentable. The polished finish is lost with time, due to tarnishing. Although there is an increasing demand

from patients for more aesthetic restorations, in the case of posterior restorations, durability is usually the most important consideration. In the early decades of their use composites were not an adequate substitute for amalgam in some instances, particularly large posterior restorations and those instances where good moisture control was not achievable. Many modern composites, however, can perform very well in these situations, as can some of the glass ionomer cements, and this will hasten the demise of amalgam as a dental material.

Mercury and Its Health and Environmental Properties

Mercury is a highly toxic substance, and its use demands the greatest of care. When amalgams were supplied as alloy and elemental mercury and were measured and mixed manually, there were elevated risks of exposure owing to spills, direct skin contact with elemental mercury due to poor handling techniques, and inhalation of mercury vapor. These days, the use of capsules greatly reduces these risks as the material should only be exposed to the air once the amalgamation reaction is well underway. In the rare event that elemental mercury could be released, for instance, due to a faulty capsule or the breakage of a capsule, it must be dealt with immediately and thoroughly. Any elemental mercury that is exposed to the air will vaporize and thence be inhaled, and exposure to mercury carries many health risks including damage to the kidneys and nervous system.

There is a suite of safety procedures that must be followed in the handling and disposal of amalgam to minimize the risk to the patient, the dental team, and the wider environment. Amalgam should always be handled using a 'no touch' technique and amalgamators should be well maintained to ensure they are operating at the stated speed and duration and have appropriate seals. Excess amalgam and removed amalgam should be stored and then disposed of using approved containers and waste disposal handlers, and amalgam separators must be used in all clinical settings to capture any amalgam from the wastewater.

> **CLINICAL SIGNIFICANCE**
>
> It is important to emphasize the safe handling of dental amalgam to the whole of the dental team, and to stay abreast of local and national regulations regarding which patient groups should receive amalgam restorations.

Amalgam and Health Concerns

There is a world of difference between the statements 'a dental material *contains* a hazardous substance' and 'a dental material *is* a hazardous substance'. The mercury, which forms a little under half of the substance of a dental amalgam, *is*, objectively, a hazardous substance, *when in its elemental form*. When bound in the amalgam, the mercury presents a very different safety profile. Extensive research has been carried out on putative links between dental amalgam and a wide range of health conditions, and the overwhelming consensus is that amalgam is a safe and effective restorative material. From the patient's point of view, there is a finite and elevated exposure to mercury during the placement of amalgam and during its removal compared to under normal day-to-day conditions, but even these are accepted to be short term and not of sufficient magnitude to present a health risk.

There have been occasions when patients have reacted badly to the presence of amalgams in their mouth, due to a delayed hypersensitivity reaction. As rare as these allergic reactions are, the symptoms can be quite severe, and the clinician should be aware of such a possibility. There have also been reports of local lichenoid-type reactions associated with amalgam fillings, and removal of the amalgam restoration is recommended when there is a clear link between the restoration and the lesion.

Besides mercury vapor inhalation, wear and corrosion will contribute to a patient's overall mercury exposure from amalgam. On average, the mercury intake into the body from dental amalgam fillings is believed to be well below the threshold recommended by the World Health Organization. Some patient behaviors, such as excessive chewing or bruxism or the use of bleaching products, can result in higher mercury release. Patients claiming to have symptoms of mercury toxicity or expressing concern about the potential health effects of new amalgam restorations should be treated with care and respect, even where the clinician is convinced that they are at no risk, and clinicians should take every care to educate themselves on the contemporary thinking regarding any health risks of amalgam so that they can present objective and evidenced guidance to the concerned patient. It was found in a recent review that the causes of so-called 'amalgam illness', where people attribute ill health to the presence of amalgam fillings, were overwhelmingly likely to be due to psychological factors or psychiatric conditions rather than elevated mercury blood levels.

> **CLINICAL SIGNIFICANCE**
>
> Patients expressing concern about amalgam safety should be treated with respect and empathy and, where possible, the clinician should seek to advise the patient using objective, scientific evidence in appropriate non-technical language to address their questions or concerns.

THE MINAMATA CONVENTION AND THE AMALGAM PHASE-DOWN

The Minamata Convention is a 2013 global agreement on mercury use in all industries and across the entire life cycle of mercury-containing products, from sourcing, processing, manufacture, and disposal. It is named after the Japanese city of Minamata, where, over a period of years, mercury was released into the local watercourses via industrial wastewater and had devastating effects on the health of people, flora and fauna in the area. The convention entered into force in 2017 and seeks to control and ultimately eliminate the use of mercury across diverse industries.

When first proposed, this presented the dental profession with some very real concerns, as at that time there were not adequate substitutes for amalgams in all of their common uses. There was an initial proposal of an amalgam *phase-out* but, following intensive discussion, the rhetoric was adjusted to describe a *phase-down* of the material. It should be stressed that this was a part of a much larger initiative to vastly reduce or eliminate the use of mercury across all industries and does not relate to any putative health risks of dental amalgam.

Some years on, we are certainly seeing a steady reduction in the use of amalgam. Some countries now use virtually none; others still recommend it for certain patient groups and clinical situations, especially where dentistry is partially or fully funded by the public purse. For instance, a 2018 report of dentists practicing in Wales, UK, indicated dentists carrying out publicly subsidized (National Health Service) dental restorations use amalgam 'often' or 'always' for over 70% of adult patients when two or more posterior restorations are required. This is because the material itself is cheaper than the composite alternative, *and* faster to use – some estimates suggest that appointment time would increase by around 60% if composites were used for restorations currently carried out using amalgam, with the associated cost rising by a similar degree.

Nevertheless, the industry is committed to a continued reduction of the use of amalgam. The World Health Organization released an analysis in 2021 of the progress of countries across the world in reducing amalgam use and concluded that a phase-down or even phase-out is possible, highlighting the need for particular support for low-income countries where caries prevalence is high and resources are very limited. A combination of the environmental arguments used in the Minamata Convention, patient pressure for natural-looking restorations, and the commitment to minimally invasive dentistry means that amalgam use is on the decline across much of the world.

ALLOY ALTERNATIVES TO AMALGAMS

The complex and divisive history of dental amalgam and the persistent (although not well-founded) concerns about amalgam safety have led to efforts to create metallic restorative materials without mercury. One approach is to replace mercury with gallium, which has the second-lowest melting temperature after mercury. When alloyed with tin and indium, a liquid is produced at room temperature. Alloy powders with a composition close to that of the alloys used in mercury amalgams are mixed with this liquid, which produces a workable mix that can be condensed into the cavity. Although the resulting alloy has physical and mechanical properties similar to those of mercury amalgam, excessive setting expansion and poor handling properties have prevented its adoption.

In another approach the use of liquid metal is eliminated altogether by relying on the cold welding of pre-alloyed silver-coated particles. Cold welding takes place where there is silver-to-silver contact between the particles. This process is promoted by exposure of the particles to a mild acid so as to remove any surface contaminants, which would interfere with the cold welding. One problem with this material is the high compaction pressure needed to consolidate the silver particles. Although a promising material in the laboratory, it has not become commercially available.

FURTHER READING

Baratieri, L.N., Machado, A., Van Noort, R., Ritter, A.V., Baratieri, N.M., 2002. Effect of pulp protection technique on the clinical performance of amalgam restorations: three-year results. Operative Dentistry 27 (4), 319–324.

Bayne, S., Petersen, P.E., Piper, D., Schmalz, G., Meyer, D., 2013. The challenge for innovation in direct restorative materials. Advances in Dental Research 25 (1), 8.

Letzel, H., van 't Hof, M.A., Marshall, G.W., Marshall, S.J., 1997. The influence of the amalgam alloy on the survival of amalgam restorations: a secondary analysis of multiple controlled clinical trials. Journal of Dental Research 76, 1787.

Lynch, C.D., Farnell, D.J.J., Stanton, H., Chestnutt, I.G., Brunton, P.A., Wilson, N.H.F., 2018. No more amalgams: use of amalgam and amalgam alternative materials in primary dental care. British Dental Journal 225 (2), 171–176.

Mahler, D.B., 1997. The high-copper dental amalgam alloy. Journal of Dental Research 76, 537.

Mjor, I.A., 1985. Frequency of secondary caries at various anatomical locations. Operative Dentistry 10, 88.

Opdam, N.J., Bronkhurst, E.M., Loomans, B.A., Huysmans, M.C., 2010. 12-year survival of composite vs. amalgam restorations. Journal of Dental Research 89 (10), 1063–1067.

Qvist, V., Poulsen, A., Teglers, P.T., Mjör, I.A., 2010. The longevity of different restorations in primary teeth. International Journal of Paediatric Dentistry 20 (1), 1–7.

Roberts, H.W., Charlton, D.G., 2009. The release of mercury from amalgam restorations and its health effects: a review. Operative Dentistry 34 (5), 605–614.

Sarkar, N.K., 1978. Creep, corrosion and marginal fracture of amalgam fillings. Journal of Oral Rehabilitation 5, 413.

Shaini, F.J., Fleming, G.J., Shortall, A.C., Marquis, P.M., 2001. A comparison of the mechanical properties of a gallium-based alloy with a spherical high-copper amalgam. Dental Materials 17, 142.

Summitt, J.B., Burgess, J.O., Berry, T.G., Robbins, J.W., Osborne, J.W., Haveman, C.W., 2004. Six-year clinical evaluation of bonded and pin-retained complex amalgam restorations. Operative Dentistry 29, 261.

Wahl, M.J., 2001. Amalgam – Resurrection and redemption. Part 2: the medical mythology of anti-amalgam. Quintessence International 32, 696–710.

The UN Environment Programme, 2021. https://mercuryconvention.org.

Resin-Based Composites

INTRODUCTION

A composite, as the name implies, consists of a mixture of two or more materials. Each of these materials contributes to the overall properties of the composite and is present in its discrete form. Resin-based composites are possibly the most ubiquitous materials in dentistry, as they are used in a huge variety of clinical applications, ranging from filling materials, luting agents, indirect restorations, and metal facings to endodontic posts and cores.

A variation on this theme is the polyacid-modified resin composite, or compomer for short. In this chapter we will first consider the resin composites and then explore how the compomers differ from the resin composites.

COMPOSITION AND STRUCTURE

The resin-based composite restorative materials ('composites' in brief) that are used in dentistry have three major components:
- an organic resin matrix
- an inorganic filler
- a coupling agent.

The resin forms the matrix of the composite material, binding the individual filler particles together via the coupling agent (Figure 2.2.1). The filler particles form the bulk of the material, making up typically 70–85% of the total mass of the material.

Resin Matrix

The resin is the chemically active component of the composite. It is initially a fluid monomer but is converted into a rigid polymer by a radical-mediated addition polymerization reaction. It is this ability to convert from a plastic mass into a rigid solid that allows this material to be used for the restoration of dentition.

The most commonly used monomers are from the methacrylate family. Specifically, most modern composites use urethane dimethacrylate (UDMA) or a closely related monomer. Less commonly nowadays, one also encounters composites that use bisphenol A-glycidyl methacrylate (Bis-GMA), which is derived from the reaction of bisphenol-A and glycidylmethacrylate. These resins have a comparatively high molecular weight compared to those used in indirect materials such as methyl methacrylate, which is one of many formulations choices that helps to minimize polymerization shrinkage (Figure 2.2.2). It is beneficial to use composites with a very low polymerization shrinkage as it is essential that the finished restoration does not pull away from the cavity walls, creating a gap that is susceptible to infiltration by bacteria. When the restoration is well bonded to the cavity walls, this can place stresses on the adjacent tissues as it pulls the tooth cusps inwards.

UDMA and Bis-GMA monomers are highly viscous fluids because of their high molecular weights; the addition of even a small amount of filler would produce a composite with a stiffness that is excessive for clinical use. To overcome this problem, low-viscosity monomers known as *viscosity controllers* are added, most commonly triethylene glycol dimethacrylate (TEGDMA). The chemical structures of some of these monomers are presented in Figure 2.2.3.

To ensure an adequately long shelf life for the composite, it is essential that premature polymerization is prevented. To this end, an *inhibitor*, such as hydroquinone, is included, usually in amounts of 0.1% or less.

The resin matrix also contains the activator/initiator systems for achieving the cure. These components depend on the type of reaction employed, which may be either chemical curing ('auto cure') or light-activated curing.

Filler

A wide variety of fillers have been employed in composites to improve their properties.
- Polymerization of monomers is usually accompanied by substantial polymerization shrinkage, as the spaces between the monomers are closed when the bonds form (Figure 2.2.2). By incorporating inorganic filler particles, the shrinkage is reduced because the amount of resin used is reduced and the filler does not take part in the polymerization process. Shrinkage is not totally eliminated and will depend on the monomers used and the amount of filler incorporated.
- Many monomers have a high coefficient of thermal expansion, whereas the inorganic fillers used in composites have a coefficient of thermal expansion similar to that of tooth tissues (8–10 ppm °C^{-1}). The net coefficient of thermal expansion of the composite is influenced by that of the two components: the more filler there is, the closer the net coefficient is to the tooth tissues.
- The fillers can improve mechanical properties such as hardness and compressive strength as these are themselves inherently hard, strong materials, and as long as well bonded to the resin component, they have a beneficial effect on the overall mechanical properties.
- The use of salts of heavy metals such as barium and strontium incorporated in the glass provides radiopacity, allowing the

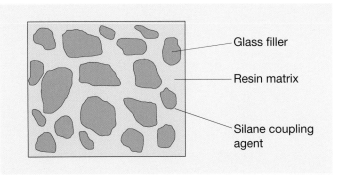

Figure 2.2.1 Schematic showing the structure of a resin-based composite.

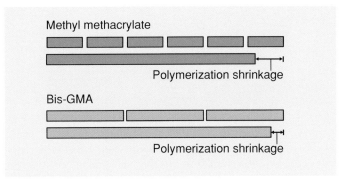

Figure 2.2.2 Schematic showing that there is less polymerization shrinkage with a larger monomer, as there are fewer new bonds formed on polymerization and thus fewer 'gaps' to be closed up.

clinician to identify the material on a radiograph and aiding in the diagnosis of secondary or recurrent caries at the margins.

- The fillers provide the primary means of controlling various aesthetic features such as color, translucency, and fluorescence.

Developments in both resin and filler technology have led to many improvements in composites, meaning that modern composites are carefully engineered, sophisticated materials with versions suitable for a wide range of applications.

Coupling Agent

In order for a composite to have acceptable mechanical properties, it is of the utmost importance that the filler and the resin are strongly bonded to each other. If there is a breakdown of this interface, the stresses developed under load will not be effectively distributed throughout the material; the interface will act as a primary source for fracture, leading to the subsequent disintegration of the composite. In short, the material is as strong as its weakest point, and without a coupling agent, that weakest point would be the interface between the filler and the resin.

The bond is achieved by the use of coupling agents that are incorporated into the resin. These coupling agents are silanes and the one most commonly used in glass-filled resin composites is γ-methacryloxypropyltriethoxysilane, or γ-MPTS for short, shown in Figure 2.2.4 (see also Chapter 1.9).

It is extremely important that there is a strong and durable bond between the resin and the filler particles. Firstly, if there is no bond, then stress transfer between the resin and glass will be inefficient and, as a consequence, most of the stress will have to be carried by the resin matrix. This will result in excessive creep and eventually fracture and wear of the restoration. Secondly, the lack of bonding between the resin and the glass filler particles will create crack initiation sites. Since the resins do not have a high resistance to the propagation of cracks, this makes the composite susceptible to fatigue failure if the bond between filler and resin is inadequate (Figure 2.2.5).

The fundamental challenge is that resins are hydrophobic, whereas silica-based glasses are hydrophilic due to a surface layer of hydroxyl groups bound to the silica. Hence the resin does not have a natural affinity to bond to the glass surface (Figure 2.2.6). The solution to the problem lies in the use of a suitable coupling agent. The silane coupling agent has been so chosen as to have hydroxyl groups on one end, which are attracted to the hydroxyl groups on the glass surface. The other end consists of a methacrylate group that is able to bond to the resin via the carbon double bond (Figure 2.2.7). A condensation reaction at the interface between the glass and the silane coupling agent ensures that the silane is covalently bonded to the glass surface (Figure 2.2.8). Improvement in the quality of the bond between the resin and the glass filler was an essential step in the development of this class of materials; without this, the composites would probably never have achieved anything like the dominant position they hold in the dental materials toolbox.

When considering how modern composites are differentiated from earlier generations, we need to focus on developments in two areas:

- resin technology
- filler technology.

Resin Technology
Polymerization Techniques

The process by which the composite paste turns into a hard material is the *polymerization* of the monomeric resin matrix.

The earliest composites employed a paste-paste system, as is seen in many other dental materials. There would be an activator, such as a tertiary amine, in one paste and an initiator, usually benzoyl peroxide, in the other (see Chapter 1.5 for details of this curing system). This same activator and initiator combination is used in certain types of composites today, although they are not mixed by hand anymore.

It was over 50 years ago, in the early 1970s, that the first light-activated composites became available. This first generation was activated by ultraviolet (UV) light, which generated free radicals to start the polymerization process. The energy of the UV light is sufficient to break the central bond of benzoin methyl ether to create two free radicals, so only a single paste was necessary, which would not set until exposed to UV light. The first truly command-cure material had arrived! However, there were some serious drawbacks to the use of UV-light-cured systems. UV light can cause soft-tissue burns and can also cause damage to the eye; hence protection needed to be used

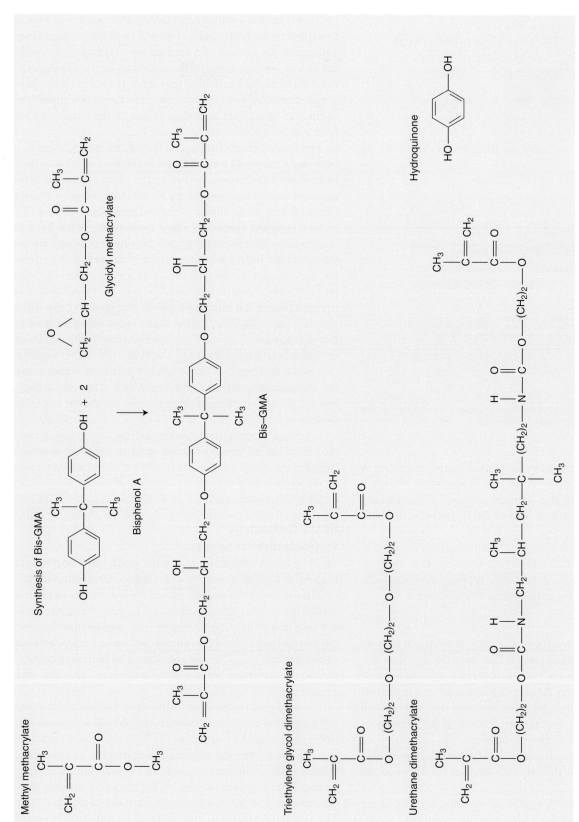

Figure 2.2.3 The chemical structure of some common monomers used in composites and other dental materials.

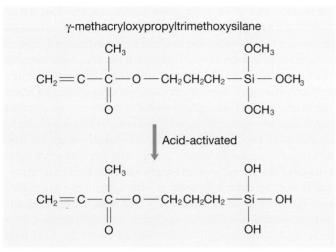

γ-methacryloxypropyltrimethoxysilane

Acid-activated

Figure 2.2.4 Structure of silane coupling agent before and after acid activation.

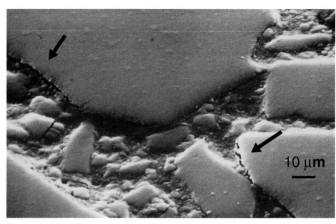

Figure 2.2.5 Scanning electron micrograph showing a failure of bonding between the resin matrix and the filler.

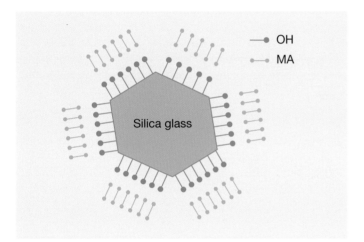

Figure 2.2.6 Schematic of resin monomer molecules being repelled by the glass surface due to the presence of hydroxyl groups on the glass.

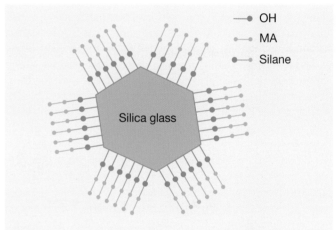

Figure 2.2.7 Schematic of silane coupling agent acting as a link between the methacrylate resin and the hydroxylated glass surface.

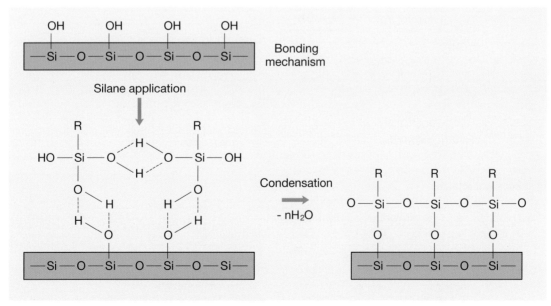

Figure 2.2.8 Application and condensation of silane onto a silica glass surface.

and generally great care needed to be exercised in the use of these light-curing units. UV is not visible to the naked eye, so in effect, you have to protect the eyes and tissues from the light without being able to actually see where the light is. The UV light source was a mercury discharge lamp, which was very expensive, and suffered deterioration as the lamp got older, meaning that the older lamps were less effective but the clinician, not being able to see the light, was unlikely to notice. Furthermore, UV-cured composites had a limited depth of cure due to the high degree of light absorption that took place as it traveled through the composite.

Three steps forward, two steps back, one might think. The first command cure composite was in existence, but it had some major limitations. Nevertheless, the practice of having a single paste, which would set hard on demand, was enthusiastically embraced by the dental profession and opened the way for the introduction of visible-light-activated (VLA) composites. VLA composites use camphorquinone as the source of free radicals. The energy for excitation is lower than that of benzoin methyl

ether such that light with a wavelength in the blue range (~460–480 nm) is required. This had the advantage that cheaper and more reliable light sources could be used; initially quartz halogen light sources dominated, and nowadays, light emitting diodes are by far the most commonly used. The light is more readily transmitted through the composite, providing a greater depth of cure. And blue light is visible to the eye, so the clinician can clearly see where the light is incident and if it is working!

It is only the blue light, in the wavelength range of 460–480 nm, that serves to initiate polymerization. Any other light, outside of this range, is of no benefit and may even cause drawbacks. For the older light sources with a broad-spectrum output, filters are used to remove UV and infrared light for the output, so as to avoid soft tissue burns and any excessive temperature rise, respectively. This is not necessary for LED light curing units(LCUs) as LEDs have a very narrow emission spectrum; this also makes them much more efficient from an energy point of view.

The curing methods are summarized in Figure 2.2.9.

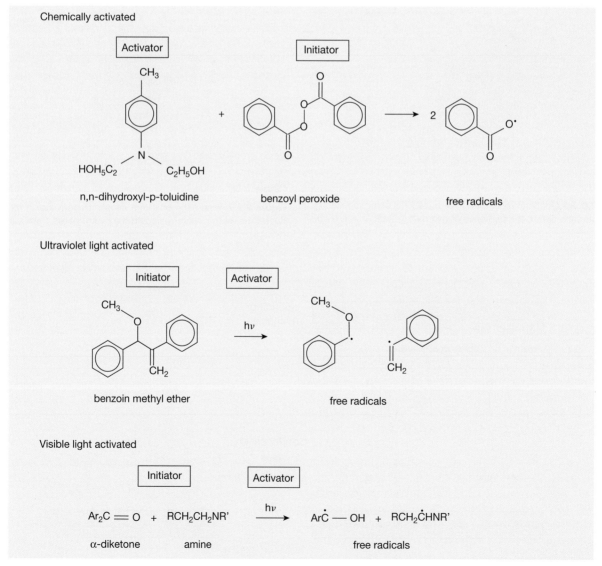

Figure 2.2.9 Methods of polymerization.

Safety. There were significant concern about the use of high-intensity UV light in the dental clinic, and this only served to increase the practitioner community's enthusiasm for visible light–cured composites. The use of the phrase 'visible light' instills a feeling of safety, since it is something that we are exposed to all the time. However, it is important to be aware that the use of high-intensity blue light can also have a significant harmful effect on the retina. Eye protection must be used, for both practitioner and patient, and assistant if present. Individual devices should detail the specification of appropriate protective eyewear and a maximum time exposure and these must be followed stringently in order to protect the eyes of all concerned.

Color perception. Another difficulty that the discerning clinician needs to be aware of is that caused by a long period of exposure to high-intensity light. Such exposure can compromise one's color perception, meaning that the selection of suitable shades of composites then becomes a real problem, especially when performing multiple restorations or when applying composite veneers.

Oxygen inhibition. Where there is an air interface with the resin, the resin will not cure and a sticky surface is left behind. This is not a problem when carrying out an incremental placement procedure, as it ensures that each layer of composite will be well bonded to the next. However, it can be a problem when the last increment is placed. When it is possible to use a matrix strip, this is usually sufficient to exclude the oxygen and the resin will be fully cured up to the surface. For most resin systems, this oxygen-inhibited surface layer is very thin and extends no more than a few micrometers below the surface. Thus it is easily wiped off, for example, when fissure sealing. However, there are some resin systems where the oxygen inhibition is considerable and a special gel needs to be used to avoid contact with oxygen in the air.

Limited depth of cure. For all light-activated composites, the conversion from a paste to a solid material relies on the ability of the light to access and initiate the curing in all parts of the restoration. The degree to which the light can penetrate the composite is finite, so the depth to which the material can be cured is limited. Another reason why the VLA composites were more successful than the UV systems is that the depth of cure that can be achieved with UV light was considerably less than that obtained with visible light.

In particular, there is a danger of incomplete curing for deep restorations, which would be a serious drawback in posterior applications. For the UV-cured composites, the maximum depth of cure is little more than 2.0 mm, while for the VLA composites, a depth of cure of at least 3–4 mm is possible with a *good light source* and *good technique*. With 'bulk cure' composites, the depth of cure is very much greater; we shall come on to them a little later.

Notwithstanding these improvements in composite engineering, the depth of cure is finite for any light-cured composite, and there is always the danger that deeper parts of the restoration will not be fully cured. This is especially problematic with the proximal boxes of posterior composites (Figure 2.2.10). All can appear perfectly satisfactory on the surface, but the bases of the boxes of composite may not be fully cured, particularly when

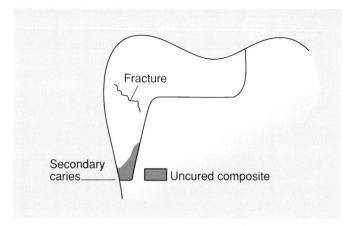

Figure 2.2.10 Lack of cure of light-activated composite material at the base of a proximal box.

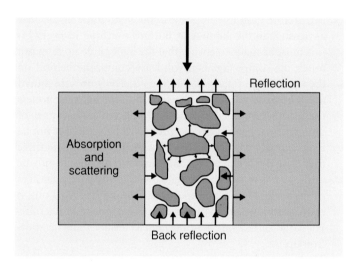

Figure 2.2.11 Reflection, scattering, and absorption of light as it enters the composite.

metal matrix bands are being used. A high degree of conversion of the C=C double bond in the resins is highly desirable to achieve the optimum mechanical properties and this relates to the curing time and the power of the LCU.

Any lack of cure provides a poor foundation for the restoration and may lead to fracture. This is due to a lack of support at the cervical margins, caused by the washout of the uncured restorative material and the development of recurrent caries.

Several factors affect the depth of cure:

- *The type of composite.* As light hits the composite, it is reflected, scattered, and absorbed as shown in Figure 2.2.11, and this limits the extent to which the light penetrates into the deeper areas of the composite. This is a function of filler particles, both the particle size distribution and the total loading, as well as the shade, as the pigments used to impart color also absorb light. This means that when all other factors are the same, a darker shade of composite may cure to less depth than a lighter shade.
- *The quality of the light source.* Camphorquinone is activated by light of wavelength range 460–480 nm, and light must be sufficiently intense at this wavelength to activate the

camphorquinone. Human eyes are very poorly equipped to estimate light intensity, and as such, it is sensible, particularly if using one of the quartz tungsten halogen LCUs still found in some surgeries, to check the intensity regularly using an appropriate intensity meter. Some quartz tungsten halogen LCUs come with these built into the cradle that holds the unit. This is not considered necessary for LED light curing units as LEDs show little deterioration in intensity over time; they either work, and work at full intensity, until one day they eventually fail and then will not work at all.

• *The distance between light guide and composite.* The tip of the light guide should be placed as close as possible to the surface of the restoration, as the curing efficiency drops off rapidly when the tip is moved away from the surface. In fact, the light intensity on unit surface area can, without focusing optics, falls with the inverse square of the distance between the light source and the resin, as shown in Figure 2.2.12. It is therefore desirable to position the light guide tip as close as possible to the composite, but not touching it! Every effort must be made to ensure that the light guide tip does not touch the composite, as it will leave composite behind on the tip and will reduce the curing efficiency on subsequent use. The material should be exposed to the light for no less than the recommended time so that there is no danger of undercuring. For large restorations, the light tip may not be large enough to cover the whole of the restoration and there may be a tendency to fan the surface. This should not be done, as it is impossible to tell how long any particular area of the surface has been exposed. If fanning is carried out, it must be followed up with further curing, one spot at a time. For large surfaces, it is important to ensure that the spots overlap.

There is a tendency on the part of some manufacturers to recommend curing times of as little as 10 or 20 seconds, as this obviously reduces the time it takes to complete a particular procedure. This may be sufficient for applications where only a very thin layer of the composite is to be applied but may be insufficient when adopted for extensive restorations. Most independent research continues to support curing times of 40–60 seconds.

In situations where light access presents a problem, such as distal boxes of a mesial occlusal distal restoration in a posterior composite, aids to curing, such as light-conducting wedges and transparent matrices, must be considered. Curing for excessively long times is, however, not a means of getting greater depths of cure. The depth of cure for a particular composite used in conjunction with a particular light source reaches a limit, which cannot be exceeded, and curing times of more than 60 seconds tend not to offer any further benefit.

Generally speaking, most if not all modern composites should yield a depth of cure of at least 2 mm if handled properly and used in conjunction with a well-maintained and appropriately wielded LCU. Many can offer more; even a 'regular' composite often achieves depths of cure of 3–4 mm in laboratory studies, and the 'bulk fill' composites that we will discuss later can provide significantly greater depths than this. Inferring clinical behavior from laboratory studies is difficult, however, as the laboratory does not present the complexities of a patient attached to the tooth! A safe approach is to cure increments of no more than 2 mm and use incremental placement for deeper restorations.

Light Curing Units

Blue-light-cured composites can be cured with LED, quartz halogen, argon laser, and xenon plasma LCUs. The latter two are very rarely used nowadays and are mostly consigned to museums! The LED LCU is by far the most commonly used, but the most up-to-date usage data available does indicate that a substantial number of dental practices still use the quartz halogen variety.

The blue-LED light curing unit has the advantage that it only emits light within a very narrow wavelength range of around 460–480 nm. There is no UV to filter out, no additional energy being consumed in creating other colors of visible light, and no generation of heat via infrared radiation. It is therefore ultra-energy-efficient and can be operated with a small rechargeable battery, meaning they are often cordless and very portable (Figure 2.2.13). They also have excellent longevity, with most LEDs working for thousands of hours without material degradation. Quartz halogen lights on the other hand are corded and the light intensity deteriorates over time, meaning that the clinician must be vigilant in checking the intensity to ensure it does not fall below the threshold specified by the manufacturer for effective curing.

Polymerization Shrinkage

As previously noted, a long-recognized drawback with composites is polymerization shrinkage. In a sense, the whole field of adhesive restorative dentistry grew from this limitation of composites, because without adhesion, there would inevitably be a marginal gap as the composite shrinks away from the cavity wall on setting (Figure 2.2.14). Despite major advances in the field of adhesive dental materials (see Chapter 2.5), polymerization shrinkage is still implicated as a primary source of interfacial breakdown. Shrinkage stresses develop because the material is constrained by the adhesion to the cavity walls. These stresses can be sufficient to cause breakdown of the interfacial bond, whereby the advantage of the adhesive procedure is lost. Gaps occurring at the margin may be invisible to the naked eye and are only visible clinically when using transillumination and

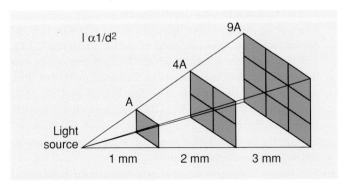

Figure 2.2.12 Relationship between intensity (I) of the light and the distance (d) from the light source to the surface.

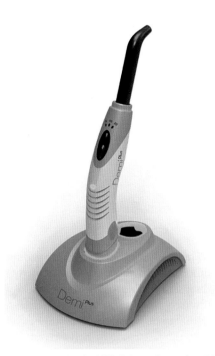

Figure 2.2.13 An example of a LED light curing unit, which is compact and often cordless, in contrast to the earlier quartz halogen units. Image courtesy of and copyright Kerr UK, with thanks.

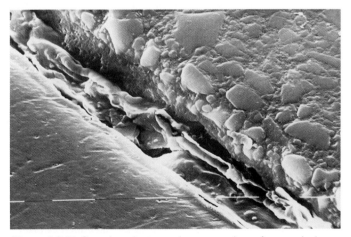

Figure 2.2.14 Scanning electron microscope view of a marginal gap formed due to polymerization shrinkage of a composite.

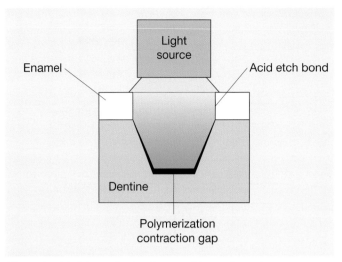

Figure 2.2.15 Schematic showing possible gap formation as a consequence of polymerization shrinkage.

magnification. This is particularly observed for the bond to dentine, which is less strong than that achieved to acid-etched enamel, and, as a consequence, the shrinkage tends to occur toward the acid-etched enamel-bonded interface if the bond to the dentine breaks down (Figure 2.2.15). The gap that forms between the restoration and the dentine will give rise to postoperative sensitivity due to the hydrodynamic effect. If any of the margins are in dentine, then the breakdown of the bond will also give rise to marginal leakage. This is especially a problem when composites are placed subgingivally in proximal boxes.

Polymerization shrinkage of modern composites is typically in the region of 1–3%; some claim or have been measured to show exceptionally low shrinkage of <1%, whereas others may exhibit shrinkage of up to 6%. It is worth reflecting that, while much development in LCUs has been focused on maximizing the degree of conversion of the monomer, this also maximizes the amount of polymerization shrinkage, as every bond made contributes to the shrinkage.

The polymerization shrinkage of a composite is dependent on the type of resin monomer(s) employed and the amount of resin present in its unpolymerized form. In general, a higher proportion of filler results in a lower final shrinkage – there is less resin to shrink! This is not always a hard-and-fast rule, though. Some composites use particles of prepolymerized resin in their formulation, and thus the label will specify a higher content of resin, but as this polymerization has already happened prior to curing, it does not contribute to the shrinkage.

Ideally, the polymerization shrinkage of the composite should be as low as possible, since this enhances marginal adaptation and reduces the possibility of breakdown of the bond to the tooth tissues, and the risk of cuspal deflection and stress on the enamel. For this reason, much effort has been made by both the scientific and commercial research communities to develop composites with low shrinkage. While fillers – content, size, nature – play their role, the biggest gains have been made in adjusting the resin component.

CLINICAL SIGNIFICANCE

Polymerization shrinkage of modern composites is, in many cases, less severe than with some earlier products, but this is not universally the case and there are still composites on the market that suffer from substantial shrinkage. There is an extent to which this can be addressed by good technique, but the practitioner must be sure they are aware of any such shortcomings and operate with an understanding of the consequences.

The use of incremental placement techniques, combined with through-the-tooth curing, is one approach that is believed will encourage polymerization shrinkage toward rather than away from the cavity walls (Figure 2.2.16) and also addresses the issues of limited depth of cure.

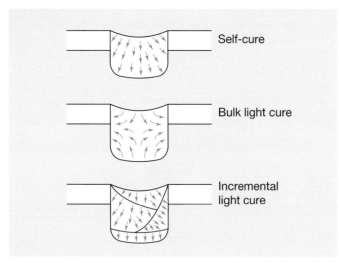

Figure 2.2.16 Various proposed options for filling a proximal box and minimizing the effects of polymerization shrinkage. The direction of the polymerization shrinkage stresses is indicated by the *arrows*.

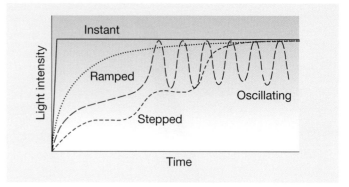

Figure 2.2.17 Light intensity profiles for slow start visible light curing units.

It is obvious that the elimination or at least a significant reduction in the polymerization shrinkage of the resin matrix is a desirable step. The steps taken to avoid or minimize the consequences of polymerization shrinkage are among the most time-consuming aspects of the procedure for the placement of composite fillings and do not really resolve the problem satisfactorily.

One potential way to address this is by the use of dentine bonding agents that act as 'stress absorbers' and compensate for the polymerization shrinkage stresses. At one time, this was thought to be a major consideration, but the data has not shown this approach to be as succesfull as had been hoped. The use of a low elastic modulus lining material to act as a stress absorber has also been postulated, but this adds another step to an already fairly lengthy and complex procedure, and the idea of using a low elastic modulus liner carries with it the penalty that stresses generated by occlusal loads cannot easily be transferred across the interface between the tooth and the restoration and may cause high stresses elsewhere in the tooth structure.

The ratio of main to diluent resin is one important factor, as the greater the proportion of small resin monomers such as TEGDMA, the greater the net shrinkage. However, a certain amount of the diluent resin is generally considered necessary to provide a suitably pliable consistency, so there is a limit to how much this can be adjusted.

It was thought at one time that a reduction in the *rate* of polymerization would allow more time for the polymerization shrinkage stresses to be dissipated by a process of flow from the free surface and stress relaxation. This led to the introduction of a variety of 'soft-start' blue-LCUs, using ramped, stepped, and oscillating light-curing profiles (Figure 2.2.17). Although these appeared to deliver promising results in laboratory studies, clinical studies yielded inconclusive results, and ultimately there was no great consensus that they offered advantages, so these LCUs are less commonly encountered than they once were. In contrast, so-called 'turbo' composite curing LCUs and protocols are increasingly found, offering shorter curing times of around

5–10 seconds. The results of these are mixed and the impact of the specific composite very significant. Particularly for bulk fill composites (discussed further below), shorter curing times do not seem to adversely affect all material properties, but there is some evidence that bond strengths may still be compromised, perhaps owing to the faster rate of polymerization and associated stress at the margins. The clinician should still bear in mind the potential relationship between polymerization rate and stress, and as the pressure on manufacturers to deliver faster and faster products results in shorter recommended polymerization times, and should always seek to consider the evidence base for the specific LCU-material combination, bearing in mind that fast curing may have a knock-on effect on stresses within and at the margins of composites.

INNOVATION IN RESIN-BASED COMPOSITES

Developments in Resin Technologies

Most of the real progress that has been made in advancing composites is through modification of the resin component of the material.

New resin monomers have proven to be effective in mitigating the effects of polymerization shrinkage, although they do tend to bring additional requirements or complexities. These include modifications of existing methacrylates such as ormocers and stress-decreasing resins as well as alternative chemistries such as siloranes. There have also been innovations in the polymerization initiation-activation system that permit a deeper cure in the 'bulk fill' composites, and a recognition that there is a place in the toolkit for 'flowable' composites, with reduced viscosity and often poorer mechanical properties, but that are still adequate for a range of applications and bring handling and aesthetic advantages.

Ormocers

Whereas methacrylate-based resin matrices consist of purely organic material, an alternative type of inorganic-organic copolymer resin was adapted for use in dental resin composite restoratives: the ORMOCER®, which stands for ORganically MOdified CERamic and is a registered trademark of Fraunhofer Gesellschaft, Germany. It consists of organic reactive species with carbon double bonds for polymerization, which is bound

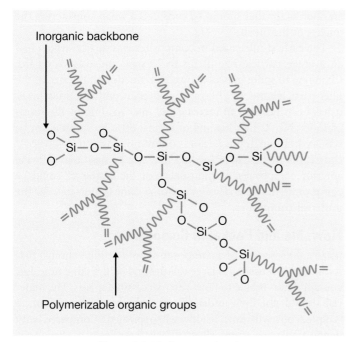

Inorganic backbone

Polymerizable organic groups

Figure 2.2.18 Ormocer chemistry.

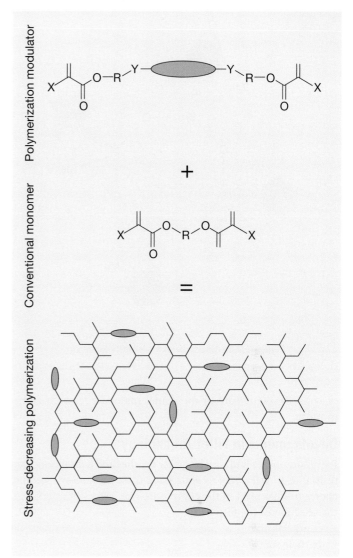

Polymerization modulator

Conventional monomer

Stress-decreasing polymerization

Figure 2.2.19 Stress-decreasing resin system.

to an inorganic Si–O–Si network (Figure 2.2.18). This inorganic-organic network exhibits a similar viscosity to Bis-GMA and thus the matrix will also contain some viscosity controllers such as TEGDMA. Admira (Voco, Cuxhaven, Germany) is a currently available ORMOCER dental restorative product.

Stress-Decreasing Resins

Some modern products incorporate a technology that has been developed in the form of what is described as a stress-decreasing resin; it is based on the incorporation of one or more moieties that acts as a means of absorbing polymerization shrinkage stress by acting as a spring/polymerization modulator (Figure 2.2.19). Based on the scientific evidence gathered to date, the 'polymerization modulator' reduces stress build-up on polymerization without a reduction in the polymerization rate or conversion. It is claimed that, by use of the polymerization modulator, the resin forms a more relaxed network and provides a significantly reduced polymerization stress. A commercially available example of this technology is a 'Smart Dentin Replacement' known as SDR™ from Dentsply, which is designed to act as a dentine substitute such that the cavity is filled up to the dentino-enamel junction with this material and then a resin composite veneer is placed over the top.

Siloranes

Unlike acrylic resins, which set by a free-radical addition polymerization, epoxy-based resins set via a quite different curing mechanism: cationic polymerization. The term 'epoxy' refers to an oxygen-containing ring molecule that contains a three-membered 'oxirane' ring. The curing process involves ring-opening, which results in a lower net shrinkage, and the delayed consumption of reactive species can provide stress relaxation throughout polymerization, which may reduce polymerization shrinkage stress. An example of this approach that, for a time, found application in dentistry is the silorane (Figure 2.2.20), which has comparable mechanical properties to existing methacrylate composites and was claimed to exhibit reduced water sorption and lower polymerization stress rates throughout curing. Unfortunately, these composites do not appear to have succeeded commercially, or at least one can infer that from the fact that they are no longer on the market. Perhaps the requirement for them to be used with a specific silorane bonding system proved too much; clinicians were willing to try a new composite but not as willing to shift from their preferred brand of the dentine bonding system.

Despite the apparent reduction in polymerization shrinkage achieved in the new resin systems, it must not be assumed that this will result in a concomitant reduction in shrinkage stress. A range of other factors such as the filler loading, elastic modulus of the resin composite and shrinkage rate have a contribution to make. Consequently, this continues to be a matter

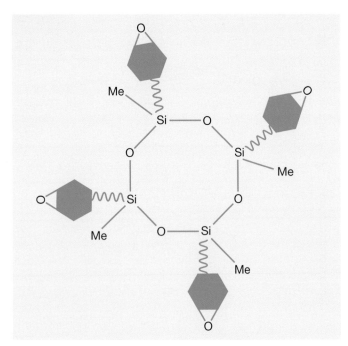

Figure 2.2.20 Structure of a silorane monomer.

of considerable debate in the dental materials research community.

Developments in Filler Technology

Early composites had rough surface finishes and a disappointing resistance to wear. Key to addressing these limitations was the choice of filler used in the composite. The factors of interest in the selection of the filler are:

- composition
- particle size.

Composition

Most composites employ one or other of a variety of quartz- and silica-based glass fillers, including colloidal silica, lithium-aluminium silicate glass, and silica glasses containing barium or strontium.

The glass formulation is critical because it has a major effect on the coloring of the composite. Its refractive index must closely match that of the resin to avoid excessive scattering of incoming light occurring, which would result in poor aesthetics and poor depth of cure.

The inclusion of barium or strontium imparts radiopacity to the composites, and this aids in the detection of recurrent caries.

Average Particle Size and Distribution

The average particle size, and particle size distribution, of the filler are important as they determine the amount of filler that can be added to the resin, without the necessary handling characteristics being lost. Particle size also has a pronounced effect on the final surface finish of the composite restoration, in that the smaller the filler particle size, the smoother the composite will be. The hardness of the filler, relative to the matrix, is

another factor that should be considered when considering the quality of the finish.

The earliest filler used in composites was quartz, which had an average particle size of up to 70 μm, and was very hard. Changing to softer glasses allowed a reduction in the size of the filler particles and, by choosing a suitable combination of sizes, it has been possible to increase the filler loading of the resins considerably. A filler loading of almost 80% by volume can be achieved, although this is more commonly closer to 60–70%. Of course, the highest filler loading may not be desirable with the anterior composites, as the quality of the aesthetics could be compromised; this is clearly not of the same importance for the posterior composites.

Flowable and Packable Composites

Ideally, the viscosity of a composite should be high enough that it can be condensed into large cavities and, at the same time, low enough that it is able to flow into inaccessible spaces. The material should not flow under its own weight so that it can be sculpted but will flow readily when pushed. Compared with dental amalgams, composites can have a tendency to stick to the instruments and this can create problems in achieving good marginal adaptation. In an effort to improve the marginal adaptation of composite restorations, so-called 'flowable' composites were introduced in the late 1990s. At the same time, 'packable' composites appeared on the market, which sought to have handling characteristics similar to that of dental amalgams by having an increased viscosity.

In order to produce flowable composites, the manufacturers typically reduce the filler loading and, so as not to have to reduce it too much, the particle size of the glass filler is sometimes also increased. Flowable composites are ideally suited for small preparations such as abrasion preparations, margin repairs, and preventive resin restorations. They may also be used as veneering or outer layers over stronger composites such as the bulk fills where aesthetics is a priority. With the reduced filler loading and larger filler particle size, these materials are usually not recommended for situations involving high levels of stress or wear.

The production of packable composites can be achieved by a slight increase in filler loading of 1–2 vol. % or a change in the rheology of the resin matrix. This is not as easy as it sounds since the filler loading of most composites has already been maximized and simply adding more filler will make the composite crumbly and cause cracking. The increased viscosity can be accomplished in a number of different ways:

- by increasing the filler particle size range, which improves the packing density, such as a trimodal particle size distribution
- by modification of the filler particle shape such that particles have a tendency to interlock, making it more difficult for them to flow past each other
- by modification of the resin matrix such that stronger intermolecular attractions are created (e.g. replacing the hydroxyl groups on the Bis-GMA with hydrogen for hydrogen bonding) and thus raising the viscosity
- by the addition of dispersants (rheological control additive), which lower the viscosity and allow an increase in the filler loading.

As with most things, there is a price to pay for the increased filler loading. These materials tend to be more opaque and have an inferior surface finish; despite the increased filler loading, the mechanical properties appear to be no different from those of the universal composites such as the small-particle hybrids. Since the aesthetics are compromised, the manufacturers provide only a limited range of shades. These materials therefore have a limited range of applications and are most suited for posterior applications, such as small to moderately sized class II preparations. Due to the high viscosity, adaptation can be a problem and there is an increased potential for trapping air, resulting in voids at the margins or in the bulk of the restoration. For this reason, it has been suggested that a thin layer of flowable composite is first placed in the base of the proximal box before the packable composite is placed.

It should be appreciated that both the flowable and the packable composites have been developed as a response by manufacturers to requests from dental practitioners to produce composites with special handling properties. Hence these composites do not represent a major advance in the context of their physical and mechanical properties. Typically, the flowable composites have inferior mechanical properties and the packable composites have inferior aesthetics compared with the universal composites.

Bulk fill composites

Bulk fill composites were introduced to address one of the significant limitations of the conventional composite: the limited depth of cure. The need to place composites in 2 mm increments, carefully positioning the successive layers and curing between each, makes larger restorations time-consuming. Bulk fill composites are designed to be placed in much thicker increments, meaning that large restorations can be completed with fewer steps, perhaps even a single layer, with increments of 4, 6, or even 8 mm.

There are several potential approaches that can be taken to achieve this, and most if not all have been trialled in commercial products.

One can reduce the filler content, which in turn reduces the scattering of light as it passes through the composite and allows more of it to penetrate through to the depths of the restoration. This is more effective if the filler size is also increased, but as we will see in later sections of this chapter, there are good reasons that many composites have high total filler content combined with at least some small filler particles, so this approach tends to have a detrimental effect on other properties.

An alternative approach is to re-think the polymerization initiation system. Most composites use camphorquinone as the photoinitiator, and this requires a certain threshold light intensity in order to stimulate sufficient polymerization to give an adequate degree of conversion. There are other photoinitiators for which the threshold intensity is lower, so even without a greater light penetration, the depth of cure can be increased if the photoinitiator responds to lower light levels. The clinician must be vigilant, however, when considering their options for bulk-fills, as some of them require special LCUs with higher intensities or even different wavelength ranges than the 'standard'; it is no good using a bulk fill that claims 8 mm cure depths if the LCU doesn't deliver the required output to achieve it, and both clinician and patient will soon be disappointed.

As with some of the luting materials we will consider later, some bulk cure composites exhibit what is often called 'dual cure', where they polymerize rapidly on exposure to light of the appropriate wavelength but *also* exhibit a slower chemical polymerization that proceeds steadily in the background. This can help to mitigate some of the potential shortcomings of bulk fill composites.

Various permutations of the bulk fill composite are found in the dental materials catalogue. There are 'true' bulk fills, which can be used for the entire restoration, although the changes made to the formulation to achieve the depth of cure may result in some minor compromise to the aesthetics, which means these are likely to be best suited to posterior restorations. Since this is where most large, deep restorations are likely to be situated, many consider this to not be too problematic.

There are 'base' bulk fills with which the aesthetics or, more seriously, the mechanical and wear properties are sufficiently limited that they require a veneering or capping layer of a different composite such as a flowable. Finally there are the 'sonic activated' bulk fills. These interesting materials are very viscous, owing to a high filler content, but when used in conjunction with a particular specification of sonic handpiece (Figure 2.2.21), they become temporarily much less viscous and can flow readily. The idea is that this aids the handling of what would otherwise be an inconveniently viscous material but that the higher filler content contributes to good mechanical properties.

CLINICAL SIGNIFICANCE

The bulk-fill composites have rapidly gained popularity with the dental community, and they do present significant advantages in terms of time and complexity of placing a composite restoration, but long-term clinical data is still fairly sparse. There are several varieties of bulk-fill materials and the clinician must ensure they understand the specific indications and limitations of the one they intend to use.

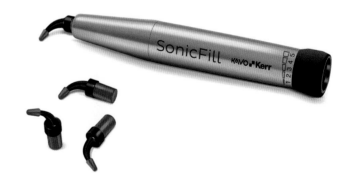

Figure 2.2.21 A bulk fill composite that exhibits a viscosity change when subjected to ultrasonic pulses, with the specialist handpiece used to generate the ultrasound. Image courtesy of and copyright Kerr UK, with thanks.

CLASSIFICATION OF COMPOSITES BASED ON FILLER PARTICLES

One useful way to categorize dental composites is according to the nature and the particle size of the filler.

Traditional Composites

'Traditional' composites contained glass filler particles with a mean particle size of 10–20 μm and a largest particle size of 40 μm. These composites had the disadvantage that the surface finish was very poor, with the surface having a dull appearance due to filler particles protruding from the surface as the resin was preferentially removed around them, as shown in Figure 2.2.22. These are no longer in use.

Microfilled Resins

Microfilled resins were the next iteration in the development of composite fillers and contained colloidal silica with an average particle size of 0.02 μm and a range of 0.01–0.05 μm. The small size of the filler particles meant that the composite could be polished to a very smooth surface finish. The very small particle size also provided a very large surface area of filler in contact with the resin, and this high surface area (compared to that of the filler used in the traditional composites) meant that it was very difficult to obtain a high filler loading, as a large amount of resin was required to wet the surfaces of these filler particles. If the filler was added directly to the resin and a reasonably fluid consistency were maintained, then the maximum filler loading that can be achieved was only of the order of 20 vol. %.

To ensure an adequate filler loading, a two-stage procedure for the incorporation of the filler was developed. A very high-filler-loaded material is first produced in a laboratory/factory environment (i.e. as part of manufacture, not in the mouth) and this material is then polymerized and ground into particles of 10–40 μm in size, which is subsequently used as a filler for more resin. Thus what is finally obtained is a composite containing composite filler particles (Figure 2.2.23). Although the filler loading of the prepolymerized particles could be as high as that of the large particle composites, the overall filler content was still considerably less (~50 vol. %).

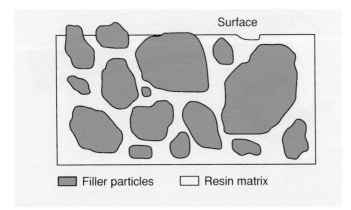

Surface

☐ Filler particles   ☐ Resin matrix

Figure 2.2.22 Filler particles protruding from the surface due to preferential removal of the resin matrix.

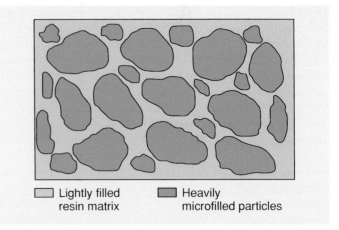

☐ Lightly filled resin matrix   ☐ Heavily microfilled particles

Figure 2.2.23 A heterogeneous microfilled resin, using prepolymerized particles that are added to the resin containing a small amount of colloidal silica.

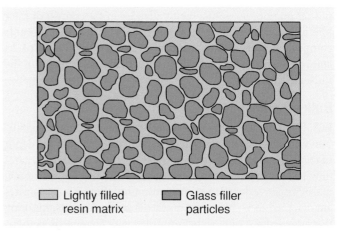

☐ Lightly filled resin matrix   ☐ Glass filler particles

Figure 2.2.24 Structure of a hybrid composite, consisting of large filler particles in a resin matrix containing colloidal silica.

Hybrid or blended composites

Hybrid composites contain large filler particles of an average size of 15–20 μm and also a small amount of colloidal silica, which has a particle size of 0.01–0.05 μm (Figure 2.2.24). These were designed to benefit from the favorable properties of the traditional and microfilled composites; the use of larger particles means the total surface area of the filler is reduced, but the smaller particles take up some of the space between the larger particles, allowing a very high total filler loading to be achieved. Most composites now contain colloidal silica, but their behavior is very much determined by the size of the larger filler particles.

Small-Particle Hybrid Composites

Developments in manufacturing methods allowed the grinding of glasses to particle sizes smaller than had previously been possible. This led to the introduction of composites having filler particles with an average particle size of less than 1 μm, and a typical range of particle sizes of 0.1–6.0 μm, usually combined with colloidal silica (Figure 2.2.25). The smaller-sized filler

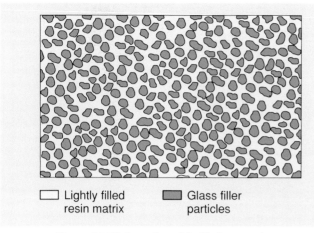

Figure 2.2.25 A small particle-filled composite.

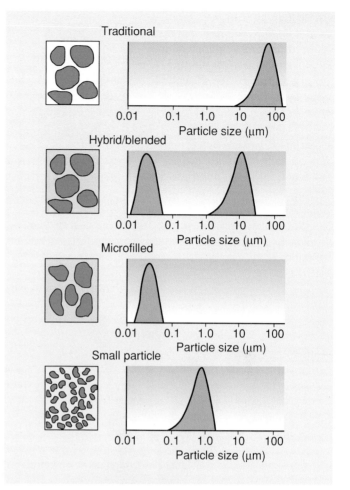

Figure 2.2.26 A classification of composites based on filler type, with the horizontal axis as the logarithmic scale of the particle size.

particles allow these composites to be polished to a smoother surface finish than those with larger particles. These composites can achieve a highly polished surface finish because any surface irregularities arising from the filler particles must be much smaller than the filler particles and therefore will be below the resolution of the wavelength of light (0.38–0.78 μm).

Nanocomposites

Since the early 2000s, there has been a vogue for the branding of materials and other products as 'nano', and there are many dental composites on the market that are described as 'nanocomposites' or as being 'nanofilled'. Nanotechnology has had, and continues to have, a profound effect on many fields, including materials science, medicine, and the food and cosmetics industries. There can be no doubt that some of the developments made possible by embracing nanotechnology have allowed academic and industrial scientists to make significant leaps forward in many areas. It is, however, important for the modern clinician to consider the evidence carefully.

Nanomaterials are defined as materials that include components with at least one dimension of the order of less than 100 nm. Practically speaking, composite filler particles are usually approximately equiaxed and thus nanocomposites contain filler particles with a diameter of 100 nm or smaller. Almost all of the composites described above – the microfilled and hybrid materials – fit this description. In one sense, the new wave of nanocomposites could be viewed as simply a rebranding of old materials.

Although a degree of skepticism might therefore be applied to dental composites with a 'nano' label, it appears that active research in this area may yet lead to some useful advances, particularly as regards the aesthetic properties of this class of material. It has been shown, for instance, that some modern composites with fillers of ~75 nm displayed superior gloss retention and reduced opacity without seriously compromising mechanical properties.

Summary

The classification described above is shown schematically in Figure 2.2.26. Since the earliest composites, it was found

beneficial to achieve a high filler loading as this provided an improvement in mechanical properties and a reduction in polymerization shrinkage. In order to increase the filler loading to its maximum, it is common practice to use fillers with two or more complementary particle size distributions. The filler with the smaller particle size distribution fills in the spaces left between the larger filler particles (Figure 2.2.27). This, combined with developments in the resin component, means that composites can provide excellent results in both anterior and posterior applications.

PROPERTIES

Handling and Presentation

Compared to other direct filling materials, the placement of composite resins is demanding, and although modern materials and techniques have allowed some simplifications, composites remain time consuming and technique sensitive. Composite resins are not intrinsically adhesive to enamel and dentine, and therefore acid etching with phosphoric acid and the application of a dentine-bonding agent is required (see Chapter 2.5). When combined with the need for incremental placement and careful attention to light-curing procedures, this means that the placement of a composite restoration can be expected to take up to

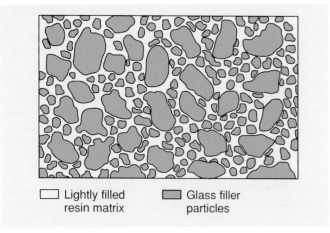

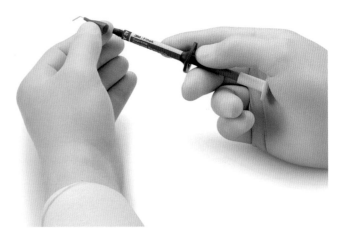

Figure 2.2.27 Bimodal particle size distribution.

□ Lightly filled resin matrix ▨ Glass filler particles

Figure 2.2.29 Flowable composites are often supplied in syringes with a fine tip as they have a lower viscosity combined with a degree of shear thinning that allows them to be placed conveniently in this way. Source: Filtek™ Supreme Flowable Restorative, Courtesy of 3M. © 2023, 3M. All rights reserved.

through a final nozzle under considerable pressure but become more viscous once dispensed. The alternative is small compules intended to deliver a single 'dose' of composite that are applied using an applicator often referred to as a 'composite gun' (Figure 2.2.30).

Biocompatibility

Composite resins are complex materials, and various components and breakdown products may be released in small quantities, when in the mouth. These include uncured resins and diluents and additives, such as UV stabilizers, plasticizers, and initiators. How much material is lost depends largely on the degree of cure that has been achieved, and since most modern composites exhibit a fairly high degree of conversion (polymerization), the data showing substantial loss of components that was published in the early years of composites is not representative of modern materials.

Some of the materials eluted from composites have been shown to be cytotoxic, but this should not be interpreted as being an indication that these materials present an unacceptable risk to the patient's health as the amounts released are very low and true adverse reactions associated with composite resins are very rare.

Some concerns have been expressed regarding the use of bisphenol-A and bisphenol-A-based monomers in composite restorative materials, as these materials have been shown to be capable of inducing changes in estrogen-sensitive organs and cells in laboratory studies. However, studies of leached components tend to show that it is the low-molecular-weight monomers, such as MMA and TEGDMA that leach out, rather than such high-molecular-weight monomers as Bis-GMA and UDMA. Hence it becomes an issue not unlike that associated with amalgams: namely, whether or not the low dose of leached components with estrogenic activity from composite resins presents an unacceptable risk to the patient. The current evidence base indicates that the safety of composite resins should not be of concern to the general public.

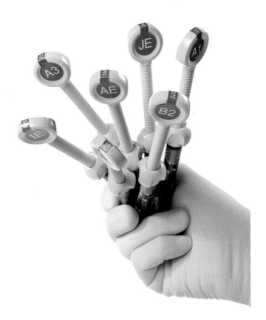

Figure 2.2.28 Composite is often supplied in syringes that dispense a blunt cylinder of material. Each syringe contains enough composite for multiple uses. Image courtesy of and copyright GC Dental Europe, with thanks.

three times as long as that for an amalgam of comparable size. The proper placement of a composite restoration is essential to ensure its longevity, and user error (or not following the instructions accurately) is a surefire way to limit the lifespan of a composite.

Composites are usually presented in one of two ways. Syringe-like devices are used which have a screw-end which, when turned, causes the composite to be extruded from the end in a 5–8 mm thick cylinder. These contain enough composite for multiple applications (Figure 2.2.28). The flowable composites are delivered in a related device which has a much finer tip, allowing precision placement Figure 2.2.29; this is possible as the flowable composites are less viscous and also often exhibit a degree of shear thinning, meaning they can be extruded

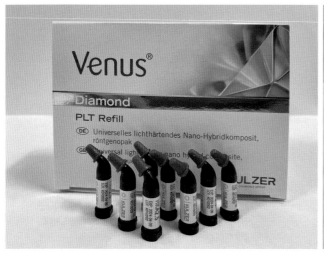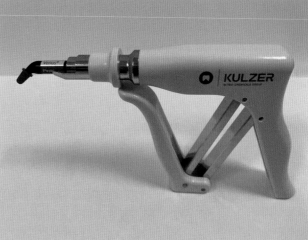

Figure 2.2.30 Composite supplied in a compule that is dispensed using a plastic applicator or 'composite gun'. Images courtesy of and copyright Kulzer Ltd, with thanks.

Water Sorption and Solubility

Water sorption should be minimized for composites because excessive water sorption has a detrimental effect on the color stability and the wear resistance. If the composite can absorb water, then it is also able to absorb other fluids from the oral cavity, which results in its discoloration.

Water sorption occurs mainly as direct absorption by the resin. The glass filler will not *absorb* water into the bulk of the material but can *adsorb* water on to its surface. Thus the amount of water sorption is dependent on the resin content of the composite and the quality of the bond between the resin and the filler. As such, it would perhaps make more sense to relate the value for the water sorption to the resin content of the composite. This would show whether or not the amount of water sorption is that predicted from a knowledge of the water sorption characteristics of the resin alone or if it is unduly high.

Data shown in Table 2.2.1 indicate that, when the filler content of the restorative material is taken into account, there is a correlation between resin volume fraction and water sorption; that is, the more resin, the more water sorption typically occurs.

TABLE 2.2.1 Equilibrium water uptake of composites as a function of the volume fraction of resin. It was assumed that the glass does not absorb water

Volume of resin (%)	Water uptake to resin ($\mu g \cdot mm^{-3}$)
28	82.4
31	41.6
31	119.0
32	63.4
36	44.4
44	37.0
47	43.6

Adapted from the data of Oysaed H., Ruyter I.E., 1986. Water sorption and filler characteristics of composites for use in posterior teeth. J Dent Res 65, 1315–1318.

There is not a linear correlation, however; the intrinsic water sorption for the resin appears to be around 40–45 $\mu g \cdot mm^{-3}$, but for two of the composites in the table, the water sorption is 2–3 times what might have been expected. The question is, 'Where does this extra water go?'

A high water sorption value for a composite (when corrected for the amount of filler present) may indicate a number of possibilities. It is possible that the material has a high soluble fraction, which dissolves and leaves a space into which the water can flow (which may be due to incomplete cure of the resin). In addition, the resin may contain air voids, introduced during mixing or placement. Another possibility is that hydrolytic breakdown of the bond between the filler and the resin has occurred, allowing adsorption on to the surface of the filler particles. This has two important consequences. First, as the bond between the filler particles and the resin is lost, the filler will lose its effectiveness as a reinforcing agent, resulting in a rapid deterioration of the restoration. Second, the filler particles lose their surface cohesion, resulting in a high rate of wear. Thus a worrying combination of features for a composite would be a high filler loading combined with a high value for water sorption.

It was once thought that the water sorption might, to some extent, compensate for the polymerization shrinkage, but water sorption is a gradual process taking many months to complete. This can be shown from a knowledge of the diffusion coefficient, D, of water in a composite, which is typically of the order of 1.25×10^{-9} cm$^2 \cdot$s^{-1}. For a sample of 2 mm thickness, the material would require 166 days to reach equilibrium, and if the sample is 5 mm thick, the time taken to reach equilibrium is in excess of 3 years. Thus water sorption cannot prevent interfacial debonding, since it cannot counteract the instantaneous shrinkage that occurs on setting. In due course, the slight swelling may well improve the marginal adaptation of the restoration, but the chances are that, by then, it will be too late.

It is important to realize that, if measurements of the water sorption characteristics are to be undertaken, it is necessary for samples to be extremely thin to be able to reach equilibrium water sorption in a realistic time. Also, for the comparison of water sorption data, the glass filler loading should be taken into account.

Coefficient of Thermal Expansion

To minimize the possibility of stresses being developed due to differential expansion and contraction in response to hot and colt stimuli, the coefficient of thermal expansion of the composite needs to be as close as possible to that of tooth tissue. The glass fillers have a low coefficient of thermal expansion, while the resin has a comparatively high coefficient of thermal expansion, so the higher the inorganic filler loading, the lower the coefficient of expansion will be. Examples of the coefficient of expansion of some commercially available composites (both regular and 'bulk fill' – see above) are presented in Table 2.2.2, illustrating the range of this property that may be encountered.

Radiopacity

When composites are used as a posterior restorative material, their radiopacity is of the utmost importance. The detection of caries under a non-radiopaque composite is virtually impossible and would allow the caries process to continue undetected for far too long. It is not clear what the optimum radiopacity for a composite is, since excessive radiopacity can potentially mask out caries lying behind the restoration, but the composite should at least be as radiopaque as the enamel.

Color match

The aesthetic qualities of composites are well recognized. The earliest composites suffered from discoloration, which can manifest itself in one of three ways:

- marginal discoloration
- general surface discoloration
- bulk discoloration.

TABLE 2.2.2 The Coefficient of Thermal Expansion (α) for Some Composites Compared with Enamel and Dentine

Material	α (ppm·°C^{-1})
Enamel	17
Dentine	11
Filtek Bulk Fill Flow*	22
Aura Bulk Fill*	23
X-tra Fill*	10
Filtek Bulk Fill Sculptable*	16
Admira Fusion*	20
Surefil SDR+*	15
Tetric Evoflow Bulk Fill*	20
X-tra Base*	16
Opus*	19
Filtek Z350XT†	18
Filtek Z350 Flow†	37

*Bulk fill composite.
†Universal/regular composite.
Data taken from Nascimento et al. Physicomechanical and thermal analysis of bulk-fill and conventional composites – PubMed (nih.gov), to nearest unit ppm·°C^{-1}.

Marginal discoloration is usually due to the presence of a marginal gap or ledge between the restoration and the tooth tissues. Debris accumulates in the gap or ledge and leads to an unsightly marginal stain; elimination of the marginal gap would completely avoid this type of staining. A good acid-etch technique should avoid a gap. The bond between acid-etched enamel and composite is sufficiently strong and durable to achieve a good marginal seal, which avoids the ingress of debris. If the bond is good, then an alternative cause of marginal discoloration may be a ridge at the interface, where material can accumulate.

General surface discoloration may be related to the surface roughness of the composite and is more likely to occur with those composite resins employing large filler particles. Debris gets trapped in the spaces between the protruding filler particles and is not readily removed by tooth brushing. Polishing with a suitable abrasive can remove this, although it is comparatively rare now that large particle composites are less commonly encountered.

Bulk, or deep, discoloration is a particular problem with some two-paste amine-cured (i.e. non-light-cured) composites. The color of the restoration changes slowly over a long time period, giving the restoration a distinctly yellow appearance. This type of discoloration arises due to both the chemical breakdown of components within the resin matrix and the absorption of fluids from the oral environment. The visible light-activated composites seem to have much better color stability, and as such this is a fairly rare occurrence now.

For many years, the approach manufacturers have taken to color matching is to provide a large selection of shades; this gives the clinician a great deal of choice, not only for a single match but for building up a complex restoration with multiple shades of different layers, for instance, to mimic a yellower dentine underneath a whiter enamel. These shades are often accompanied by different opacities, to represent the degree of opacity or translucency of different tissues and even the difference between surface, and subsurface, enamel Figure 2.2.31. In recent years an interesting trend has emerged, which is the 'universal shade' or 'chameleon' composite. The idea is that the composite reflects and transmits the color of the adjacent tooth tissue, blending in not by matching, but by transmitting that natural color to the eye. This certainly simplifies the clinician's job – far fewer shades to choose from (as few as 3

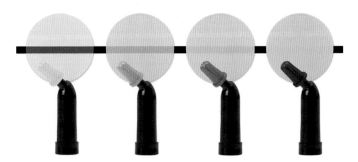

Figure 2.2.31 Composites of different shade and opacity, intended to mimic those properties of the natural tooth tissues. Left to right: 'translucent, enamel, body, and dentine' materials. The *dark line* behind the discs of composite helps to illustrate the increasing opacity from left to right. Courtesy of 3M. © 2023, 3M. All rights reserved.

with some brands, compared to 16 with the conventional approach). Are they as good? Of course, the devil is in the detail, and the outcome depends on the specific application. In narrow, but deep, cavities, they can work very well, as there is ample opportunity for them to be influenced by the adjacent tissues. With cavities that go 'through', like a class IV, they would be a poor choice, as they will transmit the dark color of the oral cavity as a whole, as that is what is 'behind' the composite as far as the eye is concerned. As with many materials, they have their place in the clinician's toolkit, but no single material is optimally suited to all applications.

MECHANICAL PROPERTIES

Compressive Strength

If one compares the compressive strengths of a number of composites and amalgams with those of enamel and dentine, the indications are that the composites are generally as strong or stronger than the tooth tissues (Table 2.2.3). It is important to know the significance of this value.

Being relatively easy to measure, the compressive strength of a material is quoted frequently. Unfortunately, it is also a property that is difficult to interpret due to the possible modes of failure under compression:

- ductile materials can spread sideways, rather like putty
- brittle materials, like glass and stone, can explode in all directions
- buckling can occur in long, thin samples.

As can be imagined, highly complex stresses are generated in the specimen when testing compressive strength.

If we ask ourselves whether restorations fail in any of the modes described above, then the answer is that this would seem unlikely. It is much more likely that the restorations will fail under tension (due to the application of bending forces), as composites have a very low tensile strength.

Thus the compressive strength is a poor indicator of a material's resistance to failure, as there is no simple relationship between a material's compressive and tensile strengths.

Diametral Tensile Strength

If restorative materials *are* more likely to fail in a tensile mode, then it would make more sense to measure their tensile

TABLE 2.2.3 Compressive Strength Data for a Variety of Materials

Material (Manufacturer)	Compressive Strength (MPa)
Molar enamel	260
Molar dentine	305
Sybralloy (Kerr)	500
Dispersalloy (Johnson & Johnson)	440
G-aenial Posterior	323
Tetric Evo Ceram	282
Filtek Bulk Fill	665
Surefil SDR Bulk Fill	1019

Composite data reproduced from Assesment of the compressive strength of the current restorative materials – ScienceDirect.

TABLE 2.2.4 Diametral Tensile Strength of Some Composite Restorative Materials

Material	Diametral Tensile Strength (MPa)
Tetric Evo Ceram Bulk Fill	49
Ceram X Mono	46
Nanoceram Bright	38
Estelite	49

Data from https://www.wjoud.com/doi/WJOUD/pdf/10.5005/jp-journals-10015-1580

strength than their compressive strength. Unfortunately, the measurement of the tensile strengths of brittle materials is extremely difficult and gives rise to a great deal of scatter in the data. The reason for this is that such materials are highly susceptible to the presence of internal flaws or small cracks in their surfaces, which are all but impossible to eliminate. As a consequence, the measured tensile strength of composites is much more dependent on the quality of surface finish than the properties of the material itself.

The *diametral tensile test* is an alternative method for measuring the tensile strength of a material (Figure 1.6.8). Again, complex stress patterns arise in the material, but the results are reasonably reproducible and it is an easy property to measure. For these reasons, the diametral tensile strength is often quoted for dental materials. It is interesting to note that this test is usually applied to brittle materials. Hence, if the diametral tensile strength is quoted rather than conventional tensile strength, this indicates that the material is brittle and therefore suffers from a lack of toughness. Typical values for the diametral tensile strength of a number of contemporary composites are given in Table 2.2.4. It is plausible that this property may provide a more useful indicator of the resistance to fracture than compressive strength.

Hardness

The surface hardness of a dental material can be measured readily by a number of techniques, resulting in a hardness value that can then be used to compare different composites. At one time, it was thought that the hardness would provide a good indicator of the wear resistance of a composite, and this is true up to a point.

The original acrylic resins were very soft materials, but their hardness and wear resistance were much improved by the addition of a filler. Measurement of the hardness initially gave some indication of the wear resistance, but this relationship unfortunately breaks down at the high filler loadings used in contemporary composites (see below).

Wear

Wear is the process by which material is displaced or removed by the interfacial forces that are generated as two surfaces rub together. Types of wear that occur in the oral environment are as follows.

Abrasive Wear

When two surfaces rub together, the harder of the two materials may indent, produce grooves in, or cut away material from the other surface. This direct contact wear is known as *two-body abrasion* and occurs in the mouth whenever there is direct tooth-to-tooth contact, in what most dentists would call *attrition*.

Abrasive wear may also occur when there is an abrasive slurry interposed between two surfaces such that the two solid surfaces are not actually in contact. This is called *three-body abrasion* and occurs in the mouth during mastication, with food acting as the abrasive agent. Toothpastes also act as abrasive slurries between the toothbrush and the tooth.

Fatigue Wear

The repeated loading of teeth produces cyclic stresses that can lead in time to the growth of fatigue cracks. These cracks often form below the surface and initially grow parallel to it before veering toward the surface or coalescing with other cracks.

Corrosive Wear

Chemical attack on composites can occur as the hydrolytic breakdown of the resin, breakdown of the resin–filler interface, or erosion of the surface due to acid attack.

It is likely that all of the above mechanisms are involved in wear of the composites. In occlusal contact areas the main wear mechanisms are two-body abrasion and fatigue, whereas three-body abrasion dominates in non-contact areas. Corrosive wear can occur in either situation and, when this takes place in combination with stressing conditions, can lead to stress corrosion cracking. This process involves the slow growth of a crack, which will eventually become sufficiently large to cause catastrophic fracture.

Since wear is such a multi-faceted process, it does not lend itself to being measured by any single parameter. The poor correlation between mechanical properties and wear has already been noted, and some of the physical properties, such as a low water sorption, can only give an indication of potential wear resistance, particularly in relation to corrosive wear.

In general, a high filler loading, a smooth surface finish, a hydrolytically stable resin, and a strong bond between the filler and the resin are desirable attributes in a composite, particularly when used in the posterior region. However, it must be recognized that, by themselves, these do not guarantee that a material will be resistant to wear.

An alternative approach is the laboratory simulation of the clinical condition. Unfortunately, it is very difficult to simulate all of the conditions in the mouth that contribute to the wear process. Although a wide variety of *in vitro* methods for measuring the wear rate have been tried, none has been found to predict, with any measure of certainty, the *in vivo* rate of wear of composites.

Another major stumbling block in the development of a reliable laboratory wear test is that one needs to be able to correlate the results with clinical wear data, which are, in themselves, extremely difficult to acquire and interpret. From the many variables that have to be taken into account, the variation in wear from patient to patient is one of the more difficult to understand.

However, it has been shown that there is a marked difference in wear rates between occlusal contact areas and non-contact areas. Thus any value quoted for a wear rate is meaningless unless it is supported with information on the methods used in determining it.

The size of the restoration can also affect the rate of wear, perhaps due to there being a greater likelihood of direct tooth-to-restoration contact with larger restorations. It must also be considered that larger restorations tend to occur more posteriorly, where the occlusal loads are higher.

Thus even *in vivo* wear data are only a guide to the ability of composites to resist wear. The situation is further complicated at present by the lack of a generally accepted method for the measurement of *in vivo* wear, and data have to be interpreted with a great deal of caution.

DENTAL LABORATORY COMPOSITES

Indirect Composite Veneers, Inlays, and Onlays

The clinical placement of multiple direct composite restorations poses a number of problems. These include the time-consuming nature of the placement itself, the difficulty of ensuring good tooth-to-tooth contact, the need to account for polymerization shrinkage, and the risk of incomplete curing of the restoration due to the limited depth of cure. One way to overcome these problems is to use indirect composites – composites cured in a laboratory or manufacturing environment rather than in the mouth – for restorations such as inlays, onlays, and veneers including veneers over other materials such as zirconium oxide.

Indirect composite restorations are constructed in the dental laboratory by a dental technician, based on an impression prepared by the dental surgeon, or alternatively in a CAD-CAM process, as with many ceramic restorations. They are well suited to those situations where there is a need to carry out multiple posterior restorations in a single quadrant or the replacement of non-functional cusps. In most other respects the indications for indirect composite restorations are identical to those of direct composites.

One advantage with this type of restoration is that much of the work in achieving good anatomical contour and tooth-to-tooth contact is done by the technician, without the time pressure of a patient sitting in the dental chair and wishing to be elsewhere. Other benefits are that full depth of cure is assured, since the curing process is carried out in the laboratory and not *in situ*. Although it is suggested that problems associated with polymerization shrinkage are reduced, the experience does not always support this. Even the thin layer of luting resin used to fix the restoration to the tooth tissue can cause sufficiently high shrinkage stresses to lead to failure of the adhesive bond, especially the bond to the dentine. Thus problems with polymerization shrinkage are not totally eliminated. There is also sometimes doubt as to the quality of the bond between the luting resin and restoration itself. The laboratory curing process for the composite inlays (or the manufacture, in the case of CAD-CAM blocks) is so effective that there are few unreacted methacrylate groups left on its surface to react with the resin luting agent.

Fiber-Reinforced Composites

Fiber-reinforced composites (FRCs) offer enormous potential for producing high-strength and high-stiffness materials but with a very low weight and are of particular interest for crowns and bridges which require these exacting mechanical properties. Fiber-reinforced resin systems for use in the dental laboratory or in the dental surgery are available in various forms, including unidirectional, mesh, and woven arrangements of the fibers. The unidirectional fibers allow the construction of long spans, while the mesh and weave patterns support stresses in different directions simultaneously. The FRCs have significantly better flexural strength and impact resistance compared with particulate-filled resins, as long as good fiber wetting and coupling by the resin and a high fiber content is achieved. The range of applications suggested for these new materials are splints, bridges, crowns, and removable dentures.

Composite or Ceramic?

One of the more recent innovations in indirect composites are those that occupy a niche at the interface between conventional dental composites and ceramic materials. These are known as the resin ceramics and borrow heavily from conventional dental composite chemistry. Further discussion of these materials can be found in Chapter 3.5.

CLINICAL CONSIDERATIONS FOR THE USE OF COMPOSITE RESTORATIONS

The indications for the use of composite restorations used to be primarily associated with their ability to achieve an excellent aesthetic result, with issues such as limitations to bonding and a restricted range of mechanical properties limiting the applications. Composites were therefore mostly suited for anterior applications, such as the restoration of proximal lesions, abrasion and erosion lesions and incisal tip fractures, and less so for larger restorations and those in the posterior area where they would experience heavy load.

Modern composites combined with contemporary bonding materials and techniques have overcome many of these limitations and the uses of composites are now very broad, including posterior and large restorations. There are still some considerations to bear in mind but these are not as extensive as they once were.

The composite restoration should always be considered as an adhesive restoration. The advantages are manifold, but principally, the reliance on adhesion rather than retention helps to conserve tooth structure, to improve the strength of the overall tooth crown, and to provide a barrier to marginal leakage. It is therefore important that these materials are used only in situations where a good-quality adhesive bond can be achieved.

Replacement of Amalgam Restorations

Composites are frequently used as a replacement for failed amalgam restorations. It is important to recognize that the cavity design has been largely dictated by the amalgam to be replaced and was designed with retention in mind, rather than adhesion. Care must be taken to achieve a good adhesive bond in all parts of the cavity, as failure to do so will lead to marginal gaps and the risk of secondary or recurrent caries. In addition, the larger the restoration, the greater the problem of polymerization shrinkage. Suitable incremental placement should be used, and/or a bulk fill composite with suitable polymerization shrinkage parameters and mitigations could be considered.

Lack of Peripheral Enamel

The acid-etch bond to the enamel of composites is extremely effective, such that breakdown of these margins is unlikely.

When a tooth is badly broken down, there will be little enamel left to bond to and the restoration has to rely more and more on the bond to the remaining dentine. Although bonding agents have improved over the years, recent evidence still suggests that to have no margins in enamel does increase the possibility of a breakdown of the marginal seal, likely due to stresses generated by polymerization shrinkage, thermal mismatch, and occlusal loading.

Ideally, resin composites should only be used when all the margins are in enamel. The only exceptions to this are restorations of abrasion/erosion lesions, which tend not to be subjected to high stressing conditions and have proved reasonably effective clinically, although adhesive failures can still present problems.

Poor Moisture Control

Since it is impossible to obtain an adhesive bond between tooth tissues and composites when the tooth surfaces are contaminated with moisture, any situation in which moisture control is not possible should be avoided and an alternative approach must be adopted.

Habitual Bruxism/Chewing

The aggressive wearing action associated with bruxism will cause any composite restoration that is in occlusal contact, or one that is in regular contact with an implement such as a pipe, to wear down extremely rapidly. Thus even incisal tip restorations, which do not normally suffer from high rates of wear, are contraindicated under these circumstances.

CLINICAL SIGNIFICANCE

The introduction of resin-based composite restorative materials has had a major impact on the practice of restorative dentistry. Many of the advances in new techniques are based on the composite materials. Their clinical applications are many and varied and will continue to grow as further improvements in their properties are achieved. However, there remain certain limitations to the use of this group of materials and it is important that these are not disregarded.

COMPOMERS (POLYACID-MODIFIED RESIN COMPOSITES)

Two of the distinctive features of glass ionomer cements (GICs; Chapter 2.3) are their ability to provide a sustained release of fluoride, and their inherent affinity for the dental hard tissues, which greatly simplifies achieving good adhesion between material and tooth. Composite resin restorative materials do not have either of these properties. Good adhesion can be achieved between a composite and a tooth, but only with careful application of appropriate intermediary materials. The addition of fluoride-containing compounds such as stannous fluoride to a composite resin will provide an initial release of fluoride over a period of a couple of weeks but this then tails off rapidly. This initial release is largely due to the presence of the fluoride compound being released from or near the surface of the restoration, but the surface layer of the restoration is rapidly depleted of the fluoride compound and the release virtually stops, as the fluoride ion cannot diffuse through the resin matrix to maintain a reasonable level of release.

Polyacid-modified resin composites, commonly referred to as compomers, are resin composite materials that have been modified to benefit from some of the properties of GICs. In particular, compomers have been designed so as to be able to release significant amounts of fluoride over an extended period.

Composition

The composition of a typical compomer is presented in Table 2.2.5. Examination of the composition indicates that the material is essentially a resin-based system, with a radical polymerization process being activated by blue light acting on camphorquinone. However, there are a number of important differences compared to composite resins.

One of the differences is the glass, which is similar to the composition of the fluorine-containing glasses used in GICs. This fluoro-alumino-silicate glass is thus susceptible to acid attack and provides the source of fluoride ions.

However, this would not be enough in itself, as some means is necessary for the fluoride ions to be released from the glass. This requires hydrogen ions able to attack and dissolve the glass in a manner similar to that occurring in the setting process of GICs. The source of these hydrogen ions is provided by a specially formulated carboxyl group (−COOH) containing polymerizable monomer, which copolymerizes with a dimethacrylate monomer such as UDMA (Figure 2.2.32). Alternatively, the methacrylated polycarboxylic acid copolymer employed in some resin-modified glass–ionomer cements (RMGICs) can be used (see Chapter 2.3).

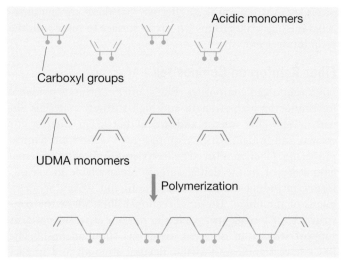

Figure 2.2.32 Copolymerization of an acidic monomer containing carboxyl groups and UDMA monomer in a compomer.

The final ingredient that is required to provide the fluoride release is water. This is not present in the starting material but comes from being absorbed into the material from the oral environment. This water sorption allows an acid–base reaction between the glass and the polycarboxyl groups on the special resin and provides the mechanism for a slow but continuous release of fluoride, which has not previously been possible with composite resins.

In order to aid the diffusion of water into the material through the matrix, and simultaneously aid the diffusion of the fluoride ions out of the matrix, some of the matrix resins used have a more hydrophilic characteristic than those normally used in composite resins (e.g. glycerol dimethacrylate).

Although compomers have both a radical polymerization and acid–base reaction, it is the former that drives the setting process of these materials. The contribution of the acid–base reaction is to provide the fluoride ions to be released over an extended period.

CLINICAL SIGNIFICANCE

It should be stressed that, although the compomer may be considered a hybrid of a resin composite and a glass–ionomer cement (GIC), it is distinctively different from the RMGIC (see Chapter 2.3). The starting material for a compomer is a composite resin, which is then modified, whereas for an RMGIC, the starting material is a GIC. Thus we have a spectrum of materials from GICs to resins, with RMGICs and compomers intermediate between those two parent materials.

Properties
Fluoride Release

Compomer products have been shown to be able to release fluoride over an extended period of time but do not typically display as high an initial 'burst' of fluoride release as is seen with GICs. Modern compomers tend to have a similar fluoride release profile to GICs and RMGICs over the lifetime of a restoration. Fluoride release is highly variable from product to product

TABLE 2.2.5 **Composition of a Compomer**	
Component	**Function**
Fluoro-alumino-silicate glass	Filler and a source of fluoride
Dimethacrylate monomer (e.g. UDMA)	Forms the resin matrix
Special resin	Provides carboxyl groups
Hydrophilic monomers	Aid the transport of water and fluoride
Photoactivators/photoinitiators	Provide cure by radical polymerization

and it is not yet known what the optimum release of fluoride is that is needed to induce an anti-cariogenic condition around the margins of a restoration – or even if this happens at all, in most circumstances. Also, the local conditions can have a significant influence on the amount of fluoride released, as some materials will be more susceptible to dissolution than others in an acid environment.

It has been shown that GICs have a capacity to reabsorb fluoride from the oral environment and release this at a later stage, at least in the earlier stages of their clinical lifetime. Compomers can also be 'recharged' with fluoride in this way, although the process is typically less efficient than with GICs. Thus the restoration can act as a fluoride reservoir that is regularly replenished when exposed to topical fluorides.

Handling Characteristics

What makes a material with good handling characteristics is a complex issue, as this is governed by multiple interrelated features including rheology (e.g. flow and tendency to slump), stickiness, and working and setting times. Nevertheless, the general consensus among dental practitioners is that compomers have reasonable handling characteristics and that compomers are easy to adapt to the cavity wall without sticking to the placement instruments, are easy to shape, and do not slump.

Adhesion

Unlike GICs and RMGICs, compomers have very little inherent affinity for enamel and dentine and have to be used in conjunction with a dentine adhesive system. In order to simplify the handling characteristics when using the dentine-bonding agent normally used with the composite resins, it is sometimes recommended that the acid etching of the enamel and dentine is omitted from the bonding procedure. This is likely to result in a lower bond strength and should only be considered when using compomers in low-stress-bearing applications. Ultimately, this statement is confusing for the dental practitioner, as it is not always easy to determine what constitutes a low-stress-bearing situation. Some compomers are provided with a proprietary adhesive, which have characteristics of the self-etching primers discussed in Chapter 2.5.

Polymerization Shrinkage

Polymerization shrinkage is similar to that of the composite resins and water sorption is not dissimilar to that of the composite resin, being in the region of 40 $\mu g \cdot mm^{-3}$. Where the compomers differ from the composite resins is in their rate of water uptake. As noted earlier in this chapter, the diffusion of water through the resin matrix is very slow and it takes many years for the composite resin restoration to achieve equilibrium water content. For the compomer, the hydrophilic resin matrix provides a more rapid pathway for the absorption of water, with equilibrium water uptake possibly being reached in a matter of days rather than years.

Mechanical Properties

The mechanical properties of compomers would generally appear to be somewhat inferior to those of the composite resins.

Although when first placed they are broadly comparable, the mechanical properties of a compomer deteriorate over time, exhibiting a reduced compressive, diametral, and flexural strength compared to composites. This precludes their use in high-stress-bearing situations, such as the repair of the fractured incisal tip. Their wear resistance is typically better than that of the GICs but inferior to that of composites. It is possible that this may be due to the use of slightly larger filler particles than normally used in composite resins, combined with a reduction in the interfacial integrity between the glass filler and the resin due to the ongoing acid–base reaction at this interface.

Applications

In order to achieve fluoride release from the compomer, it would appear that the mechanical properties have had to be compromised compared to the composite resin. Therefore the compomer does not have the same range of applications as the composite resin. Their use is usually limited to low-stress-bearing situations such as proximal and abrasion erosion lesions, permanent restorations in the primary dentition, and long-term temporaries in the permanent dentition.

Compomers have not, generally speaking, enjoyed the same commercial success as their related, but distinct, cousin, the RMGIC. They lack the adhesive properties of an RMGIC, and the early versions had some unfortunate adverse properties such as excessive water sorption. That said, they do still find favor with some clinicians and particularly so for some applications such as pediatric dentistry. A recent study of the restoration of carious deciduous teeth found that of a wide range of direct restorative materials, compomers had the lowest failure rate at 24 months.

CLINICAL SIGNIFICANCE

While compomers have a narrower range of applications than many other tooth-colored direct restorative materials, they remain a valuable component of the clinician's toolkit, and their properties are particularly well suited to some applications in pediatric dentistry.

FURTHER READING

Alasiri, R.A., Algarni, H.A., Alasiri, R.A., 2019. Ocular hazards of curing light units used in dental practice – A systematic review. Saudi Dental Journal 31 (2), 173–180.

Amend, S., Seremidi, K., Kloukos, D., Bekes, K., Frankenberger, R., Gizani, S., et al., 2022. Clinical effectiveness of restorative materials for the restoration of carious primary teeth: An umbrella review. Journal of Clinical Medicine 11 (12), 3490.

Birant, S., Özcan, H., Koruyucu, M., Seymen, F., 2021. Assesment of the compressive strength of the current restorative materials. Pediatric Dental Journal 31 (5).

Boaro, L.C., Gonçalves, F., Guimarães, T.C., Ferracane, J.L., Versluis, A., Braga, R.R., 2010. Polymerization stress, shrinkage and elastic modulus of current low-shrinkage restorative composites. Dental Materials 26 (12), 1144–1150.

Braga, R.R., Ferracane, J.L., 2004. Alternatives in polymerization contraction stress management. Critical Reviews in Oral Biology and Medicine 15, 176.

Chesterman, J., Jowett, A., Gallacher, A., Nixon, P., 2017. Bulk-fill resin-based composite restorative materials: A review. British Dental Journal 222 (5), 337–344.

German, M.J., 2022. Developments in resin-based composites. British Dental Journal 232 (9), 638–643.

Guggenberger, R., Weinmann, W., 2000. Exploring beyond methacrylates. American Journal of Dentistry 13, 82D.

Ismail, E.H., Paravina, R.D., 2022. Color adjustment potential of resin composites: Optical illusion or physical reality, a comprehensive overview. Journal of Esthetic and Restorative Dentistry 34 (1), 42–54.

Kumbuloglu, O., Saracoglu, A., Ozcan, M., 2011. Pilot study of unidirectional E-glass fibre-reinforced composite resin splints: Up to 4.5-year clinical follow-up. Journal of Dentistry 39, 871–877.

Manhart, J., Chen, H., Hamm, G., Hickel, R., 2004. Buonocore Memorial Lecture. Review of the clinical survival of direct and indirect restorations in posterior teeth of the permanent dentition. Operative Dentistry 29, 481.

Moharamzadeh, K., Brook, I.M., van Noort, R., 2009. Biocompatibility of resin-based dental materials. Materials 2 (2), 514–548.

Nascimento, A.S., Rodrigues, J.F.B., Torres, R.H.N., Santos, K.O., Fook, M.V.L., Albuquerque, M.S., et al., 2019. Physicomechanical and thermal analysis of bulk-fill and conventional composites. Brazilian Oral Research 33, e008.

Opdam, N.J., Bronkhorst, E.M., Loomans, B.A., Huysmans, M.C., 2010. 12-year survival of composite vs. amalgam restorations. Journal of Dental Research 89 (10), 1063–1067.

Oysaed, H., Ruyter, I.E., 1986. Water sorption and filler characteristics of composites for use in posterior teeth. J Dent Res 65, 1315–1318.

Pye, A., 2009. How long do fibre-reinforced resin-bonded fixed partial dentures last? Evidence-Based Dentistry 10 (3), 75.

Rueggeberg, F., 2002. From vulcanite to vinyl, a history of resins in restorative dentistry. Journal of Prosthetic Dentistry 87, 364.

van Heumen, C.C., Tanner, J., van Dijken, J.W., Pikaar, R., Lassila, L.V., Creugers, N.H., et al., 2010. Five-year survival of 3-unit fiber-reinforced composite fixed partial dentures in the posterior area. Dental Materials 26 (10), 954–960.

Wiegand, A., Buchalla, W., Attin, T., 2007. Review on fluoride-releasing restorative materials – Fluoride release and uptake characteristics, antibacterial activity and influence on caries formation. Dental Materials 23, 343.

Glass Ionomer Cements

INTRODUCTION

Glass ionomer cements (GICs), sometimes referred to as glass polyalkenoate cements, are a family of direct, tooth-colored restorative materials. In their simplest form they consist of glass particles that, through an acid–base reaction, become integrated into a network of acidic polymers that forms the continuous phase. GICs are used for a multitude of applications including as restorative (filling) materials, adhesives for orthodontic brackets, luting agents for crowns and bridges, cavity liners, and in endodontics; each application requires subtly different properties, and as such, the GIC comes in a number of different variants. The resin-modified GIC (RMGIC) was first developed a few decades after the original GICs and has proven very popular. As the name suggests, this is a GIC that has been modified in such a way as to incorporate a resin, although the resin has to be more hydrophilic than those used in composites, as we shall discuss.

GICs were first described by Wilson and Kent in 1972, and although they have evolved since the earliest formulation, they retain two key properties that make them such a useful member of the dental materials toolkit. These are their ability to bond to enamel and dentine without the need for a separate adhesive and their ability to release fluoride from the glass component of the cement. Thus GICs combine the adhesive qualities of the zinc–polycarboxylate cements with the fluoride release of the silicate cements that were popular before the introduction of the GIC. The relationship between the different materials is shown in Figure 2.3.1.

CHEMISTRY OF GLASS IONOMER CEMENTS

Composition

The principal components of a GIC are glass, polymeric acid (or 'polyacid'), and water. Additives are often used to control the rate of the setting reaction, tartaric acid being one of the most common of these. The composition and particle size of the glass can be varied, as can the polyacid component, and this gives different properties.

Glass

The glasses for the GICs are usually made up of silica (SiO_2) and alumina (Al_2O_3) as well as aluminum phosphate and various fluoride salts, typically including calcium fluoride, aluminum fluoride, and sodium aluminum fluoride, as shown in Figure 2.3.2. It is quite common to find some of the calcium salts substituted with the strontium or lanthanum equivalent to impart radiopacity to the cement. Another possible component is zinc salts within the glass, and it has been claimed these exhibit higher strengths, although recent data indicates that while the strength of zinc-containing GICs is certainly sufficient for ISO standards, it is not materially superior to many non-zinc-containing competitors.

The glass mixture is fused at a high temperature, and the molten mass is then shock-cooled and finely ground to a powder before use. The particle size of the powder is dependent on its intended application. For filling materials, the maximum particle size is typically 40–50 μm, while for the luting and lining materials, it is reduced, often to less than 15–20 μm.

The rate of release of ions from the glass (which is an important factor in determining the setting characteristics, the solubility, and the release of fluoride) is a function of the type of glass employed (see below). The glass also plays a major role in the aesthetics of the restoration, as this is dependent on both the refractive index of the glass and the presence of pigments within it.

Polyacid

While an eclectic range of polyacids has been used in experimental cements and some earlier commercial versions (Figure 2.3.3), GIC products nowadays almost exclusively employ poly(acrylic) acid or a co-polymer of acrylic and maleic acid. While higher-molecular-weight polyacids give a stronger set-cement, they also increase the viscosity of the cement prior to set, and thus there is a limit as to how high the molecular weight can be taken without creating a cement that is impractically viscous for clinical handling, and despite many forays into more exotic polyacids, the humble poly(acrylic) seems to have prevailed, at least for now. There are a few exceptions – one brand contains a co-polymer of acrylic and vinyl phosphonic acid that causes some modification to the setting rate – but not many. The optimum molecular weight has been reported to be around 11,000 units, and cements typically show an increase in compressive strength over the first 4–6 weeks owing to an extended setting reaction. Tartaric acid is also an important component of most GICs, as it has a significant influence on the working and setting times, as will be explained in the section on setting mechanism.

Presentation
Hand-Mixed GICs

GICs are often provided in two separate containers as a powder and a liquid that are measured out and mixed by hand, usually on a piece of waxed paper or proprietary mixing pad. Some

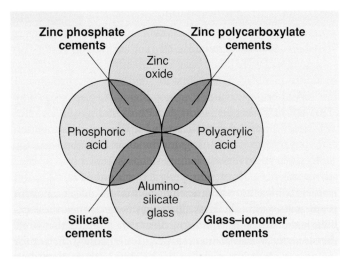

Figure 2.3.1 Schematic of the various dental cements based on powders of zinc oxide and alumino-silicate glass, and liquids consisting of phosphoric acid and polyacrylic acid.

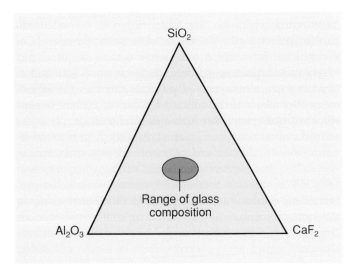

Figure 2.3.2 Composition of glass used in GICs.

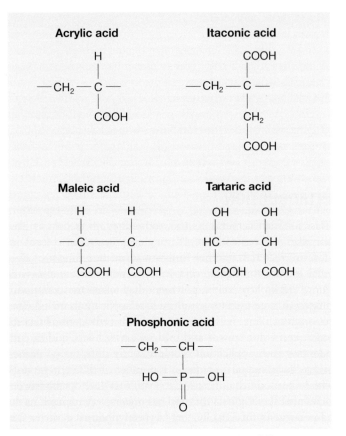

Figure 2.3.3 Acid components used in a GIC.

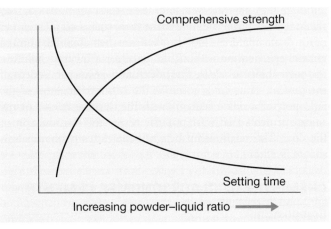

Figure 2.3.4 The effects of changes in powder–liquid ratio on the properties of GICs.

manufacturers employ an approach whereby the powder consists primarily of the glass, and the liquid is a concentrated solution of the polymeric acids, tartaric acid, and other soluble components. The liquid is quite viscous owing to the polymeric acids. Other brands are available in which the powder contains the glass *and* the acids, which have been lyophilized or "freeze dried" to form a fine powder, and the liquid component is just deionized water.

There is no clear difference in the performance or reliability of these two alternative presentations, as long as the components are accurately measured and dispensed. It can be tempting to use more of the liquid component than the instructions specify; at first glance, many inexperienced students of dental materials will comment that there is far too much powder to combine with such a tiny amount of liquid! It is very important *not* to adjust the powder/liquid ratio, as this will seriously compromise the properties of the set cement, making it significantly weaker and more susceptible to later degradation than it would otherwise be (Figure 2.3.4). With the appropriate mixing technique

and some practice, it is entirely possible to mix the liquid with the powder at the ratio specified by the manufacturer. The main challenge is mixing the components sufficiently rapidly; once the powder and liquid come into contact, the setting reaction starts, and there is only a limited time (typically around 2–3 min) during which all mixing and manipulation has to be completed.

Encapsulated GICs

Achieving the correct powder-to-liquid ratio and completing the mixing and manipulation before the setting has progressed

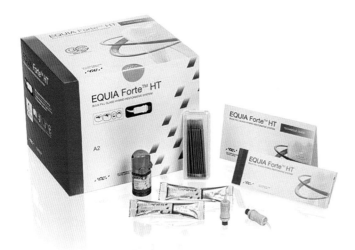

Figure 2.3.5 GICs are often supplied in capsules with pre-proportioned components that are activated by depressing a plunger or similar and then mixed in an amalgamator. Image courtesy of and copyright GC UK Ltd, with thanks.

to the point where the material is no longer pliable can be challenging. One way in which this can be overcome is by the use of encapsulated GICs.

The powder and liquid components are stored separately within internal compartments of the capsule and only come into contact when the capsule is "activated". Activation is, in this context, simply the word for breaking the seal between the two compartments to allow the components to interact with one another. For some brands, activation involves pressing a plunger or button-like device on the capsule, which physically breaks an internal membrane separating the compartments; after this, the capsule is placed in an amalgamator or similar device for a set time and speed to thoroughly mix the components (a commercial example is shown in Figure 2.3.5). For other brands a proprietary device is used to break this membrane. For other brands still there is no separate activation step; the g-force experienced when the capsule is in the amalgamator is sufficient to break the barrier between the compartments.

With any presentation option, it is important to remember that once the capsule is activated, the setting reaction will start immediately – as such, it is crucial that the user only activates when they are ready to immediately proceed to mixing in the amalgamator and then applying the material to the tooth. Any delay will lead to the GIC setting within the capsule, rendering it useless and leaving the clinician somewhat embarrassed and having to start all over again!

The formulation of encapsulated GICs is slightly different from that of the hand-mixed GICs. As the mixing is so much more vigorous for the encapsulated version, the formulation has to be adjusted to *slow down* the setting reaction, or it would set too rapidly. The mechanical properties are typically considered to be slightly more favorable for the encapsulated version with an increase in microhardness as well as flexural and compressive strength (Table 2.3.1). The other main benefit for the clinician is the convenience of the encapsulated version, but this is offset by the higher unit price and the greater waste, both of the cement itself (if the quantity in a capsule is more than is required) and of the capsule itself and the associated packaging. From a sustainability point of view, packaging and dispensing of dental materials leads to large volumes of waste, particularly single-use plastics, and the hand-mixed variety produces significantly less of this.

CLINICAL SIGNIFICANCE

The difficulty of dispensing and mixing the correct amount of powder and liquid for hand-mixed GICs means that encapsulated versions are often preferred, and while these typically offer better mechanical properties, they are also more expensive and create more waste than the hand-mixed variety.

Setting Reaction

The setting reaction of the GICs typically takes 2–3 minutes and is via an acid–base reaction:

$$\underset{\text{glass}}{MO{\cdot}SiO_2} + \underset{\text{acid}}{H_2A} \rightarrow \underset{\text{salt}}{MA} + \underset{\text{silica gel}}{SiO_2} + H_2O$$

The setting process of a GIC involves three overlapping stages:
- dissolution
- gelation
- hardening.

Property (Unit)	Hand-Mixed GIC	Encapsulated GIC	Hand-Mixed RMGIC	Encapsulated RMGIC
Microhardness (Knoop hardness number) at 1 day	40	58	33	49
Microhardness (Knoop hardness number) at 30 days	47	63	28	37
Biaxial flexural strength (MPa) at 1 day	42	56	123	136
Biaxial flexural strength (MPa) at 30 days	48	52	92	174
Compressive strength (MPa) at 1 day	159	205	165	170
Compressive strength (MPa) at 30 days	156	193	171	182

TABLE 2.3.1 Comparison of Properties of Various Formulations and Versions of Glass Ionomers

Data from Al-Taee, L., Deb, S. & Banerjee, A. An in vitro assessment of the physical properties of manually- mixed and encapsulated glass ionomer cements. BDJ Open 6, 12 (2020). https://doi.org/10.1038/s41405-020-0040-x.

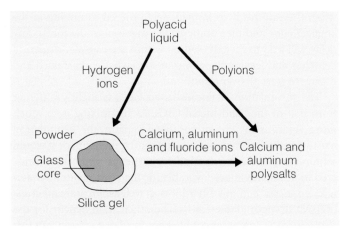

Figure 2.3.6 The variation of the rates of ion release from the glass.

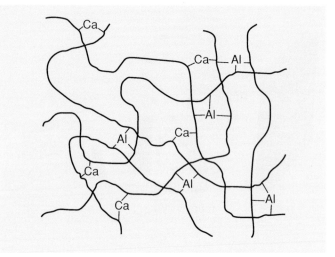

Figure 2.3.8 Gelation phase of the setting process.

This happens owing to the different rates at which the ions are released from the glass and the rate at which the salt matrix is formed (Figure 2.3.6); as is apparent from this curve, the calcium ions are released more rapidly than the aluminum ions. This is because the calcium ions are only loosely bound in the glass structure, while the aluminum ions form part of the glass network, which is more difficult to break down. It is the calcium and the aluminum ions that will eventually form the salt matrix. The sodium and fluorine ions do not take part in the setting process but combine to be released as sodium fluoride.

Dissolution

When the powder and liquids are mixed, the acid goes into solution and reacts with the outer layer of the glass. This layer becomes depleted in aluminum, calcium, sodium, and fluorine, as well as strontium if present in the formulation, so that only a silica gel remains (Figure 2.3.7). The hydrogen ions that are released from the carboxyl groups on the polyacid chain diffuse to the glass and balance the charge, making up for the loss of the calcium, aluminum, and fluoride ions.

Gelation

The initial set is due to the rapid action of the calcium ions, which, being divalent and more abundant initially, react more readily with the carboxyl groups of the acid than do the trivalent aluminum ions (Figure 2.3.8). This is the *gelation phase* of

the setting reaction. The efficiency with which the calcium ions cross-link the polyacid molecules is not as good as it might be because they are also able to link carboxyl groups on the same molecule.

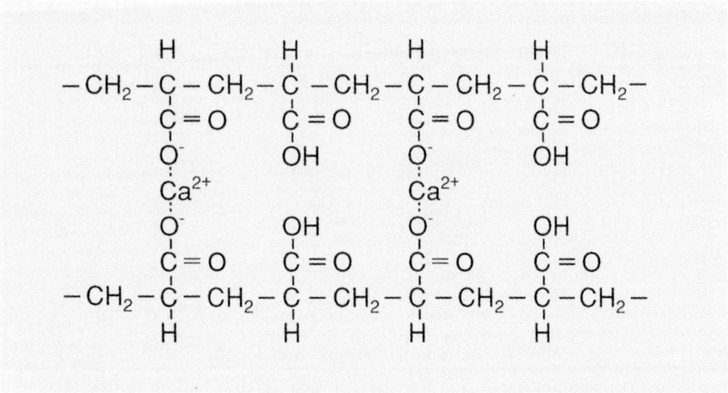

Various things can happen if the restoration is not protected from the outside environment during this critical phase. Aluminum ions may diffuse out of the material and be lost to the cement, thereby being unable to cross-link the polyacrylic acid chains. If the water is lost, the reaction cannot go to completion. In both instances a weak material will result. Alternatively, additional moisture may be absorbed, which may be contaminated with blood or saliva, leading to compromised aesthetics, with the restoration looking exceptionally dull and white. The contaminating moisture will also weaken the material and may even cause it to crumble. Hence it is essential that contamination by moisture and drying of the restoration are both avoided, at least during the initial period of setting when the material is at its most vulnerable.

Hardening

After the gelation phase, there is an extended hardening phase involving several further reactions. The most important initially is mediated by the aluminum ions, which are released more slowly than the calcium ions. It takes around 10 minutes for the uptake of aluminum ions to become significant as ascertained by spectroscopic analysis, as they start to form cross-links between the polyacid chains. In contrast to the divalent calcium ions, the trivalent nature of the aluminum ions ensures that a high degree of cross-linking of the polymer molecules takes place (Figure 2.3.9). There is a continuation of the formation of aluminum salt bridges, and water becomes bound to the silica gel, which now surrounds the residual core of each of the glass particles. This aluminum cross-linking is thought to take around 24 hours to come to completion, and during this period, not only will the hardness and strength increase, but the translucency and color of the cement may also change. This means that the color match is not always immediately apparent and the clinician must rely on shade guides to choose the color

Figure 2.3.7 The initial stages of the setting reaction in a GIC.

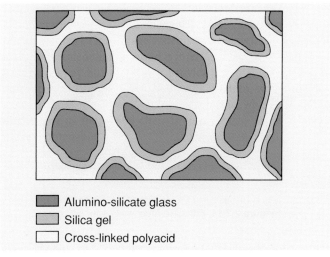

Figure 2.3.9 Hardening phase of the setting process.

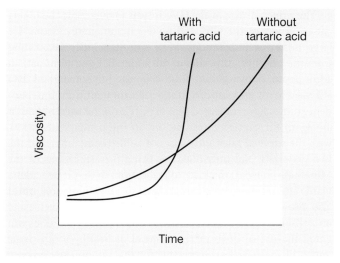

Figure 2.3.10 The effect of tartaric acid on the viscosity–time curve for a setting GIC.

and not be unduly alarmed if the restoration does not immediately appear to align with this.

The aluminum cross-linking is followed by other reactions that can continue for 4–6 weeks and contribute to further steady increases in strength, and although the mechanism of this is poorly understood, it is thought to result in the formation of a phosphate network pervading the structure. Once the cement has fully reacted, the solubility is comparatively low, but the cement is more vulnerable during its first weeks in service when the reactions are still ongoing, and most GICs benefit from protection with a compatible varnish or surface coating during this period.

From time to time, the question arises: If I coat the GIC with a varnish, will this prevent fluoride release? It is widely agreed that this is not a concern, however. For one thing, the varnish does not last very long on the surface of the GIC – probably only a few weeks, which is sufficient to protect the material during its maturation phase but is hardly a long-term fixture in the context of the lifetime of the restoration. For another, the varnish is only applied to the outer surface of the GIC, and not to those surfaces that directly contact the tooth – fluoride release direct to the dental hard tissues will not be impacted by any surface varnish.

The Role of Tartaric Acid in GIC Setting

The early GICs had reasonable properties once they were set, but the setting reaction proceeded inconveniently, in that it was slow and steady. This had a twofold negative impact. The fact that the setting started straight away on mixing meant that handling time was extremely limited. The fact that the setting didn't come to completion for a long time meant that the cement was excessively vulnerable for too long and asked too much of the patient in their home care. As a result, it was necessary to adjust the formula to first retard the setting reaction – giving a slightly longer working time – and then, after this short delay, cause it to proceed more rapidly – giving a faster progression to an acceptable degree of cross-linking and thus strength and robustness.

This was achieved by the inclusion of the optimum concentration of tartaric acid. The tartaric acid is believed to have a twofold function. First, it reacts rapidly with the calcium ions being released from the glass with the formation of calcium tartrate, which has the effect of extending the working time. This is followed by an enhancement of the rate of formation of aluminum polyacrylate cross-links, which speeds up the set (Figure 2.3.10). This is often referred to as a "snap set."

The Role of Water in GIC Setting

All of the above phases of the setting reaction require the presence of water, and water is a necessary component of the finished cement; it is this which allows ions to continue to migrate, to complete the setting reaction and also to allow the movement of fluoride, as is discussed below. Even a fully set cement contains a substantial amount of bound water.

CLINICAL SIGNIFICANCE

GICs are slow to set and need protection from the oral environment in the first few weeks of their clinical service in order to minimize dissolution or contamination.

High-Viscosity GICs

A relatively recent addition to the GIC portfolio is the high-viscosity GIC (HVGIC). These are GICs that, as the name would suggest, are more viscous than the norm; this can be achieved in a number of ways and the composition varies across different brands so is difficult to generalise. At its simplest, a higher viscosity may be achieved using a higher-than-usual powder-to-liquid ratio than with a regular GIC, but some products described as HVGIC also exhibit different particle sizes and variations in the polymer chemistry. As such, HVGIC is best thought of as a label indicating those GICs the manufacturer has intended for load bearing use and larger restorations rather than a scientifically distinct category of materials with a specified composition.

The principal aim of the HVGIC was to overcome the inherent weakness of the GIC and render it sufficiently strong for large posterior restorations while simultaneously benefitting from the adhesive properties of the material. Long-term data in adult populations will take time to amass, but some good data is available for restorations in the primary dentition. Independent studies have indicated that HVGICs *can* be used in lieu of amalgam for posterior restorations in the primary dentition, with the survival rates and causes of failure comparable for the two materials. Not only does this bring the aspirations of the Minamata convention closer to realization, in that it provides a viable alternative to amalgam, at least in this population, but it also provides other benefits, as HVGIC can be placed using an Atraumatic Restorative Therapy approach, which does not entail the use of drills or the removal of healthy tooth tissue and is likely to be less distressing for the children undergoing treatment. What data is available is also supportive of a similar approach in the permanent dentition, but of course, much longer timescales are required in order to reach the most useful conclusions.

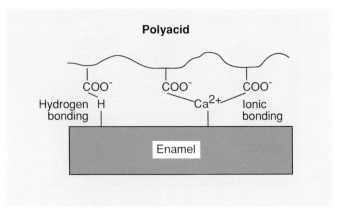

Figure 2.3.11 Adhesive mechanisms for GICs.

> ### CLINICAL SIGNIFICANCE
>
> While they are a comparably new material, the data available suggests that HVGICs may prove an appropriate substitute for amalgam in a number of clinical scenarios.

PROPERTIES

Adhesion to Tooth Tissues

One of the most attractive features of the GIC is that it is a tooth-colored, bulk placement restorative material (no need for incremental placement), which can form an adhesive bond directly to dentine and enamel without the need for a separate adhesive as in the case for composites.

As a GIC in its freshly mixed state is a hydrophilic material, it readily wets the tissue surface. Being acidic, it also causes some dissolution of the mineral, releasing ions that take part in the bonding and causing roughening of the surface, allowing for a degree of micromechanical bonding. On contact, hydrogen bonds are rapidly formed between the carboxyl groups of the polyacids and the bound water on the tissue surface. These are then gradually replaced by ionic bonds between the cement and tooth, which creates an ion-exchange layer at the interface, which is in effect part tissue and part material. The bonding, shown schematically in Figure 2.3.11, is understood to be to the mineral phase of the tissue, with the collagen in the dentine playing no part in the mechanism.

While a GIC is inherently adhesive, this does not necessarily mean that no preparation of the tooth surface is necessary. Usually, the surface is "conditioned" by the application of a solution of ~20% polyacrylic acid, which removes the smear layer from the dentine as well as any debris. The bond strength between a GIC and the tooth tissue is typically of the order of 2–10 MPa for enamel and 1–4 MPa for dentine. The bond reaches around 80% of its final strength within around 15 minutes and then continues steadily after this for several days, since, as with setting, some of

the reactions involved take a prolonged period to come to completion. Although these bond strengths are somewhat lower than those seen with some of the resin-based materials and their companion bonding systems, it is accepted to be sufficient, since the adhesive failure of GICs is very rarely observed; the material is more likely to fail cohesively than adhesively.

Aesthetics

A major requirement of any restorative material intended for use in anterior teeth is that it must blend in well with the surrounding tooth tissues. The factors governing this are the color and the translucency of the restorative material. In GICs the color is produced by the glass. This can be controlled by the addition of color pigments such as ferric oxide or carbon black, and a range of shades is available. Another aspect of the aesthetics of GICs is the observation that there is a color change during the setting process. Generally, the shade is somewhat darker after the material has fully set than at the time of placement. This darkening is believed to be associated with an increase in translucency on setting and may take up to 24 hours to develop. As such, it is important to rely on the shade guide to make the selection and to bear in mind that an apparent mismatch immediately after treatment may not be representative of the final appearance of the restoration.

Whereas color does not present a major problem, the lack of translucency of the GICs in comparison to the resin-based materials means that until recently their aesthetic appearance would certainly be considered inferior to that of composite resins. Although contemporary GICs are very much improved on the materials that were available before, and some even approach the composites in translucency (see, for instance, Figure 2.3.12), for many GICs, their opacity still limits their applications.

There are essentially two causes of the opacity of GICs:

- *Phase separation of the glass.* To some extent, this problem can be overcome by reducing the aluminum, calcium, and fluorine content of the glass, but this reduces the strength of the material and extends the working and setting times.
- *Mismatch of refractive index.* This problem can be minimized by reducing the aluminum content and increasing the fluorine content; however, the latter leads to phase separation. In general, optically good GICs tend to have poor setting characteristics.

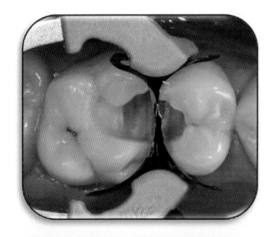

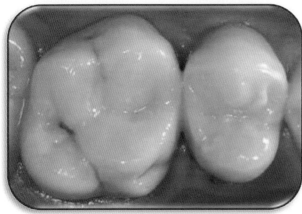

Figure 2.3.12 Two cavities restored with a modern GIC exhibiting an aesthetic match to tooth tissue that is much improved with relation to translucency compared with earlier versions of this class of material. Image courtesy of and copyright GC UK Ltd and Dr. Z Bilge Kütük, Turkey, with thanks.

The translucency of a restorative material can be described and measured by considering its inverse: *opacity*. Opacity is defined as being 0 for a transparent material and 1 for a white opaque material. For the best aesthetic results, restorative materials would be well matched in terms of translucency or opacity to the dental hard tissues. The early GICs were really quite opaque and as such, even though they were tooth-colored, their lack of translucency meant that they did not blend in well with the dentition. Modern GICs very widely in this regard; some manufacturers have invested in addressing this limitation and have produced GICs with much greater translucency, whereas others have focused, for instance, on improving strength or wear resistance and their materials are still quite opaque. As is often the case in biomaterials development, improving one property often leads to a deterioration on others. There are a small number of very recent GICs that appear to exhibit a compelling combination of mechanical properties and aesthetics, but by necessity, there is not yet a great deal of clinical data to allow clinicians to ascertain whether they stand the test of time and the rigors of the oral cavity.

It is worth noting that a very translucent material is not necessarily a good thing; in large sections these can appear darker than one would wish owing to the restricted light within the oral cavity. What this means for the clinician is that careful choice of a specific product is important, as even within the range of GICs available, there are some with much more favorable translucency than others. To add yet another complication into the mix, enamel is naturally somewhat fluorescent, and a small number of GICs have been engineered to also exhibit fluorescence as a further attempt to help them blend in the anterior zone.

Selecting the appropriate color and translucency of any restorative material is challenging, as these are affected by the optical properties of the underlying material. On some occasions, a relatively opaque material must be used in order to mask out a particularly dark substructure. In these cases the more opaque GICs can prove to be particularly beneficial.

While the initial match in color and translucency between the enamel and the GIC is important, it is also important that this close match is maintained in the challenging environment of the oral cavity. A loss of aesthetic quality of the restoration can arise from staining and, if excessive, could be considered a clinical failure and mandate replacement. Staining of the margins around GICs has been found to be less pronounced than for the composite resins. This may be a reflection of the excellent bond that can be achieved between a GIC and the tooth tissues. Another contributory factor may be that shrinkage on setting for GICs is less than that for composite resins. In effect, GICs set by an acid–base-mediated cross-linking reaction of the polyacid chains, which inherently produces less shrinkage than polymerization. Hence the local interfacial stresses generated will be less, and this may contribute to the lack of marginal staining.

Deterioration of GICs

The hydrophilic nature of the GIC and the fact that it can exchange ions with the oral environment offer several advantages, but it does also mean that GICs are somewhat soluble- more so than the resin-based restorative materials. Furthermore, GICs are susceptible to physical wear, and sometimes the dissolution and the wear combine to exacerbate the breakdown of the material.

Dissolution can be minimized and mitigated by an appreciation of the mechanisms involved and the adoption of proper clinical technique. The processes giving rise to loss of material are complex, as there are many variables involved, such as the cement composition, the clinical technique used, and the nature of the environment. The loss of material from a GIC can be classified into three main categories:
- dissolution of the immature cement
- long-term erosion
- abrasion.

Dissolution of the immature cement occurs before the material is fully set, which can take several weeks, although the dissolution rate drops after the first 24 hours. The temporary protection of a layer of protective varnish or unfilled or lightly filled resin is sufficient to minimize this. This protection must survive for at least 1 hour, as it takes this much time for the GIC to approach the properties that are achieved when it is fully set (and as such, something like petroleum jelly is inadequate for the task). Retaining the correct powder-to-liquid ratio is important in this regard. If this is not done, perhaps because the user adds more liquid to make the material easier to mix, this will exacerbate dissolution and also adversely affects the mechanical properties (see Figure 2.3.4).

Once the cement has fully set, this particular form of material loss will stop. From this point onward, loss of material can be considered long term and is a function of the conditions in the oral environment.

Loss of material in the long term may arise from acid attack or from mechanical abrasion. This is unfortunate, given that one major application of GICs is the restoration of lesions that have *themselves* arisen because of the combined effect of acid and abrasion. The potential for acid attack tends to be very marked in stagnation regions, such as around the gingival margin. Here, plaque accumulates and an acidic environment can persist due to the formation of plaque acids. GICs are also often used in areas where mechanical abrasion such as tooth brushing has caused wear to the enamel; many GICs display rather poor resistance to abrasion, which limits their application to low stress conditions and prevents their use as permanent posterior restorative materials.

Mechanical Properties

Some mechanical properties of GICs can be found in Table 2.3.1. It can be seen that for microhardness and flexural strength, there is an increase over the first 30 days post-mixing, reflecting the ongoing setting reaction during this period. GICs exhibit low diametral tensile strength in comparison to other restorative materials and thus should not be used where they are going to be subjected to high tensile loads, such as incisal tip restorations, cuspal replacement, or pin-retained cores, although HVGICs have improved mechanical properties than their predecessors. In situations where the restoration is supported all around by tooth tissue, the GIC is protected to some degree from tensile loading conditions.

The size of the glass powder particles ensures that a very high powder-to-liquid ratio can be achieved, and this is reflected in the compressive and diametral tensile strengths of these materials that are much higher than for the luting and lining cements described later. It also affects the solubility, which is reduced as the powder-to-liquid ratio is increased.

FLUORIDE RELEASE

If you were to ask a dental clinician to tell you one fact about GICs, many would respond along the lines of "GICs release fluoride." This is true: GICs *do* release fluoride. However, the interesting – and clinically important – matter is not *whether* they release fluoride. How much fluoride? When, and for how long? Under what circumstances? Does that fluoride do anything clinically useful? In this section we will consider those questions.

Mechanism and Characteristics of Fluoride Release

Fluoride salts, commonly calcium and sodium fluoride, are a component of the glass within GICs. These are solubilized by the protons released by the polyacids when they come into contact with water and the component ions are released, including the fluoride ion, F^-. Even once set, the GIC retains a significant proportion of water within its structure, and the fluoride ion can migrate by diffusion throughout the structure, moving out into the environment close to the cement and, under some circumstances, moving back in again *from* the oral environment into the cement.

The fluoride release is highest soon after the cement is placed; this is often termed a "burst" or "bolus" release and can last for up to 4 weeks. After this, the fluoride release continues but at a reduced rate, and for an extended period. It is worth noting that the profile, magnitude, and duration of fluoride release of GICs are derived from the behavior of specimens of the material immersed in water or aqueous solution under laboratory conditions. As such, it may bear some resemblance to the release of fluoride from a GIC into the oral cavity but *not* those processes that occur at the interface between the GIC and the tooth tissues, where the potential for delivering fluoride to areas at risk of secondary caries is much greater. In this location the fluid flow is very much lower than that in the wider oral cavity, and thus the fluoride will not be flushed away from the release site at anything like the same pace, and the fluoride concentration in these areas can reasonably be expected to last very much longer. It is also worth noting that, as a GIC is soluble in acid, the fluoride release is accelerated under acidic conditions. This may potentially be beneficial in that more fluoride release may occur under conditions that risk acid-mediated damage to the teeth.

It has long been claimed that GICs can absorb fluoride from the oral environment and then re-release it, and this has been demonstrated in laboratory experiments by exposing a GIC to a moderately concentrated solution of fluoride such as is found in an oral care product, and then removing the oral care product and observing a subsequent elevated fluoride release from the same GIC. Although this has been demonstrated by many researchers, the situation has become a little unclear with reports that this is only valid for *recently placed* GICs, and other studies have illustrated that GICs which have undergone maturation have reduced or even no ability to take up fluoride. The full picture is still unclear but in some senses this is of limited concern. The fluid flow at the interface between the GIC and the enamel and dentine is extremely low; one can expect high fluoride conditions to persist there for a lengthy period. In relation to the GIC surface exposed in the mouth, since the high fluoride concentrations that may or may not result in GICs absorbing fluoride will themselves provide fluoride to the surrounding tooth tissues, the outcome is elevated fluoride at the tooth surface, and whether this comes direct from the oral care product or the GIC is perhaps secondary.

Clinical Implications of Fluoride Release

The question that is of greater clinical importance is whether the fluoride releasing properties of the material are of any *clinical benefit*. It is well established that fluoride in drinking water and oral care products has a substantial positive effect on dental public health, reducing the incidence and severity of caries. The data on the benefits or otherwise of fluoride-releasing restorative materials is surprisingly muddy even several decades after their introduction.

Pit and fissure sealants have been found to significantly reduce occlusal caries in children and adolescents, but this is true whether or not they contain fluoride; the resin-based, fluoride-free fissure sealants also provide protection. That is not to say that the GIC fissure sealants aren't effective – they are – but it is not clear whether the fluoride release plays any role in this, or whether it is simply the physical covering and sealing of the occlusal surface and the exclusion of plaque and sugars from the deep fissures that provides the protection.

GICs are among those materials that can be used to bond orthodontic brackets to teeth and, since orthodontic brackets promote the accumulation of plaque and obstruct oral hygiene, it is reasonable to ask whether the fluoride release might provide any protection against the development of carious lesions in the vicinity of the brackets. Unfortunately, despite many studies, there is still no clear evidence to indicate whether this is the case. The greater ease of debonding GIC than many resin-based materials is often thought to be advantageous, in that there is less likelihood of iatrogenic damage to the teeth, but it cannot at the current time be concluded that fluoride release from GICs provides definitive protection against caries associated with orthodontic appliances.

Perhaps most surprising of all is the paucity of conclusive data in relation to the use of GICs for fillings. While there are some clinical studies that compare GICs with other materials – most commonly amalgam – many suffer from bias and other limitations, and in any case, it is not always the case that a GIC and amalgam have the same indications, and it is not good science to compare large multi-surface amalgam restoration with a small single-surface GIC restoration and then conclude that any differences are due solely to the material. When the bias and other limitations inherent in most studies are taken into account, current thinking indicates *only* that there is *weak* evidence that GIC provides better caries protection than amalgam under a handful of very specific circumstances. There are more clinical studies that show no difference in the incidence of secondary caries between the two. Given the many decades of their use and the many studies that have been carried out, it is disappointing that the data are largely unsupportive of any material protective effect.

CLINICAL SIGNIFICANCE

GIC is an intrinsically adhesive, bulk-filling material. Although it releases fluoride into the local environment once set, even after almost five decades of use, there is still little good-quality evidence of a clinical benefit of this fluoride release under most circumstances.

HANDLING

It must be appreciated that the GICs are designed to suit a wide variety of applications, their range encompassing materials with widely different properties. The tooth-colored filling materials are the focus of this chapter.

As the core subject matter of this textbook is dental materials and not clinical protocols, only broad scientific guidance is given here, and the clinician must consult appropriate sources for the specific directions for use for each material, as well as contemporary and region-specific guidance in clinical standard operating procedures.

Cavity Preparation

The adhesive quality of the GICs dictates that an ultra-conservative approach can be adopted. This means that minimal removal of tooth substance is required, and the excessive removal of tooth tissues for the provision of undercuts is not necessary. For situations where the restoration may be subjected to high stresses, it has to be stated that some undercut may be advantageous, although one should question whether the GIC is the right material to use in the case of high-stress scenarios. In the case of a replacement restoration, the original restoration should be carefully removed without removing any tooth tissues unless they are carious.

Isolation

Although the GICs are hydrophilic materials, it is nevertheless recommended that careful isolation of the field of operation is carried out. The presence of blood or saliva will not only impair the formation of a strong bond but may also lead to contamination of the restoration, thereby reducing both bond strength and aesthetics. A well-placed GIC should not fail adhesively, as the bond to dentine and enamel is at least as strong as the cohesive strength of the cement.

Preparation of the Dentinal Surfaces

The nature of the dentine surface varies from site to site, with the major distinction being between cut dentine after caries removal and sclerotic dentine.

Abrasion/Erosion Lesions

Lesions at the cervical margin need to be restored to provide direct protection of the pulp, to prevent the development of pulpal sensitivity, and to improve appearance. Since the GICs are adhesive, preparation prior to placement of the material focuses only on the cleaning and conditioning of the dentine surface. The cleaning procedure is aimed at removing any surface contaminants, such as plaque or pellicle, which obscure the dentine surface. The surface should be thoroughly washed to remove any debris. A conditioner consisting of an aqueous solution of polyacrylic acid may then be applied, which will ensure that the surface is clean, and will also result in some opening of the dentinal tubules. There is still some controversy as to the need for the prior application of polyacrylic acid to the dentine surface. Some argue that exposure of the dentinal tubules is contraindicated, as it increases the dentine permeability and thus raises the likelihood of a pulpal reaction, and that for those patients with sensitivity, acid treatment of the dentine surface should not be undertaken. Some studies have shown that this will improve the dentine bond strength, whereas others have shown that it has no effect.

Class III, Class V, and Other Carious Lesions

It is not necessary to clean the surface to the same extent when it consists of freshly exposed dentine. However, there is still the dentine smear layer to consider, which is created during any cavity preparation. While the smear layer is strongly bonded to the underlying dentine, surface debris needs to be removed in such a way as to avoid the opening of the dentinal tubules. Again, the use of polyacrylic acid is recommended.

Finishing and Surface Protection

Earlier iterations of glass ionomers had exacting finishing requirements and often necessitated a two-step process whereby the restoration was finished a day or more after it was first placed. Modern materials have done away with this requirement, and the majority can be placed and finished in a single session.

The use of a protective surface coating remains important, however, owing to the vulnerability of the GIC over the first few weeks of clinical service. The most commonly used products are proprietary varnishes or unfilled or lightly filled resin products, either of which serves the purpose – often these are similar to or the same as the light-cured dentine-bonding agents that are used with composites that provide an effective seal and last sufficiently long to offer the necessary protection. These suffer from an oxygen-inhibited set so that the surface layer remains tacky, but this can be easily removed. Coatings of petroleum jelly such as Vaseline® are to be avoided, as these rub off very rapidly owing to the action of the lips and tongue. There are materials on the market that claim not to need any surface coating, although many clinicians opt to take the precaution of applying one nonetheless; better one further minor step than risk the integrity of the restoration.

Some authors have expressed concern that the varnish or resin impedes the release of fluoride, but this is missing the point for three reasons. First, the varnish or resin will itself wear off over time, allowing fluoride release to occur. Second, if the GIC is disadvantaged by lack of protection during its maturation phase, the whole restoration may be compromised and need repair or replacement, in which case fluoride release pales into insignificance. Third, the varnish or resin is only applied to the *outer* surface of the GIC, and the GIC in direct contact with the tooth tissue will still be able to release fluoride where it really matters.

A few products claim that they do not need a coating, although the mechanism that underpins these claims is unclear and only time will tell whether they suffer as a result of failure to coat.

RESIN-MODIFIED GLASS IONOMER CEMENTS

GICs have many favorable properties, but they do have some important limitations. Their limited working time can be an inconvenience, and they suffer from relatively low tensile strength and toughness. They have to be protected from desiccation during their early weeks, and even after this time they are susceptible to acid-mediated dissolution and abrasion.

These limitations, coupled with the observation that resin-based materials perform better in these regards, gave rise to the resin-modified GIC (RMGIC). Like composites, these materials have a "command cure" and will set by polymerization of the resin component when exposed to light of an appropriate wavelength (almost always blue, 470 nm). Although sometimes also referred to as hybrid GICs or light-curing/light-cured GICs, such terms should be discouraged as they are insufficiently specific and can be confused with some other materials such as compomers or GICs with a variable particle size, which also use the term "hybrid".

Composition and Presentation

While this material can, like a conventional GIC, be presented as either a hand-mixed or encapsulated version, the latter is by far the more common for restorative materials. Some hand-mixed versions are still used, especially for luting and lining cements; in those cases the powder consists of a radiopaque fluoro-alumino-silicate glass and is supplied as with a conventional GIC; the liquid is photoactive and therefore kept in a dark glass or opaque bottle to protect it from ambient light. More popular for restorative applications are the encapsulated products, which, like a conventional GIC, contain the components separated into two compartments that come together when the capsule is activated and then mixed using an amalgamator or similar device.

The filler particles in the RMGIC are chemically the same or very similar to those in a conventional GIC. There are some products available in which the size has been adjusted – the filler consists of nanoclusters and individual nano-particles rather than the conventional micro-particles, although it is unclear whether this has any material impact on the performance of the material compared to other RMGICs on the market. Although some clinical studies have indicated that nano-filled RMGICs may show less occlusal wear – perhaps because the particles are less likely to become dislodged from the surface, or when they do, they are much smaller – other clinical studies have found the converse! This may of course relate to study design or be a reflection of minor or subtle differences between the nano- and micro-particle RMGICs.

As well as the components of a regular GIC, an RMGIC contains a resin and photoactivator system, which is what gives the material its command cure property. The polyacids may be modified, for instance, with the addition of pendant methacryloxy groups to make them better compatible with the resin. The choice of resin is dictated by the fact that GICs are water-based materials and so the resin needs to be water-soluble, both to permit the regular GIC setting reaction to proceed alongside the polymerization reaction and to permit the later transit of fluoride within and in and out of the material. The caveats given above about the clinical benefits of such fluoride release notwithstanding, fluoride release is a powerful marketing tool and an RMGIC that didn't release fluoride would be unlikely to find commercial success.

Many RMGICs contain hydroxyethyl methacrylate (HEMA) as the resin, sometimes in combination with another resin such as the UDMA which should be familiar to the reader owing to its use in composites. HEMA is a methacrylate resin like many of the resins used in dental materials but stands apart from those used in composites in that it is water-soluble. This is key to creating a resin-containing GIC without compromising the other convenient properties of a GIC such as adhesion, comparative moisture tolerance, and fluoride release.

HEMA has had some bad press in recent years, owing to concerns about the migration of the HEMA monomer out of the material and into the oral environment, and the effects it might have there. These concerns seem to be largely based on a few laboratory and small mammal studies where it has been shown (1) that HEMA monomers diffuse out of RMGICs and (2) HEMA monomers, at sufficient concentration, can cause cytotoxic effects. What has *not* been demonstrated is that RMGICs containing HEMA cause clinically adverse outcomes. It is not surprising that a material releases some of its components into the oral environment – no material is fully, truly inert in that sense. The finite release of components can be demonstrated from virtually any dental material. It is also not surprising that a particular chemical can be shown to cause adverse effects on cells in a laboratory experiment *at sufficient concentrations*. Indeed, it would be hard to find a chemical entity that didn't: table salt, sugar, and the dentist's friend sodium fluoride are all cytotoxic if enough is applied to the cells. HEMA monomers can indeed cause damage to cells, as can UDMA and TEGDMA, resins found in composites, but that is very different from demonstrating that the HEMA released from RMGIC can cause damage *in vivo*.

Doubtless, more information about the safety of HEMA-based RMGICs will become available over time, but at the time of writing, it would appear that HEMA has been the victim of misinterpretation of laboratory studies rather than any robust evidence of health risk. This is unfortunately something of a recurring theme in dental materials, and any clinician needs to fully understand the scientific basis for any such claims and be able to interpret further scientific data as it becomes available, such that they can make evidence-based choices and can properly and appropriately explain the options and evidence to their patients.

Setting Reaction

The acid–base setting reaction is essentially the same as for the GICs and is initiated when the powder and liquid are mixed. The material differs from other GICs in that this reaction is much slower, giving a considerably longer working time.

The rapid set is provided by the light activation mechanism, causing polymerization of the resin and, for the copolymer-containing materials, additional cross-linking through the pendant methacrylate groups, as shown in Figure 2.3.13. Once mixed, the material can be made to set after just 30 seconds of exposure to light. It should be appreciated that the light-activated curing reaction precedes the formation of the aluminum salt bridges. Hence these materials will continue to set via the acid–base reaction for some time after the polymerization process has been completed.

Some systems also contain a redox reaction curing process, providing an activator and an initiator, in one case using micro-encapsulation technology. This has the advantage that, if the light from the curing unit is not able to penetrate to the full depth of the restoration, the redox reaction will ensure full depth of cure of the resin component. This means that incremental

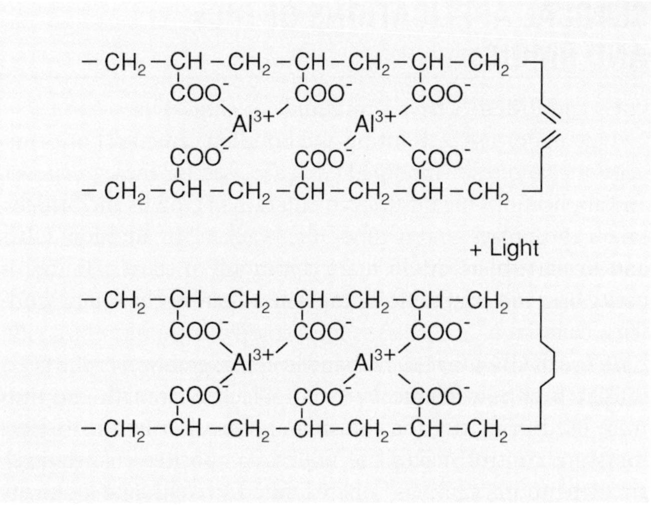

Figure 2.3.13 Combined light-activated cross-linking and hardening during the setting process for a resin-modified GIC.

placement of the RMGIC is not necessary for the redox-reaction-containing systems. One disadvantage with this system is that it cannot be provided in encapsulated form, as the shear stresses during capsule mixing, as distinct from hand mixing, are insufficient to break the glass microspheres.

Properties

The addition of resin chemistry to the GICs has significantly improved many of the properties. Using this approach, the properties of conventional GICs, such as the ability to bond to dentine and enamel and to release fluoride, are combined with a prolonged working time and a rapid set, once irradiated with visible light. The strength and resistance to desiccation and acid attack are significantly improved, and although the hardness is usually found to be somewhat lower than regular GICs, this does not seem to lead to more wear, perhaps because of the resin component. The bond to enamel and dentine is as good as, if not superior to, that of the GICs, since the resin component imparts additional tensile strength to the set cement. Like the GIC, RMGIC requires an application of a polyacrylic acid etchant prior to application. Data summarizing the differences in properties between some hand-mixed and encapsulated GICs and RMGIC are shown in Table 2.3.1.

As mentioned above, there have been concerns voiced about the biocompatibility of HEMA in relation to the leaching of uncured monomer from the finished material. While it has not been established that the amount of HEMA monomer that is released from an RMGIC, or indeed the amount of *any* monomer leaching from *any* resin-containing material, is enough to be problematic, for this and other reasons, it is important that the necessary procedures are followed to ensure that the degree of conversion is maximized and the residual monomer is as low as possible.

As a note of caution, it is important to remember that one may also inherit some of the problems associated with light-cured composites, such as limited depth of cure, which requires incremental packing, and polymerization shrinkage, which may compromise the bond to the tooth.

CLINICAL APPLICATIONS OF GICs AND RMGICs

GICs and RMGICs have a multitude of clinical uses.

One major use is as luting and bonding cements; both conventional and resin-modified GICs are used for these purposes, and applications include for cementation of crowns and bridges, inlays and onlays, and orthodontic brackets. In addition, GICs and in particular RMGICs are commonly used as a lining or cavity base material under composite as part of the "open sandwich technique."

A use of GICs that has expanded considerably over the years is as restorative cements. Early GICs lacked strength and thus were used primarily for abrasion and erosion lesions (where moisture control makes the use of composites challenging), small, temporary fillings (where limited strength and longevity were of little concern), and in the deciduous dentition (where longevity requirements are limited owing to the natural exfoliation of the teeth), and indeed these uses are still common. However, the development of HVGICs has expanded their use into larger, multi-surface load-bearing restorations in the posterior region, and the developments in aesthetics across the range but particularly in HVGICs and RMGICs have seen them move more and more into the anterior region as their ability to blend in with the natural dentition has improved. While their aesthetic appearance is rarely equal to the composites, their ease of placement in bulk, their adhesive qualities, and their fluoride release properties are seen as important advantages. As such, the range of restorative applications is now very broad.

Yet another application of GICs and RMGICs is as fissure sealants. Fissure sealants are materials applied to the occlusal surfaces of molars for the purpose of blocking out fissures and are often used where oral hygiene has proven challenging and the tooth is at risk of decay owing to the accumulation of plaque and food debris in these fissures. In some parts of the world their use is restricted largely to children and young people, although other regions are perhaps more progressive and recognize that adults can be every bit as susceptible to deficiencies in their oral hygiene regime! Dental clinicians in these countries often deploy fissure sealants as a caries-preventive measure for a much wider segment of their populations.

Fissure sealants composed of composite are also available and for a long time it was felt that the retention of composite fissure sealants was superior to the retention of glass ionomer fissure sealants. Evidence has now developed to reveal two further considerations: first, that while some GIC fissure sealants may appear to be retained for less time than composite ones, the protection they provide is at least comparable, and second, the use of HVGICs as fissure sealants appears to bring the retention times in line with those of composites. The added benefit of a GIC-based fissure sealant is that removal of all moisture from within the fissures is less important as the GIC can still adhere and provide protection in the presence of this moisture, whereas the adhesion of a composite would likely be compromised in this area.

A section on the clinical application of GICs would not be complete without mention of Atraumatic Restorative Treatment (sometimes expressed as Atraumatic Restorative Therapy), ART. This is an approach to restorative dentistry that is conducted without powered instruments, using only hand instruments. Strictly speaking, ART in its purest form does not require *any* electrical equipment and thus RMGICs – which require light curing – are excluded. ART was developed for the purpose of improving dental care in low-income countries and particularly in rural settings where electricity supply might be intermittent or nonexistent – a traveling dental clinician can manually excavate carious tissue and provide GIC restorations without the need for a drill, light curing unit, or other electrical gadgets. In the modern day, ART has also found excellent use in the treatment of anxious patients, including children and people with special educational needs, as well as that substantial proportion of the general population who exhibit dental anxiety. Doing away with the need for "the dentist's drill" and the time and hassle of stringent moisture control makes the process of restoring a tooth less distressing for these patients and can improve compliance and attendance.

SUMMARY

GICs have had a major impact on restorative dentistry. A wide variety of formulations are available, designed for a broad range of applications. They are important tools for all clinicians and are particularly popular for those situations where composites would be difficult to apply, including pediatric, geriatric, and special needs dentistry. The RMGICs offer some improvements over conventional GICs but also limitations of their own. HVGICs can increasingly provide a suitable alternative to amalgams.

FURTHER READING

Al-Taee, L., Deb, S., Banerjee, A., 2020. An in vitro assessment of the physical properties of manually-mixed and encapsulated glass-ionomer cements. BDJ Open 6, 12.

Croll, T.P., Berg, J.H., 2015. Glass ionomer restorative cement systems: an update. Pediatric Dentistry 37 (2), 116–124.

Cury, J.A., de Oliveira, B.H., dos Santos, A.P., Tenuta, L.M., 2016. Are fluoride releasing dental materials clinically effective on caries control? Dental Materials 32 (3), 323–333.

Frankenberger, R., Garcia-Godoy, F., Krämer, N., 2009. Clinical Performance of viscous glass ionomer cement in posterior cavities over two years. International Journal of Dental 2009, 781462.

Fricker, J.P., 2022. Therapeutic properties of glass-ionomer cements: their application to orthodontic treatment. Australian Dental Journal 67 (1), 12–20.

Hilgert, L.A., de Amorim, R.G., Leal, S.C., Mulder, J., Creugers, N.H., Frencken, J.E., 2014. Is high-viscosity glass-ionomer-cement a successor to amalgam for treating primary molars? Dental Materials 30 (10) 1172–1178.

Menezes-Silva, R., Oliveira, B.M.B., MagalhÃes, A.P.R., Bueno, L.S., Borges, A.F.S., Baesso, M.L., et al., 2020. Correlation between mechanical properties and stabilization time of chemical bonds in glass-ionomer cements. Brazilian Oral Research 34, e053.

Nicholson, J.W., Sidhu, S.K., Czarnecka, B., 2020. Enhancing the mechanical properties of glass-ionomer dental cements: a review. Materials (Basel) 13 (11), 2510.

Nicholson, J.W., 2018. Maturation processes in glass-ionomer dental cements. Acta Biomaterialia Odontologica Scandinavica 4 (1), 63–71.

Sidhu, S.K., Nicholson, J.W., 2016. A review of glass-ionomer cements for clinical dentistry. Journal of Functional Biomaterials 7 (3), 16.

Sidhu, S.K., 2011. Glass-ionomer cement restorative materials: a sticky subject? Australian Dental Journal 56 (Suppl. 1), 23–30.

Wilson, A.D., Kent, B.E., 1972. A new translucent cement for dentistry. British Dental Journal 132, 133–135.

Cavity Lining and Base Materials

INTRODUCTION

A wide variety of direct restorative materials are placed in dentine in close proximity to the pulp. Sometimes, it is necessary to place another material between the dentine and the main material, to create a layer to separate the two. It used to be the case that cavity liners or bases were placed under most dental restorative materials, but over the last decade or two, this practice has fallen under ever-increasing scrutiny, and there have been many challenges to the accepted norms of when to place a lining or base. Furthermore, the principles and practice of minimally invasive dentistry have led to far fewer large and deep cavities, with clinicians willing to leave behind more tissue than they might have done in years gone by, further reducing the frequency with which one would consider using a lining or base.

Many clinicians still consider that linings and bases are beneficial in particular circumstances and place them as a matter of course. After all, past experience is an important part of clinical judgment, and if they have gained good results for many years from placing linings and bases, why would they change their approach? For these clinicians, it would require very robust evidence to change an established habit that has yielded good clinical outcomes. Some clinicians are unsure whether linings and bases are really necessary but adopt a precautionary principle: 'it won't do any harm, so I'll place one just in case'. Still other clinicians interpret the data to mean that linings are *never*, or nearly never, mandated.

This is a live debate, and a detailed analysis of the evidence base falls beyond the scope of this undergraduate textbook. A number of recent systematic reviews and consensus statements suggest that there is weak, or sparse, evidence in favor of placing linings in many instances, but this is not the same as definitive evidence that it is better *not* to place these. What we will seek to do is discuss those materials that are used as linings bases, referring to the research literature where there is consensus or strong evidence, but with the primary focus on the materials science that is but one feature of the success and the properties of a lining or base.

Many of the materials used for linings and bases have been encountered elsewhere in this book, as they are used for other applications too, and where this is the case, we cover them in brief and refer the reader to the more extensive discussion in other chapters. We will give examples of their use as liners and bases in conjunction with other materials, but these are not exhaustive or intended as definitive guidance, as accepted practices change over time as the evidence base develops. For up-to-date guidance on which materials and tooth preparations require a base or a liner, the student should refer to current clinical guidelines for their country or region of practice.

While there is ongoing debate about the need for pulpal *protection* by linings and bases, these materials can serve other purposes as well. Materials might have a palliative or therapeutic effect on the dentine, and they might mitigate shortcomings of the main material such as setting shrinkage.

In earlier editions of this book this chapter was entitled "Intermediate Restorative Materials," but over the years the term *intermediate* has been used more and more to refer to *temporary* restorative materials, so to avoid confusion, in this edition we refer to them according to their use: cavity liners and bases.

DEFINITIONS AND PURPOSES OF CAVITY LININGS AND BASES

A *cavity liner* is a thin layer of a material, typically less than 0.5 mm thick, which covers the exposed dentine. A *cavity base*, on the other hand, is a thicker layer or bulk of material. The purpose depends on the restorative material it is to be used in conjunction with.

The purpose of a cavity liner or base is often casually described as 'to protect the pulp'. The question then becomes: protect the pulp *from what*? What is it that might injure, irritate, or otherwise trouble the pulp that the liner or base might provide protection from? Three possible sources of pulpal irritation can be identified:

- thermal stimuli
- chemical stimuli
- biological stimuli

Thermal Stimuli

In the intact tooth temperature changes are poorly conducted through the enamel and dentine to the pulp. The pulp contains nociceptive afferent fibers that, if thermally stimulated, elicit a pain response. Such a direct thermal stimulus of the pulp is, however, unlikely except when cutting a cavity or direct heat is generated due to an exothermic reaction on the part of the restorative material when in close proximity to the pulp. When dentinal tubules are exposed, it is possible for fluid to flow into and out of the tubules, commonly referred to as the hydrodynamic effect. This is the process responsible for exposed root surface sensitivity and is readily dealt with by sealing the root surface. The hydrodynamic effect is almost certainly also responsible for the short-latency pain produced by thermal stimulation of some minimal-amalgam restorations. If the dentinal tubules are patent and a small gap has been allowed to form under the amalgam restoration, possibly due to inadequate adaptation to the cavity wall, fluid movement down the tubules can occur because of the opening and closing action of this gap. This can happen as a consequence of the amalgam expanding or contracting when exposed to extremes of temperature or the application of an occlusal load. Thus the placement of a cavity varnish or thin lining in a cavity is done in an attempt to protect against fluid movement through the dentine. It was thought at one time that it was necessary to place a thermal insulator to protect the pulp from thermal energy transmitted from the oral cavity – hot foods and drinks – through the amalgam and onto the pulp, but this concern has largely now been dismissed given the limited temperature and duration that would be experienced under normal conditions.

Chemical Stimuli

Many of the dental materials that come into contact with dentine may release compounds that may irritate or harm the pulp because of either their organic structure or their pH.

Acrylic resins are sometimes cited as examples of materials that will cause a pulpal reaction when placed without a lining, but toxicity tests suggest that these materials are well tolerated by the soft tissues. Acrylic resins are extensively used as bone cements in hip replacements without adverse inflammatory reaction. This would suggest that other factors are responsible for the pulpal reaction associated with these materials.

In the past, many studies of the pulpal toxicity of restorative materials did not consider the influence of bacterial contamination, but it is now believed that this plays a major role in pulpal inflammation, as considered below. This does not mean that we need not worry about chemical toxicity, as the low pH of some materials, such as zinc–phosphate cements and zinc–polycarboxylate cements, may still have an effect on the pulp.

Biological Stimuli

A matter of considerable interest is the effect of *micro-leakage*. This term loosely describes the penetration of oral fluids and small numbers of bacteria and their toxic by-products between the filling material and the cavity walls. This percolation has been shown to be a potential source of pulpal irritation.

In experiments that use germ-free animals it has been shown that the pulpal response to some materials is considerably different from that seen in animals with a normal microbiological flora, suggesting that the bacteria play a role in the interaction between pulp and materials. For example, zinc–phosphate cements do not show pulpal inflammation (and may even show some dentine bridge formation) when placed on exposed pulps in the absence of bacteria. In contrast, control animals showed severe pulpal inflammation and abscess formation. Other materials do show an inflammatory response, even in the germ-free animals, demonstrating that chemical toxicity may still be an important factor in some instances.

Thus it is important that in circumstances when bacteria might reach the pulp, we provide a material that eliminates the potential for bacterial micro-leakage by the use of adhesive techniques so that no gap exists between the restorative material and the tooth and presents an antibacterial barrier to the infiltrating bacteria.

CLINICAL SIGNIFICANCE

The primary role of a lining material is to protect the pulp by providing an antibacterial barrier and preventing fluid movement within the dentinal tubules.

MATERIALS USED FOR CAVITY BASES AND LINERS

The main groups of materials that fall into the category of cavity bases and liners are:

- calcium hydroxide cements
- zinc oxide-based cements
- glass ionomer cements
- resin-modified glass ionomer cements
- visible-light-cured resins.

Calcium Hydroxide Cements
Presentation and Constituents

This material is supplied as two white or light yellow pastes. One paste consists of a mixture of calcium hydroxide (50%), zinc oxide (10%), and sulfonamide (40%). The other paste consists of butylene glycol disalicylate (40%) with varying amounts of titanium dioxide and calcium sulfate. Equal volumes of the two pastes are mixed together for about 30 seconds; the cement will then set in approximately 2 minutes. The setting process is believed to involve a chelating reaction between the zinc oxide and butylene glycol disalicylate. Alternatively it may be supplied premixed, and resin-modified versions also exist.

Properties

Calcium hydroxide cement lining materials typically have a low compressive strength of around 20 MPa, but this is sufficient to withstand the condensation pressures of dental amalgam filling materials when used as a liner, but is not suitable for use as a base.

The freshly mixed cement is highly alkaline, with a pH of 11–12. It is believed that this is responsible for an important feature of calcium hydroxide cements: their ability to cause the pulp of the tooth to lay down reparative dentine. When the paste is placed in contact with the pulp, possibly in the presence of a microscale exposures, it will cause a three-layer necrosis of some 1.5 mm thickness. This eventually develops into a calcified layer.

Once the bridge becomes dentine-like in appearance and the pulp has been isolated from any irritant, hard tissue formation ceases.

Zinc Oxide-Eugenol Cements

A number of zinc oxide-based cements are used in dentistry, and these are powder–liquid systems, with the powders being bases and the liquids being acids. When they are mixed, there is an acid–base reaction with the general formula:

$$\underset{\text{base}}{MO} + \underset{\text{acid}}{H_2O} \rightarrow \underset{\text{salt}}{MA} + \underset{\text{water}}{H_2O}$$

In these dental cements there is a surplus of powder, such that the final material consists of unreacted powder particles held together by a salt matrix.

Zinc oxide-eugenol is one example of a zinc oxide-based cement that can be used as either a cavity liner or a base material, although in the latter application RMGIC seems to be becoming more popular. Zinc oxide-eugenol cements have been used in dentistry for over 150 years, and although they have been superseded by modern materials in many applications, they still have several applications in contemporary dentistry; accordingly, there are a wide variety of different formulations for different applications. We shall discuss these in turn.

Unmodified zinc oxide–eugenol. This is supplied as a white powder, which is mainly zinc oxide, but contains up to 10% magnesium oxide that is mixed with a clear liquid, which is eugenol mixed with either olive oil or cottonseed oil. The oils are added to mask the taste of the eugenol and modify the viscosity.

The cement is mixed by adding the powder to the liquid in small increments until a thick consistency is obtained with a powder-to-liquid ratio of about 3:1. The zinc oxide initially absorbs some eugenol, which is confined to the surface layer of the powder particles and reacts to form an amorphous zinc eugenolate, as shown in Figure 2.4.1. This binds the unreacted portion of the powder together. A trace of water is needed to initiate the reaction, but once started, it is a by-product of the setting reaction. The set material contains both unreacted zinc oxide and eugenol.

The material is available as a slow-setting or a fast-setting cement. The slow-setting cement takes some 24 hours to set hard, with the fast-setting cement taking as little as 5 minutes, although this depends on the nature of the powder, its particle size, and the addition of accelerators such as zinc acetate or acetic acid.

The set cement has a pH of 6.6–8.0 and releases eugenol, which has an obtundent effect on the pulp, and reduces pain that may be associated with the antibacterial properties of the cement. One of the main failings of zinc oxide–eugenol cements is their high solubility in the oral environment. As the eugenol is continually released, the cement gradually disintegrates. It also has poor mechanical properties, with a compressive strength of only 15 MPa. This, combined with the high solubility, makes it unsuitable as a cavity base or liner material.

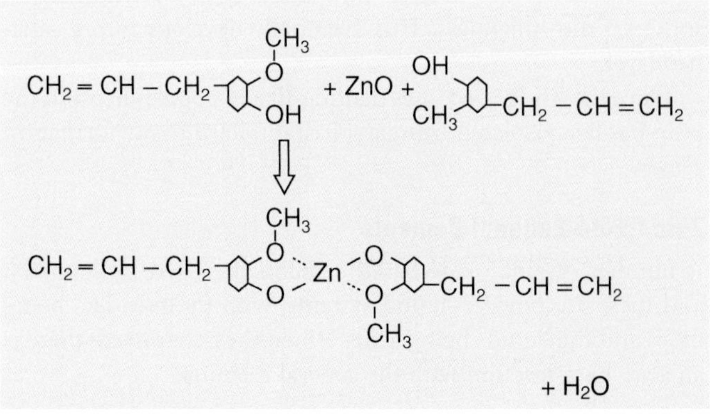

The slow-setting version is most commonly used as a root canal sealing material, with its various modifications being discussed in more detail in Chapter 2.6. The fast-setting version is mainly used in periodontal dressings. The eugenol is also known to inhibit the set of resins, so eugenol-containing cements cannot be used in conjunction with resin-based restorative materials.

Modified zinc oxide–eugenol. Modified versions of zinc oxide-eugenol were developed to overcome some of the shortcomings of the original version. The principal aims were to raise the compressive strength and reduce the solubility. These modifications take the form of resins added to the powder and/ or the liquid, such as:

- hydrogenated rosin 10%, which is added to the powder
- polystyrene or methyl methacrylate, which is dissolved in the liquid.

The added resin raises the compressive strength substantially (around 40 MPa). This is sufficiently high for the material to be used as a cavity base or liner. The material can also be used as a temporary filling material, since it is less soluble in the oral cavity than the unmodified cements.

EBA cement. EBA cement is another modified zinc oxide–eugenol cement, presented as a white powder and a pinkish-colored liquid. The powder consists of zinc oxide (60–75%), fused quartz or alumina (20–35%), and hydrogenated rosin (6%). The liquid is 37% eugenol and 63% ethoxybenzoic acid (EBA). The EBA encourages the formation of a crystalline structure, which imparts a further improvement in the compressive strength (60 MPa) and a reduction in the solubility. This makes EBA cements suitable for use as liners and bases as well as temporary filling materials.

Glass Ionomer and Resin-Modified Glass Ionomer Lining Cements

While there was a time when calcium hydroxide and variations of zinc oxide-eugenol cement dominated the base and lining market, GICs and, in particular, RMGICs have gained widespread acceptance and, for many clinicians, are now the preferred option.

A wide selection of glass ionomer lining cements are available, and these are broadly similar to the restorative GICs that were discussed in detail in Chapter 2.3. These materials are all radiopaque, which is useful when used at the base of a cavity. GIC can be used under amalgam and composite, and is able to bond to the dentine. When used under a composite restoration, the composite can be bonded to both the GIC and the etched enamel.

It is important to know what quality of bond between the GICs and the composites can be achieved. The research literature would suggest that it is advisable to etch the GIC prior to applying the composite to aid retention and bonding, but not to excess. The best method of etching is to employ a viscous etchant gel in a syringe. This would usually be applied carefully to the enamel surfaces for a period of 20 seconds; thereafter, the whole surface (including the GIC) is exposed to the etchant for

Figure 2.4.1 Chelating reaction of zinc oxide with eugenol to form a zinc eugenolate

an additional 20 seconds. Excessive exposure of the GIC to etchant will cause crazing of the surface and acid penetration that is impossible to remove on washing; this may develop into pulpal pain or sensitivity. It can also cause extensive fractures and is best avoided. It is preferable to use a low-viscosity resin in order to obtain a good bond between the composite and the GIC.

The practical problems generated by the need for differential etching can be avoided completely by using RMGIC liners, which do not require etching in order to achieve a bond to the composite resin. These liners have the added advantage that they provide a stronger adhesive between the tooth and the composite resin due to their greater cohesive strength compared to the GICs. The RMGIC has become so popular that it is now far more commonly used for this purpose than the conventional GIC.

Visible-Light-Cured Resins

A variety of miscellaneous 'resin-based' cavity bases and liners are also available on the market, although their compositions and specific roles seem somewhat obscure. The objective with some of these materials seems to be to combine the advantages of light activation with some of the therapeutic effects of calcium or fluoride release, although evidence in support of the latter having any beneficial effect for specific products is scant at best. As time passes, these materials are becoming scarcer, replaced largely by the RMGICs.

CHOICE OF CAVITY AND BASE MATERIALS

The choice of which material to use in which situation has changed over the years as new, or clearer, evidence has emerged. Nowadays, the first question is often not *which* material to use, but whether to use a lining or base at all! Different customs are adopted in different regions and according to whether the dentistry is supported by the state, in which case health economics necessarily plays a strong role, or is privately funded by the individual or an insurance company, in which additional factors play a role. Where the student wishes – and has the authority – to make their own decision about whether and when to line, they are advised to consult the guidelines that govern their own specific region and model, as well as systematic reviews and consensus statements such as those that can be found in the further reading section of this chapter. The discussion herein is limited to a brief overview of some of the principal arguments and some of the reasons why one might line a cavity, with direction for further reading.

Amalgams

Amalgam is not an adhesive material, and as such, unless an intermediate is used, there will necessarily be a microscopic gap between material and tooth tissue, certainly when first placed. Bacteria are inconveniently small – our old adversary *Streptococcus mutans*, one of the principal causative agents of dental caries, is a little under a micrometer in diameter – and as such can find their way into very tiny gaps such as those around an amalgam restoration. Fluids can also move in these small spaces and trigger the hydrodynamic effect.

The question of whether, when, and how to line under an amalgam has therefore been posed repeatedly for decades. Sadly, there is still no definitive answer. Certainly it is necessary to take into account the size of the restoration and the proximity to the pulp – how much tissue remains to protect the pulp and itself 'line' the cavity. Several systematic reviews have explored clinical studies with the hope of answering the questions 'whether to line' and 'what to line with', but time and time again, the answer that is reached is 'the data are insufficient'. Certainly, it would seem that many clinical studies can find no, or minimal, differences in outcome when different lining strategies are used (including no lining at all). This does not tell us definitively that there *is* no difference or no benefit to lining with particular materials under particular circumstances, only that we cannot say with certainty whether and when this is the case.

Of course, given that amalgam has been used with the 'older' lining materials such as calcium hydroxide for many decades, if there were a clear benefit of doing this or doing it with a certain approach, one might argue we might have found it by now – millions of such restorations have been placed and many are still in service today.

Composites

If a composite is applied in the appropriate manner, then it should achieve a good adhesive bond to the enamel and dentine. As such, some of the rationales for applying a liner under an amalgam do not apply, as there should not be a marginal gap through which fluids and bacteria can penetrate the base of the cavity. That is not to say no marginal leakage can occur – but with good technique and modern adhesive materials, this should be minimized.

Why therefore might one apply a liner under a composite at all? Many different reasons have been put forward, such as the limited micro-leakage that may occur and the leaching of any uncured monomer from the composite. In fact, while the debate continues, it seems that the most, possibly only, compelling reason to line under a composite is if the liner is intended to deliver some specific therapeutic effect, as might be the case in calcium hydroxide stimulating the production of reparative dentine. Doubtless, further data will be forthcoming; the real test is whether this data is robust and free of bias and can thus be used to make definitive guidance to practitioners.

Glass Ionomer Cements and Resin-Modified Glass Ionomer Cements

The same arguments as outlined above for GIC and RMGIC lining materials apply to the filling materials. A liner is not generally required, except in cases where the cavity is very deep and there may be the possibility of micro-exposures of the pulp, in which case a calcium hydroxide cement may be indicated (see Chapter 2.6).

CAVITY VARNISHES

Cavity varnishes were once commonplace but are now rarely used. They consist of a clear or yellowish liquid that contains natural resins such as copal, colophony, and sandarac or synthetic resins such as polystyrene. The resins are dissolved in a solvent such as alcohol, ether, or acetone and are applied to the cavity floor, and then the solvent is allowed to evaporate, leaving behind a thin coating of the resin. The varnish that *is* still in frequent use is fluoride varnish, which is applied to deliver a high and sustained dose of fluoride, although this is not commonly used as a cavity varnish but rather as a preventive treatment for the reduction or prevention of caries in children.

FURTHER READING

Arandi, N.Z., 2017. Calcium hydroxide liners: A literature review. Clinical, Cosmetic and Investigational Dentistry 9, 67–72.

Arandi, N.Z., Rabi, T., 2020. Cavity bases revisited. Clinical, Cosmetic and Investigational Dentistry 12, 305–312.

Baik, A., Alamoudi, N., El-Housseiny, A., Altuwirqi, A., 2021. Fluoride varnishes for preventing occlusal dental caries: A review. Dental Journal 9 (6), 64.

Baratieri, L.N., Machado, A., Van Noort, R., Ritter, A.V., Baratieri, N.M., 2002. Effect of pulp protection technique on the clinical performance of amalgam restorations: Three-year results. Operative Dentistry 27 (4), 319–324.

Hilton, T.J., 2016. Sealers, liners and bases. Journal of Esthetic and Restorative Dentistry 28 (3), 141–143.

Nasser, M., 2011. Evidence summary: Which dental liners under amalgam restorations are more effective in reducing postoperative sensitivity? British Dental Journal 210 (11), 533–537.

Schenkel AB, Peltz I, Veitz-Keenan A. Dental cavity liners for Class I and Class II resin-based composite restorations. Cochrane Database of Systematic Reviews 2016, Issue 10. Art. No.: CD010526. DOI: 10.1002/14651858.CD010526.pub2.

Schenkel, A.B., Peltz, I., Veitz-Keenan, A., 2019. Dental cavity liners for Class I and Class II resin-based composite restorations. Cochrane Database of Systematic Reviews 10 (10), CD010526.

Schwendicke, F., Göstemeyer, G., Gluud, C., 2015. Cavity lining after excavating caries lesions: Meta-analysis and trial sequential analysis of randomized clinical trials. Journal of Dentistry 43 (11) 1291–1297.

Enamel and Dentine Bonding

INTRODUCTION

Adhesive dentistry is central to many modern materials and processes. The modern clinician would barely recognize the pre-adhesive age, where retention of restorations was predicated on mechanical interlocking (e.g. undercut cavities for amalgam) and careful 'single path of entry' design (e.g. for crowns). That is not to say those approaches no longer have their place, but the modern clinician has a very much greater range of options available to them.

A wide variety of adhesive systems have been introduced over the past five decades. Some of these have prevailed and are still used today; many others have been superseded by further materials and products that claim to offer a more reliable bond, a stronger bond, a faster bond. Some of the modern products actually deliver poorer, or more inconsistent, results than their predecessors! It is also often said that the sheer range and variety of products available make adhesion one of the most confusing areas for dental clinicians; how on earth to compare all of these different products, each of which promises to be better than the rest?

In this chapter we will seek to dispel some of that confusion. We will first discuss the steps – scientifically – that have to occur in order to achieve a good bond, and some of the parameters that can be used to define what 'good' means. Then we shall consider some of the major categories of modern materials and how these map to those underlying scientific principles.

Stepping back from the detail for a moment, let us first consider the bigger picture. What must a dental adhesive achieve if it is to deliver for both clinician and patient? It must:

- provide a high bond strength to enamel and dentine
- provide an immediate bond
- provide a durable bond
- prevent the ingress of bacteria
- have an acceptable biocompatibility and safety profile
- be simple to use, and not more time-consuming or complex than is necessary.

Why some materials and techniques should have survived and others waned is due to the requirement that the adhesive needs to be able to bond to a variety of materials (e.g. composites, metals, ceramics) and to two very different substrates: namely, enamel and dentine.

The principles of adhesion have already been discussed in Chapter 1.9, and the adhesive aspects of GICs have already been dealt with in Chapter 2.3. In this chapter we will focus on the methods of bonding composites and other resins to enamel and dentine.

ENAMEL BONDING

Structure of Enamel

Enamel is the most densely calcified tissue of the human body and is unique in the sense that it is formed extracellularly.

It is a heterogeneous structure, with mature human enamel consisting of 96% mineral, 1% organic material, and 3% water by weight (Table 2.5.1). The mineral phase is made up of millions of tiny crystals of hydroxyapatite, $Ca_{10}(PO_4)_6(OH)_2$, which are packed tightly together in bundles, often called 'rods' or 'prisms', held together by an organic matrix. Due to ionic substitution (e.g. fluoride), the enamel apatite does not have the calcium-to-phosphate ratio of theoretically pure hydroxyapatite (1.6:1) and is usually in the ratio 2:1 by weight.

The rods or prisms are long, rod-like shapes of approximately 5 μm in diameter, having a distinctive cross-section with a head and a tail, often described as resembling a keyhole. The prisms are aligned perpendicular to the tooth surface, as shown in Figure 2.5.1.

The crystals of hydroxyapatite are flattened hexagonals, as shown in Figure 2.5.2, and because of their structure, it is not possible to obtain a perfect packing. The spaces left between the crystals are occupied by water and organic material. Much of the water is tightly bound within the enamel structure and not easily removed on drying. The surface layer of enamel tends to have a higher organic content than the deeper layers and is protected by a layer of salivary pellicle, which is about 1 μm thick.

Acid-Etch Technique

Due to its composite structure, the surface of enamel can be modified by the application of acids. The importance and potential exploitation of this was first appreciated by Buonocore in 1955, when he found that he could make the surface of enamel more amenable to adhesive techniques by modifying it with the application of a solution of phosphoric acid. Thence, the acid-etch technique for the bonding of composite restorative materials to enamel was developed. Its main effect is that of increasing the surface roughness of the enamel at the microscopic level (Figure 2.5.3) and raising the surface energy, which improves wettability (see below).

A major shortcoming of composites is that they have no intrinsic adhesive qualities to tooth tissues, as the resins are essentially

TABLE 2.5.1 **Typical Composition of Enamel and Dentine**				
	ENAMEL		DENTINE	
	Wt %	Vol. %	Wt %	Vol. %
Organic	1	2	20	30
Inorganic	95	86	70	45
Water	4	12	10	25

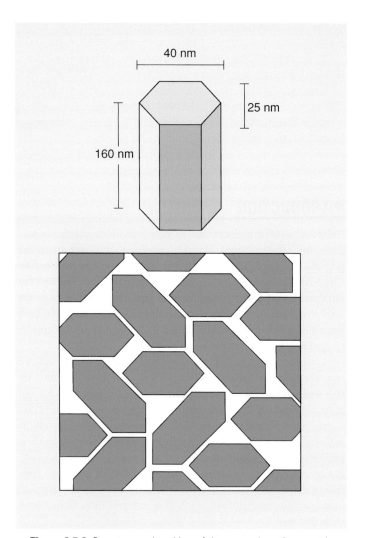

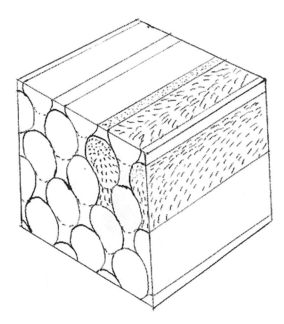

Figure 2.5.1 Schematic showing the structure of enamel, illustrating the keyhole-shaped 'prisms' and the approximate alignment of the hydroxyapatite crystallites

Figure 2.5.2 Structure and packing of the enamel apatite crystals

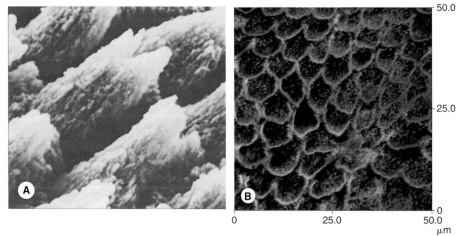

Figure 2.5.3 The enamel surface after acid etching. (a) Scanning electron micrograph image showing a predominant loss of prism periphery; (b) atomic force microscopy image showing a predominant loss of prism core.

non-polar. The acid-etch modification of the enamel surface allows the formation of an intimate micro-mechanical bond between enamel and the resin component of the composite, as long as there is close adaptation at the molecular level.

This discovery allowed the introduction of a wide variety of restorative techniques that were not previously possible, such as fissure sealants, directly bonded orthodontic brackets, resin-bonded bridges, and laminate veneers. The acid-etch technique is firmly embedded as an integral part of restorative procedures using composites.

The application of a strongly acidic solution (such as phosphoric acid) to enamel has the effect of modifying the surface characteristics. It does this in two important ways.

- The etching process increases the surface roughness of the enamel. When the phosphoric acid is applied to the enamel surface, an acid–base reaction is initiated, which causes the hydroxyapatite to go into solution and different surface features can develop. These include a predominant loss of enamel prism periphery (Figure 2.5.3a), a predominant loss of prism core constituents (Figure 2.5.3b), and a pattern in which there is no specific evidence of a prism structure. These etch patterns are shown schematically in Figure 2.5.4. The overall effect is that of increasing the surface roughness and hence the bonding area. It is possible to bond to this surface by a process of micro-mechanical interlocking. The increased surface roughness provides the added advantage that the surface area for bonding by chemical means, be it only through secondary bonding, is much enhanced.
- The acid has the effect of raising the surface energy of the enamel by removing surface contaminants. This provides for a better wettability of the enamel by the adhesive (see Chapter 1.9). Typically, the surface tension of an adhesive resin is in the range of 34–38 mJ·m^{-2}. Untreated enamel has a surface energy lower than this, and thus the conditions for perfect wetting to take place are not complied with. Normally, the surface of enamel is covered with a layer of pellicle, which has an extremely low surface energy (28 mJ·m^{-2}). This layer is removed by the acid and exposes the underlying surface of the enamel with its high surface energy and thus high reactivity (42 mJ·m^{-2}). The resin will adapt well to this high surface energy surface, as long as it is thoroughly dry. The micro-mechanical interlocking will ensure

that the resin will not separate from the enamel. Thus the acid-etch bond to enamel is essentially mechanical in nature.

Clinical Procedure

The features of increased surface roughness and raised resin wettability using the acid etching of the enamel surface combine to offer the opportunity for an excellent bond between a composite and the enamel. However, as with any seemingly simple technique, mistakes are easily made unless the operator adheres strictly to the rules for achieving a bond. The various stages of the acid-etch technique can be identified as follows:

- patient factors
- enamel prophylaxis
- application of the etchant.

Patient Factors

The first rule of achieving a good adhesive bond is that the surfaces to be bonded to must be kept free of contaminants. If the surface becomes contaminated with water or saliva, a good bond between the composite and enamel will not be obtained. The highly polar nature of the surface contaminants will prevent the non-polar resin from closely adapting to the enamel surface.

This means it is essential to consider whether appropriate moisture control can be achieved prior to selecting the material that is to be used. This includes consideration of the particular patient and also the location in the mouth. Regarding the former point about patient selection, if the patient were to find it difficult or impossible to remain calm and compliant during the whole procedure, then this is a risk to moisture control. This might be the case for some pediatric or geriatric patients, and people with conditions or needs that make receiving dental treatment a challenging experience for them. Regarding the latter point about the location in the mouth, there are areas in the mouth that are easier to keep (temporarily) dry than others, and both the anterior/posterior positioning and the proximity to the gingival margin are important considerations.

CLINICAL SIGNIFICANCE

The acid-etch technique should not be attempted with patients for whom the procedure is too time-consuming or when patient compliance is compromised.

Enamel Prophylaxis

As with any other adhesive joint, it is important that the surface of the substrate is thoroughly clean. The surface of enamel is covered with a layer of pellicle and possibly a layer of plaque as well. Such layers need to be removed before the etching process.

Whereas a thin layer of pellicle may be stripped off by the acid, it is not possible to remove thick deposits of plaque in this way. If this is not addressed, the resin will effectively bond to the surface contaminants and not the enamel. Cleaning of the enamel surface is best performed with a slurry of pumice and water, applied with a bristle brush for some 30 seconds. It is best to avoid brands of prophylactic pastes that contain oils, which can be left behind on the enamel surface. These will have the effect of reducing the wettability of the enamel surface by the

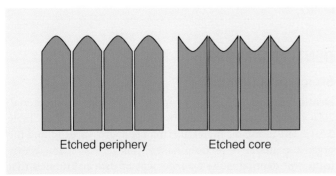

Etched periphery   Etched core

Figure 2.5.4 Schematic showing the common effects of phosphoric acid on enamel etching, where either prism periphery or core is preferentially removed

resin. Once the surface has been cleaned, it should be thoroughly washed and dried to remove all the debris.

Application of the Etchant

Considerable research has been undertaken to evaluate the best method of etching the surface of enamel.

With the teeth dried and properly isolated from the saliva, the aqueous solution of phosphoric acid-etchant can be applied to the enamel with a suitable brush, pledget, or other implement. An interesting and important observation is that there is an inverse relationship between the effectiveness of the etching and the concentration of the phosphoric acid. High, and low, concentrations of phosphoric acid are not as effective at producing the ideal etch pattern as intermediate concentrations. The optimum concentration appears to be in the range of 30–40%. Excessively high concentrations of phosphoric acid tend to show minimal change of the enamel surface, possibly because the low pH causes a rapid and indiscriminate (not patterned as in Figure 2.5.3) dissolution, which then leads to saturation of the solution with the reaction by-products, slowing down the rate of dissolution. Hence the use of phosphoric acid solutions supplied with zinc–phosphate cements should not be used, as the concentration is too high (approximate acid concentration 65%).

It is important that the surface of the enamel is not rubbed during the etching process, as the enamel prisms that stick up from the surface are extremely friable and will break under even the slightest load. A rubbing action will have the effect of breaking all of these prisms, and the crevices and cracks for resin tag formation will be lost.

It is also important that all of the phosphoric acid and the reaction products produced during the etching process are removed. Too often, this is dealt with in a cursory and dismissive manner. The procedure to adopt is to wash the enamel surface with copious amounts of water and to follow this with a water–air spray for no less than 20 seconds. If cotton rolls are used to isolate the teeth, these will have to be replaced in order to ensure a dry field. The drying process is equally critical, as the objective is to achieve a perfectly dry enamel surface.

> **CLINICAL SIGNIFICANCE**
>
> Since water is highly polar, the non-polar resin will not adapt to a wet enamel surface.

The removal of surface hydroxyl groups in the drying procedure will enhance the wettability of the resin on the surface and allow it to flow readily over the surface and into all the little cracks and crevices generated by the etching process. It is important to ensure that the air-hose that is used for drying is free of any contaminants such as oils and water. The etched and dried enamel should have the appearance of a dull, white, slightly frosted surface finish.

Application of Unfilled Resins

When resin is applied to a dry and well-etched enamel surface, it will readily invade all the surface irregularities and form resin tags that penetrate the enamel to a depth of up to 30 μm. This produces a very effective bond, by the mechanism of micro-mechanical interlocking.

Although opinions are divided, some maintain that a low-viscosity resin (i.e. either an unfilled resin or one of the many dentine adhesive resins) is applied to the enamel surface prior to placement of the composite. The rationale for the use of such an intermediate bonding resin is that the low viscosity of the bonding agent facilitates a better penetration into the microscopic spaces in the etched enamel than would be achieved by the direct placement of the composite.

The wettability of the resin composite is as good as that of low-viscosity resin, but the high viscosity of the composite, due to the presence of filler particles, prevents it from spreading easily over the surface of the enamel. Also, the viscosity of the composite is sufficiently high that it can actually bridge across the recesses in the enamel and cause entrapment of air. This has the dual effect of creating a zone of inhibition of the cure of the resin and an interfacial defect, which may be the source of subsequent bond breakdown.

Bond Strength

If the above procedure is carried out with diligence, an extremely effective bond between the enamel and the composite is created. In those situations where failure of the adhesive bond has occurred, it can usually be ascribed to poor clinical technique.

Clinically, bonding to enamel should not present a problem. The intimate micro-mechanical interlocking between the etched enamel and the resin will be such that it should be impossible to separate the resin from the enamel without causing the resin or the enamel to fracture. However, this does not mean that failure of enamel bonded restorations will not occur, since cohesive failure of the adhesive or the restoration can still take place. Equally, metallic or ceramic restorations can fail adhesively due to a lack of bonding between the resin and these restorative materials. When a bond failure occurs, it is very important to establish where the fracture has arisen, as this will tell you which component represented the weakest link in the bonding system.

> **CLINICAL SIGNIFICANCE**
>
> If bond failure occurs along the adhesive interface between the enamel and the resin, then this is most likely to be due to contamination of the enamel surface prior to placement of the resin.

DENTINE BONDING

Structure of Dentine

Dentine is composed of approximately 70% inorganic material, 20% organic material, and 10% water by weight (see Table 2.5.1). The inorganic material is mainly hydroxyapatite, and the organic material is predominantly collagen. A characteristic feature of dentine is the arrangement of dentinal tubules that traverse its entire thickness. The presence of these tubules makes the dentine permeable to drugs, chemicals, and toxins, which can diffuse through the dentine and injure the pulp.

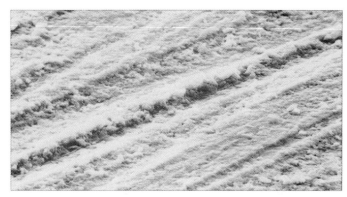

Figure 2.5.5 Scanning electron micrograph (SEM) showing the dentine smear layer

The heterogeneous composition of dentine makes it a particularly difficult substrate to bond to with an adhesive. A second problem is that the differential pressure between the pulp and the dentine floor causes fluid to pump out of the dentinal tubules, such that it is not possible to create a dry dentine surface. Excessive desiccation of the dentine is likely to result in irreversible damage to the vital pulp and is thus not an option.

In the case of an abrasion/erosion lesion the dentine surface usually consists of sclerotic dentine that is covered with a layer of pellicle, plaque, and possibly calculus. It is important that these surface contaminants are removed prior to the use of a dentine-bonding procedure. This removal is readily achieved with the application of pumice and water. A surface is then available that should be free of any contaminants and ready for the bonding procedure. However, the dentine surface is still covered with a layer of disorganized dentine known as the smear layer (Figure 2.5.5).

The smear layer consists of a gelatinous surface layer of coagulated protein, some 0.5–5 μm thick. It is generally highly contaminated with bacteria from the caries process and contains cutting debris. It is quite tightly bound to the underlying dentine – tightly enough that it cannot be removed simply by wiping or rubbing it, but not so tightly that it can be left in place and the composite bound to it!

The problems with dentine bonding can thus be summarized as follows:
- dentine is hydrophilic, whereas most adhesives are hydrophobic
- dentine cannot be dried in the same way as enamel
- dentine is a vital tissue
- dentine consists of both inorganic and organic material
- dentine is covered by a smear layer.

Perspectives on Traditional and Contemporary Dentine Bonding Agents

Dentine bonding agents have evolved a great deal since they were first introduced. As we shall see in the sections that follow, the earliest dentine bonding agents consisted of three separate products, which were applied to the dentine one at a time and in a specific sequence, and each of which had a unique and well-defined purpose. These worked very well. In fact, they still work very well, and some of the independent research continues to illustrate that this simple stepwise approach gives the best results. However, time is one of the clinician's most precious commodities, and the time taken to apply three separate products one at a time constitutes a significant portion of the total time to apply a composite restoration. One could be cynical and say 'time is money' – the clinician wants their procedure to be as fast as possible – and that may be true, but that would be missing the fact that the patient, also, does not typically want their treatment to be more prolonged than it needs to be. Furthermore, the need to apply three products, each of which will have slightly different, but similar, instructions according to the brand used (leave in place for 10 seconds? 20 seconds? 30 seconds? Air dry or not air dry? Light cure for 10 seconds, 20 seconds, or not at all? Rinse or not rinse?), all under the pressure of the busy clinical schedule, meant that errors were common. If the products are not applied exactly as specified by the manufacturer – a rinsing step is missed, or a light cure is not applied at the right stage or for the right duration – then the bond, and thus the whole restoration, will be compromised.

As such, while the early dentine bonding systems could deliver excellent results, they fell victim to the dual pressures of time and complexity. Modern dentine bonding systems are 'simplified' – at least, simplified as far as the clinician is concerned – as they require fewer individual steps. From the scientific point of view, they are actually more complicated!

We will start in this section by considering the processes that are going on at the interface between dentine and material – what is it that needs to happen in order for the bond to be achieved. We will do this in the language of the original three-stage bonding systems, as *these three stages still happen in modern systems*. The difference in the modern system is that some of the stages happen *in parallel rather than in series*.

Once we have discussed the steps that occur as part of dentine bonding, we will consider how these are now presented to the clinician and how modern products relate back to the earlier step-by-step procedure.

Traditional Dentine Bonding Systems

Based on the concepts of primers and coupling agents, as discussed in Chapter 1.9, dentine bonding systems can be considered to consist of three essential components, namely:
- a primer
- a coupling agent
- a sealer.

In the dental literature and in product marketing the primers are commonly called *dentine conditioners* and consist of a variety of acids that alter the surface appearance and characteristics of the dentine. The coupling agents are, in effect, the components that do the bonding but are generally described in the dental literature and by the manufacturers as *primers*. The function of the *sealer* is to flow into the dentinal tubules and seal the dentine by producing a surface layer rich in methacrylates that will ensure bonding to the resin in the composite. This component is variously referred to as the bond, the resin, or the *adhesive*. This last term is especially confusing since it is the coupling agent that provides the bond. This mixing of terminology for the various components of dentine bonding agents adds to the general confusion surrounding them. In further discussions of dentine bonding agents we will use the terminology that is commonly used in the dental literature – dentine conditioners, primers, and sealers – so as hopefully not to add to the confusion. Besides, later we will discuss how these various components can be mixed up in order to produce formulations that are easier to use.

Dentine Conditioners

The role of the dentine conditioners is to modify the smear layer that is formed on the dentine due to the cutting action of the bur when preparing a cavity or during exposure to abrasives such as toothpastes in smooth surface caries and abrasion/erosion lesions. One of the major distinguishing features of dentine bonding agents is the variety of dentine conditioners that have been used over time. These include maleic acid, EDTA (ethylenediaminetetraacetic acid), oxalic acid, phosphoric acid, and nitric acid. What these substances have in common is that they are all acids and they modify the smear layer to varying degrees. The

application of an acid to the dentine surface induces an acid–base reaction with the hydroxyapatite. This causes the hydroxyapatite to be dissolved and results in an opening of the dentinal tubules and the creation of a demineralized surface layer of dentine that is generally up to 4 μm deep (Figure 2.5.6). The stronger the acid, the more pronounced these effects, up to a point. Thus, for EDTA, which is a weakly acidic chelating agent, only partial opening of the tubules occurs (Figure 2.5.7), whereas, for nitric acid, which is a stronger acid, extensive opening of the dentinal tubules occurs (Figure 2.5.8). The effect of this is shown schematically for a cross-sectional view of the dentine in Figure 2.5.9.

Dentine conditioners used for composite placement are nowadays almost always 35-40% phosphoric acid, in an aqueous gel which is colored to help the clinician see where they have placed it and when it is all fully rinsed away. It is usually the same product that is used to etch the enamel, although with some procedures, it is necessary to apply it to the two tissues for different durations (differential etching).

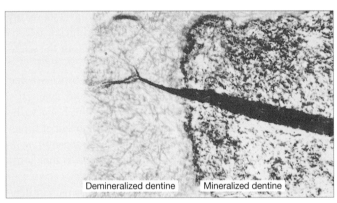

Figure 2.5.6 Transmission electron micrograph (TEM) of dentine after application of a nitric acid primer to the surface. Observe the surface layer of demineralized dentine – where the hydroxyapatite has been depleted or dissolved entirely – and the underlying sound dentine

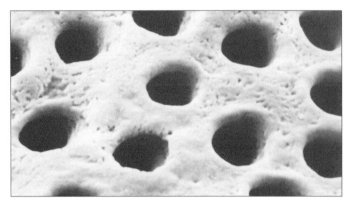

Figure 2.5.8 SEM of the dentine surface after application of a nitric acid primer. Note that the dentine tubules are fully open or 'patent' as nitric acid is a more aggressive etchant than EDTA

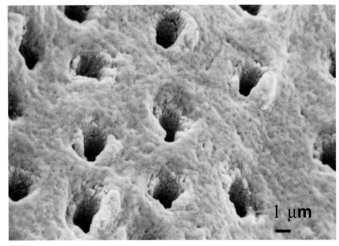

Figure 2.5.7 SEM of the dentine surface after application of EDTA primer. Note the partial opening of the dentine tubules, as EDTA is a comparatively mild etchant

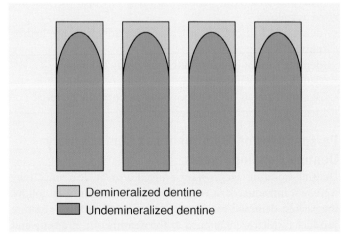

Figure 2.5.9 Schematic showing a cross-sectional view through dentine after application of an acid primer

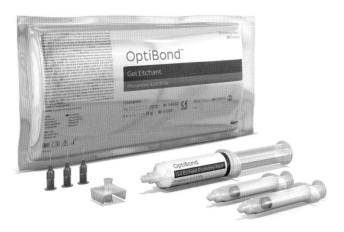

Figure 2.5.10 An example of a commercial dentine conditioner or etchant composed of a 37.5% solution of phosphoric acid in a colored gel. Image courtesy of and copyright Kerr UK, with thanks.

TABLE 2.5.2 Polarity Patterns in Some Common Functional Groups	
Compound Type	**Functional Group Structure**
Alcohol	$-\overset{\displaystyle\backslash}{\underset{\displaystyle/}{C}}{}^{\delta+}-OH^{\delta-}$
Amine	$-\overset{\displaystyle\backslash}{\underset{\displaystyle/}{C}}{}^{\delta+}-NH_2{}^{\delta-}$
Carboxylic acid	$-C^{\delta+}\overset{O^{\delta-}}{\underset{OH^{\delta-}}{\Vert}}$
Aldehyde	$-C^{\delta+}\overset{O^{\delta-}}{\underset{H}{\Vert}}$

It is often supplied in a bottle or a syringe for easy dispensing (Figure 2.5.10).

Some dentine conditioners contain glutaraldehyde. The incorporation of glutaraldehyde is also aimed at modifying the dentine. Glutaraldehyde is a well-known cross-linking agent for proteins, including collagen. The cross-linking process is said to produce a stronger dentine substrate by improving the strength and stability of the collagen structure. One reservation about the use of glutaraldehyde is that tissue necrosis has been observed in other areas where it has been used.

Primers

The role of the primer is to act as the adhesive in dentine-bonding system since it provides a means of bonding hydrophobic composites and compomers to hydrophilic dentine. The conditioner simply served the purpose of getting the dentine ready for the adhesive step. Primers act as an intermediary and consist of bifunctional monomers dissolved in a suitable solvent. The bifunctional monomer is, in fact, a coupling agent that is able to combine with two distinctly different materials. The situation is analogous to that of bonding resin to glass in the composites, where a silane coupling agent is used (see Chapter 1.9). The general formula for the coupling agent in dentine primers is as follows:

Methacrylate group-Spacer group-Reactive group

M-S-R

The methacrylate group (M) has the ability to bond to the composite resin and provide a strong covalent bond. The methacrylate group must be able to provide a satisfactory means for polymerization with the resin of the composite.

The spacer group (S) must be able to provide the necessary flexibility to the coupling agent to enhance the potential for bonding of the reactive groups. If the molecule is excessively rigid (due to steric hindrance), the ability of the reactive group to find a satisfactory conformational arrangement may be jeopardized,

leading, at best, to a strained bond arrangement and, at worst, to only limited sites for bonding being available.

The reactive groups (R) are polar pendant- or end-groups. A variety of polar functional groups are shown in Table 2.5.2. The bond polarity is a consequence of asymmetric electron distribution in the bond. Polar reactions occur as the result of attractive forces between positive and negative charges on the molecules (see Chapter 1.2). Thus the polar pendant- and end-groups on the coupling agent can combine with similar polar molecules in the dentine, such as hydroxyl groups on the apatite and amino groups on the collagen. The attraction may be purely physical but can, in some instances, result in the formation of a chemical bond. The nature of this reactive group will determine whether the bond will be to the apatite in the dentine or to the collagen. In some cases both may be involved.

Although all of the coupling agents used in dentine primers have polar reactive groups, these vary from one dentine bonding agent to another. All have the objective of producing a strong bond to the dentine, but manufacturers and researchers are not agreed on which coupling agent may be the best. A small selection of these coupling agents is shown in Table 2.5.3, with hydroxyethylmethacrylate (HEMA) in particular being a popular choice.

HEMA is able to penetrate the demineralized dentine and bond to the collagen via the hydroxyl and amino groups on the collagen. The action of the coupling agent in the primer solution is therefore to create a molecular entanglement network of poly(HEMA) and collagen.

It is very important that the primer is able to penetrate fully into and saturate the demineralized collagen layer. If this does not happen, then a thin layer of demineralized collagen will remain. This layer will not be reinforced by the resin and will form a weak interfacial region. In order to achieve good depth of penetration, the coupling agent is therefore dissolved in a

TABLE 2.5.3 Coupling Agents Used for Dentine Bonding

Hydroxyethylmethacrylate (HEMA)	$CH_2{=}C(CH_3){-}C({=}O){-}O{-}CH_2{-}CH_2{-}OH$
Dimethacryloxyethyl phenol phosphate (MEP-P)	$CH_2{=}C(CH_3){-}C({=}O){-}O{-}CH_2{-}CH_2{-}O{-}P({=}O)(OH){-}C{-}$ (phenyl)
N-Phenylglycine glycidyl methacrylate (NPG-GMA)	$CH_2{=}C(CH_3){-}C({=}O){-}O{-}CH_2{-}CH(OH){-}CH_2{-}N(phenyl){-}CH_2{-}C{-}OH$

solvent, such as ethanol or acetone. The solvents are extremely effective at seeking out water and displacing it ('water-chasing'), carrying the coupling agent along with it as it penetrates the demineralized dentine. This delivers the primer molecules into the demineralized zone (Figure 2.5.11) and allows them to form a layer that is chemically bonded to the dentine and provides functional groups that can then react with the resin sealer. It is important that the dentine is not excessively demineralized, as the depth of demineralization may become too much for complete penetration by the primer to occur.

In order to saturate the demineralized dentine, it is important that enough of the dentine-bonding agent is applied to the dentine surface. This may require multiple applications, and sufficient time should be allowed for the primer to penetrate and absorb. Many products recommend only limited or no air drying with an air-stream, as it is best to evaporate the solvents gently and not over-dry the dentine itself.

Many self-etching products employ 10-MDP (10-methacryloyloxy decyl phosphate) as the adhesive monomer, which interacts with the hydroxyapatite in the dentine to form a resilient bond that seems particularly resistant to degradation over time. 10-MDP has an interesting dual interaction with the hydroxyapatite. It is particularly acidic compared to some monomers and is thereby effective in etching the hydroxyapatite, and it also forms an ionic bond to calcium that is liberated from the hydroxyapatite in the acidic conditions, forming a stable, nanoscale layered structured at the material-hydroxyapatite interface. It is thought that this nanolayered structure might help the bond resist degradation over time.

CLINICAL SIGNIFICANCE

The method of application of the primer will largely determine whether or not micro-leakage will develop.

Sealers

The earliest dentine sealers were simply light- or dual-cured unfilled Bis-GMA or UDMA resins. Although the direct application of an unfilled resin such as Bis-GMA to an acid-treated dentine surface would result in the formation of resin tags, this has been shown not to result in an adequate bond between the resin and the dentine. The major difference is that, by not using the primer, the hydrophobic resin will adapt poorly to the hydrophilic dentine. When a primer is employed, its action is to make the dentine surface more hydrophobic, thus preventing the resin from shrinking away from the walls within the dentinal tubules, and ensure the formation of a tightly fitting resin-tag structure. For example, the methacrylate ends of the HEMA coupling agent are available for bonding to the resin sealer when this is subsequently placed onto the prepared surface of the dentine.

The dentine surface is thus thoroughly sealed with a resin, which is bonded to the dentine via the coupling agent in the primer. This sealer will now readily bond to the composite resin. The resulting inter-penetrating layer of dentine and resin

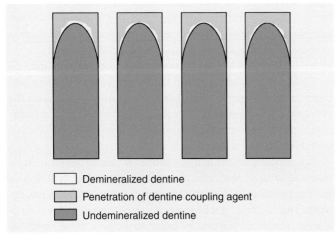

☐ Demineralized dentine
▨ Penetration of dentine coupling agent
▨ Undemineralized dentine

Figure 2.5.11 The penetration of the coupling agent into the demineralized dentine

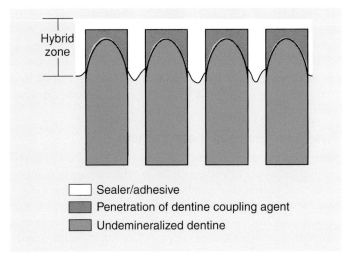

Figure 2.5.12 The hybrid zone created with a dentine-bonding agent

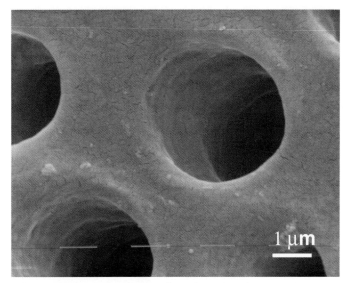

Figure 2.5.13 Demineralized surface of dentine after air drying. Note that the collagen layer is dense and impenetrable

is commonly referred to as the *hybrid zone,* as shown schematically in Figure 2.5.12.

One of the most common formulations of standalone dentine sealers is a mixture of Bis-GMA and HEMA. This helps to improve the adaptation of the sealer to the dentine surface. Rather than being entirely unfilled, some sealers are lightly filled, commonly with nanoscale silica particles. Larger, 'micro' filler particles such as those used in some composites and GICs would not be appropriate for dentine sealers, as they would interfere with the penetration of the dentine tubules and collagen network by the resin. It is plausible that the addition of nanoscale filler particles to dentine sealers would increase the compressive strength of these materials, although it is not yet clear what clinical advantage this offers.

CLINICAL SIGNIFICANCE

Penetration of the sealer down the dentinal tubules provides some micro-mechanical bonding, but it is mainly the chemical bond achieved with the primer that will determine the quality of the final bond.

Wet Dentine Bonding

The coupling agent component of the dentine bonding agents is carried in a volatile solvent such as ethanol or acetone. Such solvents are very effective at displacing the water in the dentine and, in the process, pull the adhesive into the dentine with them. Therefore it is not necessary – in fact, it may be detrimental – to dehydrate the dentine surface excessively. If the dentine is dried excessively, the consequence of this is that the demineralized collagen layer will collapse down onto the mineralized dentine, producing a dense structure that is difficult for the primer to penetrate Figure 2.5.13. If the demineralized collagen layer is kept moist, a porous structure is maintained and the primer can readily infiltrate this layer and form a molecular entanglement bond Figure 2.5.14. Thus it is considered usually only necessary to remove excess surface moisture.

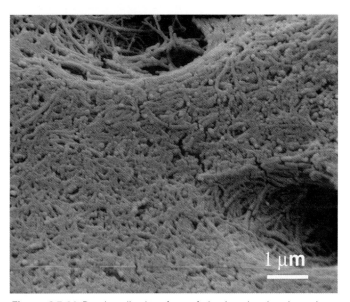

Figure 2.5.14 Demineralized surface of dentine that has been kept moist to prevent the collapse of the collagen structure

It is interesting, however, how thinking shifts over time. Thoroughly drying dentine was never an option. For many years, wet or 'glistening' dentine was advocated for the reasons given above and certainly some clinicians still proceed in this way. Now, it is felt this is less important than was once thought and that an intermediate, not-dry-but-not-wet dentine is probably optimal, as long as one agitates the adhesive on the dentine surface to help it penetrate the collagen layer. Furthermore, some primers contain water as a carrier and for those it is possible that the demineralized collagen will rehydrate sufficiently after drying for the primer to penetrate the collagen structure. This serves to illustrate how important it is to adhere to the prescribed clinical protocol for the specific material – wet or partially dried dentine, agitate or don't agitate – for the best results.

Total-Etch Technique

When dentine bonding agents were first introduced, there was concern about etching the dentine surface. Before the advent of dentine bonding agents, the dental practitioner's experience was that, when the phosphoric acid from the enamel etching procedure was allowed to flow onto the dentine, patients would return complaining of postoperative sensitivity. It was thought that this was due to the increased permeability of the dentine after acid etching resulting in the hydrodynamic effect and possibly penetration of the acid into the pulp. Hence there was a reluctance to etch dentine.

The development of dentine bonding agents meant that the dentine surface could be sealed and postoperative sensitivity due to the hydrodynamic effect could be avoided as long as the bond between the dentine and restoration was maintained. Gradually, it was also realized that the use of a solution such as 35% phosphoric acid resulted in minimal penetration of the dentine (4–5 μm) and thus it was unlikely that the acid would contact the pulp. As confidence increased, a differential etching technique was introduced, which involved etching the dentine separately with a low concentration of phosphoric acid or using a mild acid such as EDTA. However, this process of differential etching was cumbersome and time-consuming. Eventually, the concept of the total-etch technique evolved; this involves etching both the enamel and the dentine simultaneously, typically for 10–15 seconds with a 35-40% phosphoric acid solution. This procedure is only applicable to freshly cut enamel, and unprepared enamel still needs to be etched in the conventional way.

MODERN PRESENTATION OF DENTINE BONDING AGENTS

Three-Stage Etch and Rinse Systems

These are effectively the presentation described above, with a separate container of condition, primer, and sealer (noting the above comments that the naming is not consistent, so conditioner might be called etchant, acid etch, or just etch; the sealer might be called sealant or resin; and the primer has been given all kinds of fanciful names). The dentine conditioner is generally the 35–40% phosphoric acid solution, while the primer either can be a single-component, light-activated, bifunctional monomer in a solvent or may require the mixing of two components to be chemically cured. The dentine sealer also may be a single-component, light-activated resin or chemically and often dual-cured. Thus the number of syringes/bottles can be as many as 5, and once the application, rinsing, curing, and drying steps are added up, the process can have 10 or more individual steps.

The problem with these three-stage bonding systems was that they involve many bottles, which can be confusing, and many bonding steps, which are time-consuming and high-stakes, as missing any one will compromise the whole restoration. Both dental practitioners and the manufacturers wanted to see a reduction in the number of steps involved in the bonding process while still allowing each individual and necessary interaction between material and dentine to occur. This has resulted in a plethora of two-stage and even 'one-stage' dentine bonding agents.

Two-Stage Etch and Rinse Systems

Since the three-stage systems consist of a dentine conditioner, primer, and sealer, one way of reducing the number of components, and possibly the number of steps, is to combine the action of some of these components. In order to simplify the presentation and use of dentine bonding agents, essentially two different approaches can be adopted. Two-stage dentine bonding agents were developed, where in some cases the primer and sealer are combined, or the dentine conditioner and primer are combined. The former are frequently referred to as *one-bottle bond* systems and the latter as *self-etching primers*.

The one-bottle bonding systems continue to use a separate acid-etch step before infiltration with the primer/adhesive. In this instance the objective is for the process of hybridization of the demineralized dentine and the sealing of the dentinal tubules to take place simultaneously. In order to achieve this, many of the one-bottle bonding systems require multiple applications of the primer/adhesive. This will ensure complete saturation of the demineralized dentine with the mixture of resins provided in the primer/adhesive.

The benefits of one-bottle bond systems are that:
- The dental practitioner only needs to consider two components ('one bottle' and acid-etchant), compared with the myriad of bottles associated with the three-stage bonding systems.
- The order in which the components are to be used is less likely to be confused.
- Inventory control is kept very simple.

One limitation of the one-bottle bonding systems is that they cannot be used in situations where access to the light from the light-curing unit is compromised, such as for resin-bonded posts or amalgam bonding.

Some manufacturers have proposed that, when the one-bottle bonding systems are used in conjunction with compomers, it is possible in certain low-stress-bearing situations to omit the acid-etch step and thus use the one-bottle bond systems directly on the enamel and dentine. Although this approach may not be too detrimental to the bond to the dentine, it will compromise the bond to enamel.

At least one manufacturer has produced a dentine conditioner to be used with compomers, which consists of an aqueous solution of itaconic and maleic acid, and does not require to be rinsed off. This two-stage system has the advantage of reducing the steps involved but has the disadvantage that it still has to compete with other dentine adhesives used with compomers that are single-stage systems (see below). Clinical studies have revealed that the bond is inferior to products that must be rinsed away but that it can provide acceptable bonding in quite specific situations, specifically in children, where the restoration does not have to last too long and when the child's discomfort in the dental chair is sufficient to make a longer process untenable.

Two-Stage Self-Etching Systems

The self-etching primers work on the premise that these will carry out both the demineralization and the infiltration process simultaneously and thus form the hybrid layer. This has the advantage that the ambiguous drying step for the dentine is avoided. The second-stage application of the unfilled resin(s) will ensure that the dentinal tubules are sealed and a methacrylate-rich surface layer is formed. It has been suggested that the two-stage self-etching systems should be further subdivided into a 'strong' (pH < 1), an 'intermediately strong' (pH ≈ 1.5), a 'mild' (pH ≈ 2), and an 'ultra-mild' (pH ≥ 2.5) self-etch approach, depending on the self-etching or demineralization intensity. The strongest, or most acidic, of these might be thought to be most effective but, in fact, have been shown to result in a rather unstable bond, with the slightly less acidic ones now favored. The self-etching systems do not involve a rinsing step and thus the dissolved calcium phosphates remain in the hybrid layer. The lower the pH, the more intense the dissolution process, such that more of the calcium phosphates remain embedded in the hybrid layer. Since these calcium phosphates are rather soluble, they may leach out and compromise the long-term durability of the bond to dentine. However, it is possible that the bond to enamel is better with the low pH systems due to the more aggressive etching of the enamel.

Single-Stage Self-Etching Systems

The simplest adhesive would be the one that is applied in a single-stage procedure. The manufacturers have not quite gone to the lengths of simply putting all the components into a single bottle. Although this might seem to be the logical next step, lack of compatibility between the components does not allow this. Some single-stage dentine bonding agents are presented as two components that have to be mixed prior to application to the enamel and dentine surface, without the prior need to treat the enamel or dentine, while other systems are based on a combination of ingredients in a single bottle. The ingredients used by each manufacturer are quite varied and complex, and it is not possible to give a generic composition. The bonding procedure involves up to four steps, consisting of (1) dispensing and/or mixing the two components, where appropriate, (2) application to the enamel and dentine surface, (3) drying, and (4) light curing. The advantage with this approach is not only its simplicity but also the avoidance of the ambiguous drying step for the dentine.

The single-stage dentine bonding agents are generally indicated in low-stress-bearing areas, as the bond strength to enamel in particular and, to a lesser degree, to dentine is possibly not as good as that obtained with the three-stage or two-stage bonding systems. Since the bond to enamel may be inferior, it is recommended that, in situations involving a significant amount of enamel, selective etching of the enamel with phosphoric acid is carried out. Single-stage dentine bonding agents can also be used to overcome sensitivity by simply painting them onto the affected surface.

Universal Adhesives

The dental adhesives described so far are designed to be used in either the etch-and-rinse or self-etch mode, which may involve three, two, or a single application step. The increasing demand for yet simpler, faster, easier-to-use and less technique-sensitive dental adhesives has led to the introduction of a class of adhesives termed *universal adhesives* (UAs) (Figure 2.5.15). These multi-mode adhesives may be used as etch-and-rinse adhesives, self-etch adhesives, or self-etch adhesives on dentine and etch-and-rinse adhesives on enamel, a technique commonly referred to as selective enamel etching. They are also used in conjunction with indirect materials such as ceramics and alloys.

At present, the available clinical evidence is sparse, and one must turn to laboratory data. The UAs appear to perform well in in vitro studies, in some cases surpassing the earlier generations of bonding systems, but such data is of limited relevance to clinical performance and does not support the claim that UAs can be used with any adhesive strategy. While it is true that they can chemically bond to various tooth and direct/indirect restorative substrates, the stability of this bond is material dependent and subject to the procedure used. For example, phosphoric acid etching creates a more pronounced and retentive etching pattern in enamel than self-etch systems, and therefore etch-and-rinse bonding systems are often preferred for indirect restorations and when large areas of enamel are still present. If UAs are to be used when enamel is present, differential etching should be carried out to ensure the enamel is sufficiently

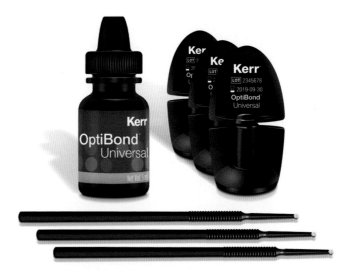

Figure 2.5.15 An example of a commercial "universal adhesive", which contains a proprietary adhesive monomer as well as both acetone and ethanol, to aid penetration and the formation of a hybrid layer. Image courtesy of and copyright Kerr UK, with thanks.

etched. Conversely, self-etch adhesives provide an excellent bond to dentine and are, consequently, indicated for direct composite resin restorations, especially when predominantly supported by dentine. UAs are a recent addition to the range of bonding agents, which means that there is a lack of long-term data regarding their clinical performance, which further complicates clinical decision-making.

Summing Up

A classification of dentine-bonding agents is provided in Table 2.5.4. It must be stressed that different dentine-bonding agents have distinctive and different detailed instructions on how they should be used to best effect. It is not possible here to cover each and every one of the subtleties and nuances of the application procedure for each, but we have sought to establish *why* it is crucial to follow the detailed and product-specific instructions. Dentine bonding is an intricate process governed by several factors, and however 'simple' the product, it can only deliver if it is applied in precisely the correct way. It should be clear from the above description of dentine-bonding agents that there is no universal technique for producing a bond to dentine and that each system has its own unique procedure.

CLINICAL SIGNIFICANCE

It is extremely important that careful note is taken of the instructions for the use of individual dentine bonding agents, as these will differ widely, depending on the components used and how these are presented to the user.

Selection of a Dentine Bonding Agent
Biocompatibility

The way in which the pulp may react to the procedure adopted (particularly the application of acid to dentine) is an important consideration. It is apparent that these dentine adhesives rely, to varying degrees, on the formation of resin

tags in order to achieve a bond to dentine. One potential problem is that opening the dentinal tubules can cause fluids from within the tubules to rise to the surface under the influence of the pulpal pressure. This will prevent good bonding, as it prevents the adhesive from penetrating the dentinal tubules and from adapting to the dentine surface. While this may be overcome by thorough drying of the dentine surface prior to the application of the bonding agent, excessive desiccation of the dentine is likely to result in postoperative pulpal sensitivity and a poor bond.

Concern has also been expressed about the possible pulpal response to the application of acids to the dentine surface. Some consideration is given to this with regard to direct pulp capping in Chapter 2.6.

In the case of sclerotic dentine, as is found in cervical abrasion lesions on mature patients, the application of acids to the dentine is felt to be acceptable, as the dentine is highly mineralized and an open pathway to the pulp is not created. In fact, sclerotic dentine does not etch very readily at all, and in some instances it is necessary to roughen the surface mechanically to aid retention. There could be greater concerns with carious dentine, but a number of studies have indicated that dentine bonding agents and their associated acid primers will not have an adverse effect on the pulp.

Thus pulpal inflammation will only occur if there is a bond failure resulting in bacterial leakage. Whether or not this is likely to happen depends on the strength and durability of the bond to dentine, how easy it is to achieve this bond clinically, and the restorative material used. Most dentine bonding agents do not have any intrinsic antibacterial activity to counter the bacterial invasion, although in some cases attempts have been made to incorporate antibacterial agents.

CLINICAL SIGNIFICANCE

A very important point to appreciate is that should the adhesive bond fail, there is a ready route for bacterial invasion through the permeable dentine.

With all dentine bonding agents, it is important to avoid direct skin contact with the primer/adhesive liquids, as regular contact may result in a type IV sensitization (delayed allergic reaction) or contact dermatitis.

Strength and Durability

A breakdown of the adhesive bond can have serious consequences, as it allows the reintroduction of bacteria and debris into the cavity margins. This will cause unsightly marginal staining and can result in the development of pulpal sensitivity. Alternatively, the restoration may simply be lost due to a lack of adhesion, unless some form of retention has been provided.

There are a number of potential causes for the breakdown of the bond between the restoration and the dentine:
- polymerization shrinkage
- differential thermal expansion and contraction
- internal stresses from occlusal loading
- chemical attack, such as hydrolysis.

The possible consequences of polymerization shrinkage of the composites have been discussed already (see Chapter 2.2).

TABLE 2.5.4 **Classification of Dentine-Bonding Systems**	
Stage	**Bonding Steps**
Three-stage etch and rinse	1. Application of etchant and washed off to create demineralized dentine layer 2. Application of primer 3. Application of sealer
Two-stage etch and rinse	1. Application of etchant and washed off to create demineralized dentine layer 2. Application of primer and sealer in single solution
Two-stage self-etching	1. Application of self-etching primer 2. Sealer applied separately
Single-stage self-etching	1. Self-etching primer and sealer applied as a single solution
Universal	Etch and rinse or self-etch

As it can take up to 24 hours before the full bond strength for the dentine bonding agents is achieved, the polymerization shrinkage may cause disruption of the bond before it has had a chance to establish itself.

CLINICAL SIGNIFICANCE

It is prudent to recommend to patients that they try to place minimal stress on a newly bonded restoration, at least for the first 24 hours.

The breakdown of the dentine bond due to polymerization shrinkage is also dependent on the cavity shape. This is defined by the so-called C-factor, which is the ratio of bonded surface area to the free surface area. If the free surface for contraction is very small compared to the surface area of the interface between the tooth and the restoration, then disruption of the composite/dentine bond is favored over contraction toward the surface. This means that a bond may only be achievable on a flat surface or in very shallow cavities, unless the bond is sufficiently strong to resist the stresses generated by the polymerization contraction of the resin. Should this be the case, then the cusps of the tooth will need to deform to compensate for the shrinkage effect.

In situations of heavily undermined cusps, as may be the case in large mesial occlusal distal restorations, this could result in fracture at the base of the cusp. Even if this does not occur, the stress generated within the tooth crown may give rise to pulpal sensitivity.

In situations of stress-induced lesions, such as cervical abfraction lesions, the application of eccentric or high occlusal forces can cause the restoration to debond and eventually to be dislodged. It has been suggested that this problem can be overcome to some degree by employing a restorative material with a low elastic modulus (e.g. micro-filled resins), since this prevents stresses from being transferred across the tooth–restoration interface. However, this does mean that the stresses have to be supported elsewhere in the tooth structure and this may not be the most benign situation.

Number of Bonding Steps

If the choice between dentine bonding agents were simply based on their complexity of application, then the single-stage agents would be the preferred option. However, fewer steps do not necessarily mean better performance. Furthermore, the actual number of steps is not always what it would first appear upon reading the marketing material; some 'one-step' bonding agents might require three or four actual steps to be carried out.

CLINICAL SIGNIFICANCE

The rapid development of dentine bonding systems, with new and modified products launched onto the market with bewildering rapidity, makes it all the more difficult to gather meaningful clinical data on their relative merits and the longevity and robustness of the bond.

There are situations in which some of the dentine bonding agents would be inappropriate. For example, when a dentine bonding agent is to be used in conjunction with an indirect restoration, those that have to be light-cured immediately can give rise to problems of seating of the restoration, as there is a ten-dency for the resin to pool at the internal line angles. In those situations a dentine bonding agent with a two-component, chemically cured primer would be indicated. As mentioned previously, in situations where access to light is a problem, such as resin-bonded metal posts and amalgam bonding, a chemically cured primer is also indicated.

Clinical Performance

Composites and bonding systems have both evolved a great deal over the past four or five decades. As such, clinical data is hard to come by. The dental materials researcher can take one of two approaches.

They can look at a specific combination of materials – a specific composite used with a specific bonding system and methodology – and observe how these fare over time – how many fail, how many require remediation, how many are still in good service after a given period has passed. Patients are carefully screened for confounding factors; the site, nature, and scale of the restoration have to meet strict eligibility criteria; and the clinicians are carefully trained and calibrated to ensure their approach is consistent. Ideally this would be comparative – more than one set of material and procedure conditions would be compared, to allow the clinician to make an informed choice about the most appropriate selection for their needs. There are several problems with this approach.

One is that by the time the study is designed, funding is secured, ethical approval is sought and given, research-engaged clinicians are recruited, patients are consented and recruited, restorations are placed, and records are combined, months or years will have passed. Then if you add the time over which the restorations must be observed to give any meaningful insight – at least 2 years and preferably 5 – we are probably at least 6–8 years from the original conception of the study. Add another year to finish the follow-ups, write the paper, and have it published – we could easily find ourselves 10 years older at this stage. Over that 10-year period, it is highly likely that the materials that were used will have been superseded by the next generation of composites and bonding systems – probably even more than one generation. However robust the data, it is of limited merit to the practicing clinician who can now say for sure which obsolete product was better than which other obsolete product – not a terribly practical insight.

The alternative approach that a dental materials researcher might take is to step back and look at the bigger picture. To compare two *categories* of material/procedure combination rather than to look to specific products. To use data from a very large number of patients and clinicians. One can imagine a study where the survival and state of restorations was compared where they were divided by the nature of the bonding system – was it three-stage? Two-stage etch and rinse? Self-etching? This has the benefit that even if specific products have been withdrawn by the time the data become available, at least one might gain insights into the relative merits of the different approaches, by looking across lots of products.

One of the problems with this approach is that it would be very expensive. Dental materials research is not well funded; medical research funding bodies have many demands on their resources, and how long a filling lasts does not (quite reasonably) attract the same support and attention as cancer treatments or cardiovascular disease. To do this properly would be a major investment, and who is going to make that investment? Dental materials manufacturers sometimes fund research, but they are not likely to be keen to fund research where their materials are lumped in with everybody else's. They might be better, but the data will never let us find out!

Another problem is the diversity of products – if we aggregate data across a lot of different bonding systems, even those in the same broad category may perform very differently, resulting in data that may have differences buried within but, in aggregate, show everything to look pretty much the same. A third problem is the diversity of the restoration itself, across many patients without strict entry criteria. Yet another problem is the use of many clinicians without standardization and calibration – what if skilled, ambitious, or well-resourced dentists favor one form of dentine bonding system and the more humble, less confident, or less well-resourced practitioner favors another? If one performs better than the other, was that the effect of the clinician's circumstances, or the material?

What this adds up to is a problem for today's modern dental clinician. We are all taught to ensure our practice is evidence-based, but what if the evidence is not available? Ultimately there is no simple answer. Some clinicians are by nature 'early adopters', keen to try out new technologies. For these, the best advice we can give is to critically and thoroughly scrutinize the marketing claims of any new bonding products and weigh them up against your understanding of the science – is what they say plausible? Is there anything that is important about the performance of dentine bonding systems they *don't* mention? If so, you might wonder why. Other clinicians are 'late adopters' or even what is – in technology terms – unflatteringly termed 'laggards'. Those of us who sit in that category lean toward the 'I've used this for years and it has served me well, so I shan't change just because there is something new for sale'. This approach has merit, not least because older products at least have some data available to augment our own personal experience. But of course, this approach might also hold us back from trying something that could turn out to be quicker, easier, better. Ultimately, the clinician must make the best use of the data they have, combined with their scientific understanding of the underpinning principles and mechanisms, to make the most informed choice they can.

SUMMARY

There are many different dentine adhesive systems, and it is not always straightforward to choose between them. However, since the early days of dentine bonding systems, their clinical performance has significantly improved, such that clinical success with adhesive restorations has become more predictable.

CLINICAL SIGNIFICANCE

When selecting a dentine bonding system, the clinician should look to the data that is available, scrutinize the claims made with a scientifically educated, critical eye, and place value on their own clinical experiences.

FURTHER READING

Armstrong, S.R., Keller, J.C., Boyer, D.B., 2001. The influence of water storage and C-factor on the dentine-resin composite microtensile bond strength and debond pathway utilizing a filled and unfilled adhesive resin. Dental Materials 17, 268–276.

Elkaffas, A.A., Hamama, H.H.H., Mahmud, S.H., 2018. Do universal adhesives promote bonding to dentin? A systematic review and meta-analysis. Restorative Dentistry & Endodontics 43 (3), e29.

Fehrenbach, J., Isolan, C.P., Münchow, E.A., 2021. Is the presence of 10-MDP associated to higher bonding performance for self-etching adhesive systems? A meta-analysis of in vitro studies. Dental Materials 37 (10) 1463–1485.

Perdigao, J., 2020. Current perspectives on dental adhesion: (1) Dentin adhesion – not there yet. Japanese Dental Science Review 56 (1) 190–207.

Peumans, M., De Munck, J., Mine, A., van Meerbeek, B., 2014. Clinical effectiveness of contemporary adhesives for the restoration of non-carious cervical lesions. A systematic review. Dental Materials 30, 1089–1103.

Tay, F.R., Sano, H., Carvalho, R., Pashley, E.L., Pashley, D.H., 2000. An ultrastructural study of the influence of acidity of self-etching primers and smear layer thickness on bonding to intact dentine. Journal of Adhesive Dentistry 2, 83–98.

Van Meerbeek, B., Peumans, M., Poitevin, A., Mine, A., Van Ende, A., Neves, A., et al., 2010. Relationship between bond-strength tests and clinical outcomes. Dental Materials 26 (2), 100–121.

van Noort, R., Noroozi, S., Howard, I.C., Cardew, G., 1989. A critique of bond strength measurements. Journal of Dentistry 17, 61–67.

Endodontic Materials

INTRODUCTION

Endodontics is concerned with the morphology, physiology, and pathology of the human dental pulp and periradicular tissues. Endodontic treatment is aimed at saving the tooth when injury to the pulp and associated periradicular tissues has occurred. Treatments involving the use of dental materials include capping of an exposed vital pulp, sealing of the root canal space when the pulp has had to be removed, and, in the case of badly broken down teeth, reconstruction with endodontic post and core systems (Figure 2.6.1).

VITAL PULP CAPPING

Two main causes of pulpal exposure are:
- dental decay and tooth wear
- accidental exposure during operative procedures or due to trauma.

In each of the above instances remedial treatment is necessary. Clinical treatment planning and the processes that relate to diagnosis and options appraisal are covered in other textbooks relating specifically to endodontics. In this chapter we will briefly define some of the key phrases and then focus on those materials that are used in the various common procedures that the dental student will encounter.

Indirect and Direct Pulp Capping

Sir John Tomes stated in 1859, 'It is better that a layer of discolored dentine be allowed to remain for the protection of the pulp rather than run the risk of sacrificing the tooth'. He had observed that discolored and demineralized dentine could be left behind in deep cavities of the tooth before restoration, often with highly satisfactory results. The removal of this dentine may lead to exposure of the pulp, thus impairing its prognosis. It has been shown that demineralized dentine, if it is free of bacteria, will re-mineralize once the source of the infection has been eliminated. The diagnosis of the presence of demineralized dentine that is caries-free can be assisted by using a caries-disclosing solution. The placement of a suitable material directly on this demineralized dentine is commonly called *indirect pulp capping* (IPC) and a range of materials are available for this purpose, principally variations on mineral trioxide aggregate (MTA) as well as resin-based materials such as resin-modified MTA and resin-modified GIC.

While IPC involves placing material on top of demineralized dentin, direct pulp capping involves the placing of material onto exposed pulp without an intervening layer of dentine. As such, a pulp-capping material has to be suitable to behave as a wound dressing for the pulp. It must not only protect the pulp but stimulate it to produce reparative dentine, thus creating a protective barrier. This is in effect an irritation but, unlike with most materials, it is an irritation that we seek to achieve, as it causes the pulp to do something constructive. While doing so, it must of course only have these irritant effects locally and must have no systemic effects or have sufficient local irritancy such that it compromises the pulp's vitality. The formation of the reparative dentine will take some time and in the interim the capping material must also protect the pulp from bacterial ingress.

> ### CLINICAL SIGNIFICANCE
> The irritant properties of certain dental materials used in direct pulp capping can stimulate the pulp to form a protective layer of dentine.

PULP-CAPPING MATERIALS

Here we consider the main classes of materials used for indirect and direct pulp capping, from the traditional (but still widely used) to the more recent.

Calcium Hydroxide Cements

Calcium hydroxide has been used as a direct and indirect pulp capping material for over 100 years, with some of the earliest attempts being to simply apply calcium hydroxide powder directly to the pulp. It is still considered by some to be the gold standard, or at least the standard comparator, for direct pulp capping. Since its first, very simple, formulation, the product has evolved and is usually supplied either as a powder to be mixed with water or, for convenience, ready-mixed in a syringe dispenser. As well as $Ca(OH)_2$ and water, calcium hydroxide cements often contain a salicylate ester chelating agent and a toluene sulfonamide plasticizer, as well as heavy metal salts such as barium sulfate to provide radiopacity. Resin-modified versions are also available, which consist of calcium hydroxide-filled dimethacrylates, polymerized by blue light in a similar way to the dental composites.

Although the calcium hydroxide cements used today are somewhat more complex than the simple material used in the 1920s and 1930s, the underlying concept is the same. Calcium hydroxide is strongly alkaline, and the high pH irritates the pulp. Ordinarily when a clinician learns that a material is irritating to

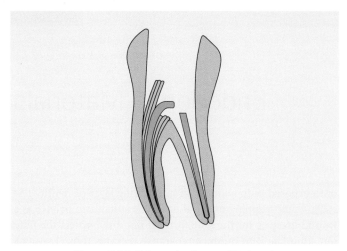

Figure 2.6.1 Schematic of a root-filled tooth

the biological tissues, they would look for an alternative material! Not so with calcium hydroxide – the level of irritation is just what is required to stimulate the formation of a 'bridge' of reparative dentine. When the paste is brought in contact with the pulp, it causes a layer of necrosis some 1.0–1.5 mm thick, whereupon the pulpal cells differentiate and secrete extracellular matrix, which ultimately mineralizes to form dentine. Experiments using radioactive calcium in the paste have shown that the calcium salts necessary for the mineralization of the bridge are not derived from the cement but are instead supplied by the tissue fluids of the pulp. Once the bridge has become dentin-like in appearance and the pulp has been shut off from the source of the irritation, the hard tissue formation ceases. Reported success rates of this approach vary quite widely, although it does appear that pulp exposed by mechanical intervention (trauma, or during surgery) is more amenable to treatment in this way than pulp exposed due to caries.

Silicate Cements

Di- and tri-silicate cements are bioactive materials that also stimulate the formation of reparative dentine due to their high pH and release of calcium ions. Some studies appear to indicate that the thickness of the dentine bridge formed due to these materials is thicker and more uniform than that formed adjacent to calcium hydroxide, with less associated pulpal necrosis. The current products contain primarily two ceramic compounds: tricalcium silicate and dicalcium silicate. Many are based on a mixture commonly known as mineral trioxide aggregate (MTA), a cement composed of tricalcium silicate, dicalcium silicate, tricalcium aluminate, tetracalcium aluminoferrite, calcium sulfate, and bismuth oxide as well as calcium, sodium, and potassium oxides. Its composition is not unlike that of Portland cement (used as a building material in the production of concrete), with the addition of bismuth oxide to impart radiopacity. MTA-based materials are used for a wide range of procedures in endodontics, including root-end filling, repair of perforations and apexification, as well as direct and indirect pulp capping.

MTA is very alkaline (pH ~12.5) and has biological and histological implications similar to those of calcium hydroxide cement. It has been shown that MTA can induce bone deposition with a minimal inflammatory response and is less cytotoxic than reinforced zinc oxide–eugenol cements, which were commonly used prior to the widespread adoption of MTA. The early products were supplied as a powder that was mixed with sterile water to provide a grainy, sandy mixture to be packed into the desired space. Some of the more modern equivalents are supplied in a cartridge with a static mixer tip (similar to those used for silicone impression materials, although much reduced in size). Hand-mixed powder-liquid varieties and versions that can be mixed in an amalgamator or similar device are also used. MTA requires moisture to set, such that absolute dryness is not only unnecessary but also contraindicated. As such, it is important that the instructions for the specific product are followed in relation to tooth preparation; some materials have water as part of the formulation but some do not, and will only set effectively if they can absorb water from the oral environment. For these materials, if the canal is dried to too great a degree, the set will be compromised.

One drawback of MTA is that it can cause discoloration of the teeth, especially if used coronally. Various explanations exist for the cause of the discoloration, including oxidation of bismuth oxide, Bi_2O_3, to the brown-colored salt Bi_2O_4, or alternatively the formation of bismuth carbonate due to reaction with the collagen, or even the oxygen-poor environment leading to the bismuth oxide being converted into metallic bismuth. Whatever the precise mechanism(s), the consensus would appear to be that it is the bismuth oxide that is the culprit, and varieties that contain alternative radiopacifying agents such as calcium tungstate or zirconium oxide go some way to getting around this undesirable outcome.

Since the early days of the use of MTA materials in endodontics, there have been attempts to modify the materials and build on the successes of the initial Portland cement-like materials to address some of their shortcomings. In particular, the use of synthetic silicate salts rather than naturally derived ones offers the opportunity to modify the properties of the finished material as the manufacturer is not limited by what natural materials are available in sufficient quantity and consistency to make them suitable for manufacturing purposes. Synthetic materials allow the manufacturer to have greater control over the composition including what trace elements are present. In formulating these next-generation MTA-like materials the principal focus would appear to have been on handling properties, with many exhibiting a faster setting process than the more conventional MTA materials.

Resin-Based Pulp Capping Materials

Resin-based dental materials first found widespread adoption in dental composites and, as has been discussed elsewhere in this book, their properties were sufficiently favorable that they have since been introduced to other materials in the hope that these would also benefit. This is the case with MTA, and resin-containing varieties have developed. While the resin-modified MTA offers some predictable benefits such as reduced solubility and a degree of on-demand curing, unfortunately, data appears to indicate that these materials stimulate less, or at least delayed, formation of reparative dentine than the more conventional resin-free materials. As such, it remains to be seen whether these materials stand the test of time as they are and/or are developed further to elicit a more favorable pulpal response.

There was much excitement a few years ago about the prospect of using dentine bonding agents as pulp capping materials. After all, these materials are designed to adhere to the relevant tissues forming a lasting bond with excellent sealing; it is not surprising that someone thought to apply this in endodontic practice. Unfortunately, this initial excitement was comparatively short-lived as a series of studies in the early 2000s comparing commercial dentine bonding agents with calcium hydroxide found that they were inferior to calcium hydroxide in this regard, and most attributed this to the cytotoxicity of the monomers used in the dentine bonding agent and the adverse effects of these on the pulp. These monomers can have an acute effect prior to and during to setting, when they are present as the majority of the resin, but they can also have a chronic effect, as even a polymerized resin has a finite degree of conversion and some monomers will remain. These monomers can under some circumstances leach out and thus continue to irritate the pulp. As such, dentine bonding agents have not found as much application as pulp capping materials as was once hoped.

Another resin-based material has emerged as a promising candidate. Methyl methacrylate (MMA), familiar as the starting component of denture base resin polymethyl methacrylate (PMMA), finds extensive use in another application requiring somewhat more stringent biocompatibility properties. Bone cements, used for both structural purposes and for delivering antibiotics to the site of an orthopedic intervention, are largely based on MMA. MMA-based materials have been reported to elicit less of a cytotoxic effect than the resin monomers used in most dentine bonding systems and as such may prove a more suitable basis for a resin-based pulp capping material, but at the time of writing, calcium hydroxide and the MTA or MTA-like materials dominate the market.

Failure After Direct Pulp Capping

Failure after direct pulp capping can be due to three reasons:
- *Chronically inflamed pulp.* There is no healing effect on inflamed pulp, and in such situations a full pulpectomy is indicated.
- *Extra-pulpal blood clot.* Such a blood clot prevents contact between the healthy pulpal tissue and the cement and interferes with the wound-healing process.
- *Restoration failure.* If the restoration fails to provide a bacterial seal, then coronal ingress of bacteria can lead to failure.

It is important to distinguish the last of these failures from the others, as it is not, strictly speaking, a failure of pulp capping. The outcome of direct pulp capping with calcium hydroxide cement can be unpredictable, which may be related to the importance of achieving direct contact between the sealant and the pulp tissue without any intervening blood clot. It has been found that iatrogenic pulp exposures treated with MTA and related bioactive cements are generally free from inflammation

one week after placement and a hard tissue bridge will form over a period of about 3 weeks. Thus it would appear that these cements generally have excellent sealing abilities and prevent pulpal inflammation by providing a predictable secondary barrier under the surface seal provided by the restorative material.

CLINICAL SIGNIFICANCE

The long-term success of direct pulp capping not only depends on the reactions induced locally to the pulp by the pulp-capping material but also is crucially dependent on the practitioner being able to make certain that micro-leakage will not occur and the marginal seal is maintained.

ROOT CANAL FILLING MATERIALS

The objectives of non-surgical endodontic treatment are:
- *to provide a clean canal.* The aim is to produce a reduction of bacteria to a non-pathogenic level.
- *to provide an 'apical seal'.* This prevents the ingress of fluids at the apex of the root, such that it prevents the entry of nutrients that would sustain any remaining canal bacteria, and also prevents irritants from leaving the canal and entering the periapical tissues.
- *to provide a 'coronal seal'.* This prevents recontamination due to the ingress of oral microorganisms.

A wide variety of materials have been used in an attempt to produce an impervious seal of the tooth root apex. The most widely used root canal–sealing materials are a combination of root-obturating points and canal-sealer cements.

Obturating points
Gutta percha

Gutta percha is a naturally derived material: a rubber that is tapped from trees of the *Palaquium* genus and sourced from tropical regions including the Malay peninsula, Indonesia, and Sumatra, as well as parts of South America. It was introduced into the UK in 1843 and has been used in dentistry for almost 180 years. Rubbers are polymers of isoprene (2-methyl-1,3-butadiene), and isoprene is a geometric isomer, which means that it can have different structural arrangements despite having the same composition, as depicted in Figure 2.6.2. When the CH_3 group and the H atom are positioned on the same side of the isoprene mer, this is termed a *cis* structure and the resulting polymer, *cis*-isoprene, is known as *natural rubber*. When the CH_3 group and the H atom sit on opposite sides of the isoprene mer, this is termed the *trans* structure and *trans*-isoprene polymer is commonly referred to as *gutta percha* Figure 2.6.3. The effect on the properties of these different configurations of the polymer is quite profound. In the *cis* form the hydrogen atom and methyl group prevent close packing such that the natural rubber is amorphous and consequently soft and highly flexible, whereas the gutta percha crystallizes and usually becomes about 60% crystalline, forming a hard, rigid polymer.

The natural rubbers are soft and tacky unless they are hardened by *vulcanization,* a process discovered by Charles Goodyear in 1839. Vulcanization involves heating the polymer with a few percent by weight of sulfur. The hardening occurs because

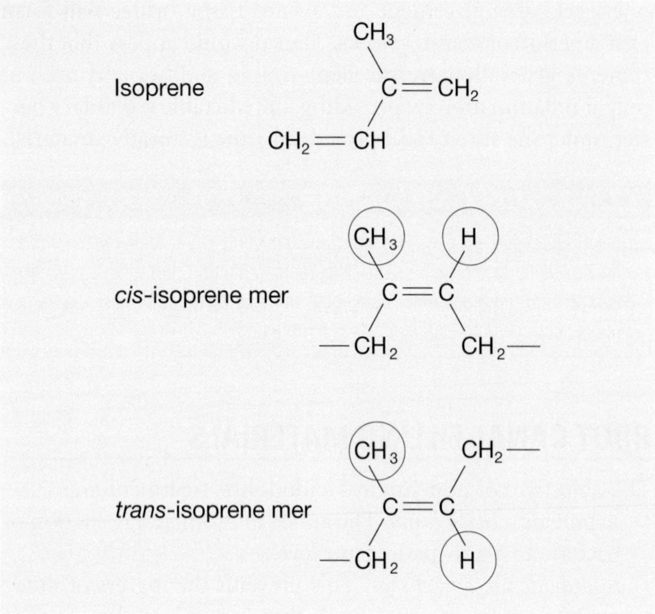

Isoprene

cis-isoprene mer

trans-isoprene mer

Figure 2.6.2 The structure of isoprene and the *cis*-mer and *trans*-mer of isoprene, on which natural rubber and gutta percha are based

sulfur bridges or *cross-links* form between the polymer chains, preventing the polymer molecules from slipping over one another.

Gutta percha is a thermoplastic material and softens at 60–65°C; it will melt at about 100°C, so it cannot be heat-sterilized. Some gutta percha points are supplied pre-sterilized; if necessary, disinfection can be carried out in a solution of sodium hypochlorite (5%). The use of solvents such as acetone or alcohol should be avoided, as these are absorbed by the gutta percha, causing it to swell. Eventually, the gutta percha will return to its unswollen state, thus compromising the apical seal. On exposure to light, gutta percha oxidizes and becomes brittle. It is therefore important to check that the points have retained their flexibility before using them.

The gutta percha can take up two distinct conformations. At high temperatures, the gutta percha chains take on an extended conformation, which can be preserved if cooled rapidly so that it forms the crystalline β-phase, whereas when the gutta percha is cooled more slowly, the denser α-phase is formed (see Figure 2.6.3). The α-phase gutta percha has better thermoplastic characteristics and is therefore preferred for use in hot gutta percha application systems, where heat-softened

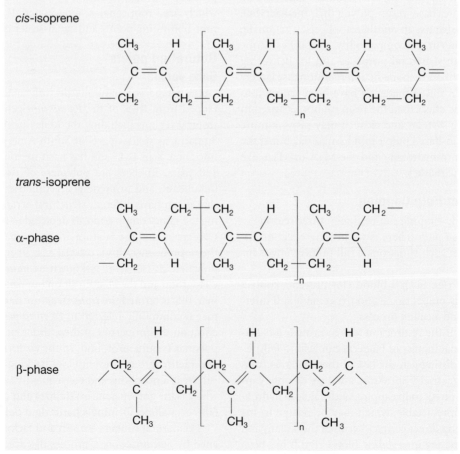

Figure 2.6.3 The structure of cis-isoprene (natural rubber) and the α-phase and β-phase of trans-isoprene of gutta percha

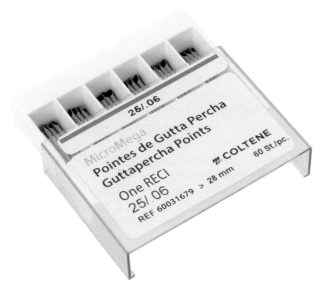

Figure 2.6.4 Gutta percha points. Image courtesy of Coltene Group with thanks.

TABLE 2.6.1 **Composition of Gutta Percha Points**		
Constituent	**Amount (%)**	**Purpose**
Gutta percha	19–22	Rubber
Zinc oxide	59–75	Filler
Heavy metal salts	1–17	Radio-opacifier
Wax or resin	1–4	Plasticizer

gutta percha is injected into the root canal filling, often using injection guns to aid the delivery of softened gutta percha. However, in the presence of a patent apical foramen, there may be a predisposition for extrusion of filling material beyond the apex.

While injectable gutta percha has its uses, the material is mostly employed in the form of gutta percha *points*: long, thin, tapered lengths of material available in an array of sizes to suit the canal (Figure 2.6.4). The points are softened and compacted by warm vertical and lateral condensation. The composition of commercially available gutta percha obturating points will vary from product to product, but typical values are shown in Table 2.6.1. The additional ingredients are added to overcome the inherent brittleness of the rubber and to make it radiopaque.

Other Materials Used for Endodontic Points

In an interesting departure from gutta percha, which has been around for a very long time, a root canal point consisting of a thermoplastic polyester polymer became available in the early 2000s and elicited a flurry of research. The central thesis was that a pair of mutually compatible materials, a point and an associated sealer, would set to form a 'monoblock', a single continuous phase to seal well to the tooth and prevent any ingress of bacteria. It was sometimes referred to as 'resin percha'. Unfortunately, the material did not stand the test of time as it was found, first *in vitro* and ultimately *in vivo*, to break down over

time and compromise the integrity of the root canal restoration. As such, the material, while showing early promise, failed to take hold and is no longer available. A salutary lesson when considering new and exciting dental materials: sometimes they fulfill their potential, but sometimes the tried-and-tested is the best option.

A wide range of metals and alloys, including gold, tin, lead, titanium, and silver, has also been used as root canal filling materials. Silver points were used extensively for a period because of their bactericidal effect. However, the rigidity of alloys made it impossible to adapt the points closely to the canal wall and greater reliance had to be placed on the cements used to provide the seal. The silver, the most popular and widely used of the metal options, also tended to corrode, which could give rise to apical discoloration of the soft tissues, and they were problematic to remove. These and other metal points have now largely been withdrawn from use.

Root Canal Sealer Cements

Obturating points are used in conjunction with sealer cements, which fill the spaces around the points and form as tight a seal as possible, preventing the ingress of fluids or bacteria to the root canal. It is recognized that a fully hermetic seal is probably an unrealistic expectation, and as such it has proven necessary to also incorporate a degree of antibacterial properties to sealer materials, to mitigate against infection. Sealers also lubricate the gutta percha points during compaction and fill canal irregularities and lateral canals. The use of root canal cements *without* obturating points is contraindicated, since when used in bulk, the cements either are too soluble or shrink excessively on setting. Additionally, it is difficult to gauge when, or if, the canal is adequately filled, and there is a danger that the cement may pass beyond the root apex into the surrounding tissues.

Along with the standard properties required of almost any dental material; that is, that they should be easy and convenient to store, handle, and use and that they should be biocompatible and radiopaque; it is also necessary for root canal sealing materials to have suitable viscosity to flow as a thin film, to not be prone to producing bubbles when mixed or dispensed, and to not be soluble in the root environment such that the seal could be compromised over time. It is also necessary for the material to have some degree of antimicrobial properties, as even with the most stringent cleaning, the root is very unlikely to be free of bacteria altogether, and those remaining must not be permitted to thrive and multiply.

A wide variety of materials are used as root canal sealers. We will discuss some of the most commonly used materials in detail and briefly summarize some of the alternatives that have emerged more recently and show promise.

Zinc Oxide–Eugenol-Based Cements

Zinc oxide–eugenol cements have been used as root canal sealers for many decades and, as such, represent one of the most tried-and-tested options available to the clinician. The reader is familiar with some uses of cements based on zinc oxide and eugenol, as discussed in Chapter 2.4, and these materials require some modification for use as root canal sealers, in order to impart antibacterial properties, provide radiopacity, and improve adhesion to the walls of the root canal.

As with zinc oxide–eugenol cements used for cavity liners and temporary fillings, some of the sealers are presented as a powder and a liquid which are to be mixed to form the cement. The complete list of ingredients of one widely used material (based on a formulation originally proposed in 1931!) is presented in Table 2.6.2. The powder is predominantly zinc oxide, to which silver is added to increase the radiopacity. The resin acts as a plasticizer and the iodide as an antibacterial agent.

The problem with this formulation is that the silver is prone to causing discoloration of the dentine. This is problematical particularly in the coronal access cavity and affects the appearance of the tooth. Formulations such as Grossman's Sealer (Table 2.6.3) replace the silver with barium or bismuth compounds.

The particle size of the above preparations is fairly large and tends to produce a gritty texture to the resultant mix unless it is thoroughly spatulated. To overcome this, paste–paste systems have been developed and are very popular. The typical constituents of such a root canal sealer are presented in Table 2.6.4. The zinc oxide–eugenol-based materials remain popular even after many decades of use owing to their predictable performance,

due in part to their antibacterial properties, long working time, and low cost.

Resin-Based Sealers

The attraction of resin systems is that these materials can readily be formulated in such a way that they have a rapid setting time and yet maintain a sufficiently long working time. Also, these products do not contain coarse powders, so they have a very smooth texture.

One example is an epoxy–amine resin (AH Plus, DeTrey, Germany), for which the composition is shown in Table 2.6.5. The resin sets by an addition polymerization reaction after the two pastes are mixed. The diepoxide, a diglycidyl ether of bisphenol-A, and an amine, either 1-adamantane amine or N,N'-dibenzyl-5-oxanonane-diamine-1,9, react to form oligomers with epoxy and amino end-groups, which can then react with other monomers or oligomers, as shown in a simplified form in Figure 2.6.5. This produces a highly flexible thermoplastic polymer of high dimensional stability, although still subject to polymerization shrinkage. The addition polymerization reaction takes several hours and thus provides a long working time. The radiopaque fillers ensure that the material has a high radiopacity, even when applied in thin layers. Viscosity is controlled by

TABLE 2.6.2 Composition of a Zinc Oxide–Eugenol Cement Based on Rickert's Formulation

Powder	%	Liquid	%
Zinc oxide	34–41	Oil of cloves	78–80
Silver	25–30	Canada balsam	20–22
Oleoresin	16–30		
Dithymoliodide	11–13		

TABLE 2.6.3 Composition of Grossman's Sealer (Grossman)

Powder	%	Liquid	%
Zinc oxide	42	Eugenol	100
Staybelite resin	27		
Bismuth subcarbonate	15		
Barium sulfate	15		
Sodium borate	1		

TABLE 2.6.4 Composition of Tubli-Seal (Kerr Mf. Co, USA)

Base	%	Catalyst
Zinc oxide	57–59	Eugenol
Oleoresin	18–21	Polymerized resin
Bismuth trioxide	7.5	Annidalin
Thymol iodide	3–5	
Oils and waxes	10	

TABLE 2.6.5 Composition of AH Plus (Dentsply DeTrey GmbH, Germany)

Paste A	Paste B
Epoxy resin	1-adamantane amine
Calcium tungstate	N,N'-dibenzyl-5-oxanonane-diamine-1,9
Zirconium oxide	Tricyclodecane (TCD)-diamine
Aerosil	Calcium tungstate
Iron oxide	Zirconium oxide
	Aerosil
	Silicone oil

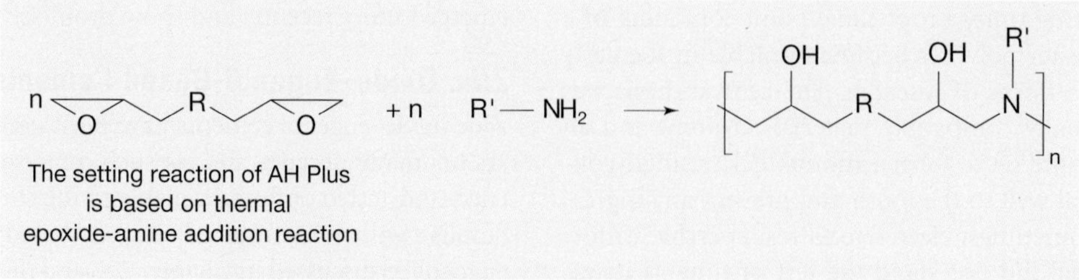

The setting reaction of AH Plus is based on thermal epoxide-amine addition reaction

Figure 2.6.5 The setting reaction of AH Plus

TABLE 2.6.6 Composition of Sealapex (Kerr Mf. Co, USA)			
Base Paste	**%**	**Catalyst Paste**	**%**
Calcium hydroxide	46	Barium sulfate	39
Sulfonamide	38	Resin	33
Zinc oxide	12	Isobutyl salicylate	17
Zinc stearate	2	Colloidal silica	6
Colloidal silica	2	Titanium dioxide	4
		Iron oxide	<1

the amount (>76% by weight) and type of filler. Filler particle size averages out at less than 10 μm to ensure a thin film thickness and provide a smooth consistency. The main problem with these resins is the amount of shrinkage that takes place on setting, which can compromise the apical seal.

Calcium-Hydroxide-Containing Cements

Calcium hydroxide-containing sealer cements are usually presented in a paste–paste form and contain a resin similar to those used in the two-paste resin composites, to which calcium hydroxide is added as a filler in place of the more usual glass fillers. The composition of one of these materials is presented in Table 2.6.6.

Calcium hydroxide–containing cements present something of a quandary in terms of endodontic materials. For the calcium hydroxide to have any beneficial effects in terms of antibacterial effects and stimulation of the formation of reparative dentine, it must dissolve, releasing its hydroxyl ions, which are the cause of the high pH. However, we require root canal sealers to be *insoluble* – a sealer that is soluble is of no use, as the seal is broken as soon as the material starts to dissolve. As such, calcium hydroxide–containing root canal sealer cements must contain some form of insoluble component, but this then compromises or prevents the release of OH⁻ ions.

The data on calcium hydroxide-containing root canal sealer cements is somewhat limited; much of it is *in vitro* and provides conflicting evidence. As such, it is still unclear to what extent the need to balance OH⁻ release and insoluble properties has compromised the clinical usefulness of these materials.

Glass Ionomer Cements

GICs were discussed at length in Chapter 2.3. Briefly, therefore, they consist of a fluoro-alumino-silicate glass, which is reacted with a polycarboxylic acid. Since GICs show low shrinkage on setting and possess the ability to bond directly to dentine and enamel, it is entirely logical that these were explored as potentially very good root canal sealers.

The GICS used for restorative and lining purposes needed to be modified to render them suitable for endodontic applications. The restorative materials have too short a working time for root canal purposes, and their handling properties make them difficult to transport the material to the root canal and adapt it to the root canal wall. There are products available that overcome these difficulties largely by adapting the particle size distribution as well as aspects of the formulation chemistry, with suitable viscous flow properties and setting times in the region of a few hours rather than the under 2 minutes typically seen with restorative glass ionomer materials.

Polydimethyl Siloxanes

This root canal sealer is essentially a variant on the addition-cured polyvinylsiloxane impression materials, consisting of a polydimethylsiloxane, silicone oil, paraffin-base oil, a platinum catalyst, and zirconium dioxide (see Chapter 2.7). The delivery system ensures a homogeneous mix, free of air bubbles, and the rheology can be carefully controlled by the addition of the appropriate amount of filler. The small filler particle size ensures that this material has excellent flow properties and can achieve a film thickness of 5 μm, which allows the sealer to flow into tiny crevices and tubules. As with the impression materials, the root canal sealer is insoluble and dimensionally stable and has excellent biocompatibility. One concern is that this root canal sealer has neither the ability to bond to dentine nor any antibacterial properties. It relies for its seal on the ability to adapt to the root canal wall and, according to the manufacturer, undergoes a slight expansion (0.2%) on setting. Further studies, especially clinical data, are needed to confirm the suitability of this product as a root canal sealer.

Di- and Tri-Calcium Silicate Cements

Di- and tri-calcium silicate cements were discussed in detail in the context of pulp capping materials, and these same materials can be used to good effect as a root canal sealant. These materials tend to exhibit more solubility than the resin-based materials, although the international standards do permit some slight dissolution and whether the silicate cements exhibit more than this threshold is not yet clear.

IMPORTANT PROPERTIES OF ROOT CANAL MATERIALS

Most dental materials are in contact with oral tissues, but these are protected by epithelia. Root canal materials are in contact with living biological tissue that is *not* protected by any epithelial layer, and as such, the biocompatibility requirements are even more stringent than for other dental materials. Their physical properties, relevant to the production of an apical seal, are also a major consideration.

Biocompatibility

It is easy to assume that for a material to be biologically acceptable, it must be as inert as possible. However, as we have already seen elsewhere in this book, this need not always be the case. Some materials are inert in the oral environment, but others are bioactive, interacting with the tissues and fluids of the mouth in such a way as to elicit a favorable or useful response. This is very different from complete lack of interaction in the case of an inert material. For a bioactive material, we must consider both the nature of the interaction in the specific context of the use of the material (e.g. the difference between applying the material in the crown or the root) and also the effect of the interaction *on the material itself*. In relation to the latter point, it is all very well if a material releases ions that stimulate the formation of reparative dentine, for instance, but if in releasing the ions, the material loses integrity and starts to crumble or dissolve away, this may render it useless. We must consider both the interaction and the implications of this for the biological system *and* the material itself.

When a sealer is placed at the apex of a root canal, it will be in contact with vital tissue. It is important that the material does not elicit an inflammatory response in the tissues, as this may induce irritation, pain, or tissue necrosis. All of these responses are likely to lead to the loss of the tooth, which is just the opposite of the intended outcome. A possibly beneficial response would be the formation of an intermediate layer of hard tissue that not only isolates the foreign material from the living tissue but also helps to improve the quality of the apical seal.

A perennial problem in endodontic treatment is the likelihood of recurrent infection due to the presence of bacteria at the apex of the tooth. Thus another feature one seeks in a root canal sealer is the ability to kill bacteria.

As might be imagined, it is difficult to reconcile these two requirements, as they would require a high degree of selectivity in the biological response. In general, materials that show antibacterial properties also induce some inflammatory response in the local tissues, while those that do not elicit an inflammatory response are, at best, bacteriostatic.

If it is accepted that a perfect seal *cannot* be achieved, the materials used must have sufficient antibacterial activity to prevent bacteria from infiltrating the canal space and proliferating. However, the antibacterial property of a material should not be achieved at the expense of its biocompatibility.

Gutta percha is a highly biocompatible material, having such a low cytotoxicity that it is the cements that are used with it that will determine the tissue response.

The zinc oxide–eugenol-based cements are all inclined to induce some inflammatory reaction in the tissues, probably due to the presence of free eugenol. It is therefore important that measures are taken to ensure that the cement does not leak beyond the apex and into the vital tissues.

The resin systems should have comparatively excellent biocompatibility, as none of them contains the eugenol that contributes to the poor biocompatibility of the zinc oxide cements. Resins are known to be slightly toxic during the setting period but, once they have fully set, any inflammation rapidly recedes, a fact often ignored when interpreting research findings that focus on the very initial phase of use of the material, and not the longer term.

For the calcium-hydroxide-containing resins, it is claimed that, in addition to the excellent biocompatibility, the material promotes cementum formation, similar to that observed for the pulp-capping agents based on calcium hydroxide. However, as noted above, the data on these materials is not yet conclusive.

Sealing Properties

One of the difficulties in interpreting the information available on sealing properties is the lack of any standardized approach to the methods of measurement adopted, as this limits the value of the data available. This is particularly so for studies of the sealing properties, whether in vivo or in vitro, where so many methods have been used that direct comparison is unreliable, and only a general assessment is possible.

First, it is noticeable that there is no clear distinction between the zinc oxide–eugenol cements, the resin-based materials, and the silicate cements. Different studies show one may be better or worse than another, but no clear trend has been demonstrated, and the conditions and models used by researchers differ to a significant degree.

However, it should be appreciated that so much depends on the technique adopted that an acceptable result can most probably be obtained with any of them. As already noted, it is probably more important that an antibacterial seal is achieved than a physical seal, although both would be desirable. A physical seal by itself may not be good enough if the sealant does not provide an antibacterial barrier.

Physical Properties

Since the results of endodontic treatment are so dependent on the operator, it is important to choose a material that has the handling characteristics that most suit the particular individual. The working and setting times and flow properties of the cements determine their handling characteristics, while the film thickness, the solubility, and the dimensional stability are important factors in determining their sealing ability. Viscosity and handling properties vary enormously from product to product, and setting times can be as short as a few minutes or as long as several hours. Even within a category of endodontic sealing materials, there is still likely to be a range of products available with handling and setting properties to suit the individual clinician.

SUMMARY

The ideal of a hermetic seal of the root apex has been abandoned in favor of an antibacterial seal for most of the root canal sealers. Perhaps only the GICs, with their intrinsic dentine-bonding capability, can possibly achieve a hermetic seal. For the present, the view is that an antibacterial seal can be achieved only by the combined use of gutta percha obturating points and root canal sealer cements.

Failure can be due to the presence of residual bacteria as a result of inadequate chemomechanical debridement, especially in inaccessible canals in multi-rooted teeth, and in unsealed lateral canals, or due to the coronal ingress of bacteria. With the currently available materials, it should be possible to obtain an adequate antibacterial seal.

POST AND CORE SYSTEMS

Extensive loss of tooth structure often requires endodontic treatment and, as a consequence, little may be left of the tooth crown. It is sometimes considered that, to rebuild such a tooth, there is a need for some form of reinforcement for the core. The most commonly used methods for reinforcing badly broken down and endodontically treated teeth are pin-retained cores or post and core systems (Figure 2.6.6). However, with regard to post and core systems, there has been passive acceptance of

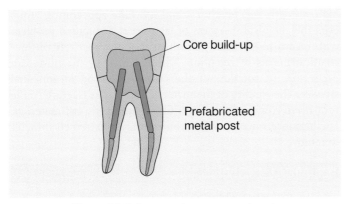

Figure 2.6.6 A post and core restored tooth

- Core build-up
- Prefabricated metal post

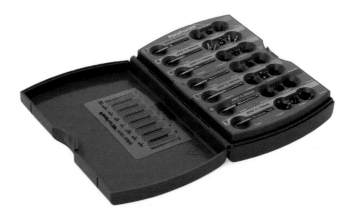

Figure 2.6.7 A set of commercial posts of different sizes. Image courtesy of Coltene Group with thanks.

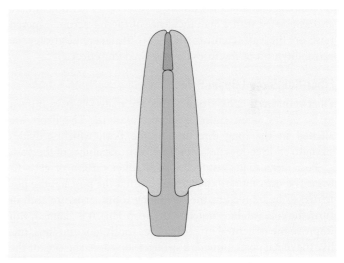

Figure 2.6.8 A cast post and core with ferrule, which is a lip of metal extending back over the preparation.

traditional concepts that have surprisingly little backing; more and more, the status quo is being challenged and some dentists are now asking if a post is really necessary, or if the factor that weakens the tooth is actually the extensive removal of tooth tissue in preparation for that post. It is not a consequence of embrittlement of the dentine, as was once thought, since the root dentine does not significantly change in properties. The fractures often associated with endodontically treated teeth are simply a consequence of the removal of tooth tissue, weakening the tooth structure such that it is no longer able to withstand the forces exerted on it. Although one will often see the post and core system referred to as a means of strengthening the tooth, this is possibly only the case when the post and core are effectively bonded to the tooth tissues such that the structural integrity of the tooth is improved. It is debatable how many, if any, of the current systems can claim to provide this benefit. Hence the function of a post and core system is not primarily to strengthen the tooth but to provide support for the retention of crown or other coronal superstructure, when a significant amount of coronal tooth structure has been lost. If there is sufficient remaining coronal tooth structure, there may be no need for a post and core build-up. However, if most of the supragingival tooth structure is missing, then a post and a core become a prerequisite to crown preparation for anterior teeth; posteriorly, it may still be possible to use a pin-retained core.

The desirable features of a post and core system are that:
- the system provides maximum retention with minimal removal of tooth tissue
- the core provides a means of transferring stress from the restoration to the post and tooth
- the post can transfer the stresses to the remaining tooth structure without creating high stresses that may otherwise cause the tooth to fracture
- the post is retrievable in the case of failure
- the post and core system is aesthetically compatible with the restoration.

Types of Post System

Posts are either prefabricated or cast. In the case of the prefabricated post the core can be built up with one of a range of core materials (amalgam, composite, GIC, RMGIC). For the cast post, it is usual to use a prefabricated plastic blank, and the core

can be incorporated with the blank such that the post and core are cast as a single unit. Whereas, at one time, a cast post and core would have been the system of choice, these days, many dentists prefer some form of prefabricated post (Figure 2.6.7). The advantage is that the procedure is much quicker, simpler and cheaper than providing a cast system. The latter takes two appointments to complete and also requires the production of temporary restorations. However, cast post and core systems act as a single unit and can be cast with a ferrule (Figure 2.6.8), which supports the tooth against wedging forces and helps to prevent tooth fracture.

Prefabricated Posts

The types of prefabricated posts available are:
- metal posts
- fiber-reinforced resin posts
- ceramic posts.

Metal Posts

Metal prefabricated posts are made from stainless steel, nickel-chromium, or titanium. The choice of these metals reflects the desire to use metals that have good corrosion resistance and a high yield strength. The posts come in a wide variety of designs and may be parallel sided or tapered, and threaded or non-threaded.

It is impossible in a textbook such as this to cover in detail all the different designs of post systems that are available. Briefly, the post should be as long as possible without infringing on the apical 4–5 mm of the root canal seal. The post diameter should be as narrow as possible to minimize the removal of tooth tissue while also being sufficiently strong not to fracture. At the same time, the post should be stiff enough not to flex, as this will compromise the marginal seal. Increasing the post diameter will weaken the tooth and make it more liable to fracture. Retentive features, such as threads or surface roughening, can help but it should be noted that threads can give rise to local stress concentrations, which can contribute to tooth fracture. In this context self-threading posts have excellent retention but are also associated with a high incidence of tooth fracture. Tapered posts are the least retentive; the greater the taper, the greater the possibility of root fractures due to a wedging effect.

Fiber-Reinforced Resin Posts

Fiber-reinforced epoxy resin composite materials have proven to be useful as an endodontic post material. The fibers are aligned in the long direction of the post, which provides strength and yet does not compromise the flexibility of the post.

Posts are usually reinforced with either carbon or glass fibers. The use of a resin matrix means that the post has the potential to be bonded to the remaining tooth structure and, in turn, the core can be bonded to the post. This, it is claimed, will improve the structural integrity of the tooth root and thus, unlike the metal posts, provide a stronger support structure for the crown with less chance of root fractures. This alters the requirements of the posts compared to metal posts, since the system acts as a single unit for supporting the crown. Whereas in the case of metal posts, a high stiffness is important in preventing bending, as noted earlier, in the case of fiber-reinforced resin composite posts, the aim is to produce a restoration that, being bonded, acts as a homogeneous unit. The way to achieve this is to use a material with an elastic modulus similar to that of dentine. This would allow a more even stress distribution and should reduce the incidence of tooth fractures.

The carbon-fiber-reinforced posts are black, unless specifically coated to mask the black color. Glass-fiber-reinforced posts have the advantage that, being essentially white or white/translucent, they can produce superior aesthetic results when used in conjunction with all-ceramic restorations.

Ceramic Posts

From the point of view of aesthetics, ceramic posts would seem to show considerable promise. One of the materials that have become popular for such posts is zirconia because of its reputed high strength and toughness and its white appearance. However, the chemical inertness of zirconia is a potential problem with regard to retention and these systems must rely on mechanical means of retention. Dislodgement of the posts can occur due to rotation of the crown, resulting in torsional stresses. The rigidity of the material also makes fracture of the root more common than with fiber-reinforced post materials. Furthermore, once placed, zirconia posts are extremely difficult to remove.

CLINICAL SIGNIFICANCE

With the increasing use of all-ceramic restorations, it is likely that the demand for aesthetic post and core systems will increase. At the current time, it would appear that the fiber-reinforced posts seem to offer the most favorable balance of properties. Metal posts are more tried and tested, while ceramic posts present some fairly significant limitations.

FURTHER READING

rde-45-e35.pdf (nih.gov).

Goracci, C., Ferrari, M., 2011. Current perspectives on post systems: a literature review. Australian Dental Journal 56 (Suppl. 1), 77–83.

Komabayashi, T., Zhu, Q., Eberhart, R., Imai, Y., 2016. Current status of direct pulp-capping materials for permanent teeth. Dental Materials Journal 35 (1), 1–12.

Komabayashi, T., Colmenar, D., Cvach, N., Bhat, A., Primus, C., Imai, Y., 2020. Comprehensive review of current endodontic sealers. Dental Materials Journal 39 (5), 703–720.

Shanahan, D.J., Duncan, H.F., 2011. Root canal filling using Resilon: a review. British Dental Journal 211 (2) 81–88.

Payne, L.A., Tawil, P.Z., Phillips, C., Fouad, A.F., 2019. Resilon: assessment of degraded filling material in nonhealed cases. Journal of Endodontics 45 (6), 691–695.

Mohammadi, Z., Karim Soltani, M., Shalavi, S., Yazdizadeh, M., Jafarzadeh, M., 2014. Calcium hydroxide-based root canal sealers: an updated literature review. Compendium of Continuing Education in Dentistry 35 (5), 334–339.

Mohammadi, Z., Shalavi, S., 2012. Clinical applications of glass ionomers in endodontics: a review. International Dental Journal 62 (5), 244–250.

Browne, R.M., 1988. The *in vitro* assessment of the cytotoxicity of dental materials – does it have a role? International Endodontic Journal 21, 50–58.

Duarte, M.A.H., Marciano, M.A., Vivan, R.R., Tanomaru Filho, M., Tanomaru, J.M.G., Camilleri, J., 2018. Tricalcium silicate-based cements: properties and modifications. Brazilian Oral Research 32 (Suppl. 1), e70.

Olsson, H., Petersson, K., Rohlin, M., 2006. Formation of hard tissue barrier after pulp capping in humans: a systematic review. International Endodontic Journal 39, 429–442.

Primus, C.M., Tay, F.R., Niu, L.N., 2019. Bioactive tri/dicalcium silicate cements for treatment of pulpal and periapical tissues. Acta Biomaterialia 96, 35–54.

Impression Materials

INTRODUCTION

Impression materials are used to produce a detailed replica of the teeth and tissues of the oral cavity. From this replica, or impression, a model can be made that is used in the construction of full dentures, partial dentures, crowns, bridges, inlays and other prostheses and devices. While physical impressions remain the dominant choice, digital impressions are increasing in popularity as systems for taking and using these become cheaper and easier to use. We shall cover digital impressions later in this chapter but will first turn our attention to impression *materials*.

Over the years, a wide variety of impression materials and associated techniques have been developed, all striving to achieve the optimum desirable characteristics. Impression materials can be classified as *elastic* or *rigid* (Table 2.7.1). The rigid impression materials cannot engage undercuts that may be present on the teeth or the bone. Consequently, their use is restricted to edentulous patients without bony undercuts. The elastic impression materials are subdivided into *hydrocolloid* and *elastomeric* impression materials. Both can engage undercuts and may be used in edentulous, partially dentate, and fully dentate patients. The choice will depend on the particular requirements of each individual case.

The choice of impression material may also be affected by the technique to be adopted, with a major consideration being the selection of a stock tray or special tray. These trays are needed to support the impression material when it is still fluid so that it can be carried to the patient, inserted in the mouth, and removed once it is set. The trays also provide support when the model is poured from the impression.

The variety of applications of and techniques used with the impression materials are presented in Table 2.7.2. The choice of impression tray is determined, to some extent, by the viscosity of the impression material.

An impression material that is very fluid when it is first mixed cannot be used with a stock tray, and a close-fitting special tray needs to be produced. This can be done either by constructing a special tray from a preliminary model, or by using a high-viscosity material, which is placed in a stock tray; once this has set, a special tray is produced. Some impression materials such as zinc oxide–eugenol are not available in a sufficiently high-viscosity version for use in a stock tray. Most materials in common use are now available in formulations that *can* be used with a stock tray.

REQUIREMENTS OF AN IMPRESSION MATERIAL

The important characteristics of impression materials can be identified from the point of view of the patient or the clinician (Table 2.7.3).

Accurate Reproduction of Surface Detail

An impression material needs to capture sufficient information about the oral tissues such that the prosthesis that is ultimately made using it can serve its purpose. Quite how accurate that needs to be depends on the application: a crown or bridge requires a higher degree of accuracy than a sports mouthguard or whitening tray. However, *any* application requires a certain minimum level of accuracy; otherwise, the end result will be unsatisfactory.

The accuracy of the reproduction of the surface detail depends on the viscosity of the material and the ability of the impression material to adapt closely to both the soft and the hard tissues. A low viscosity is desirable as this will flow into the smallest of features, but it should not be so low that the material is not easily contained within the impression tray.

Some materials are hydrophobic (water-repellent) and will be repelled by moisture on the surface. If this should happen in a critical area, then important surface detail may be lost as a blow hole is formed on the impression surface due to trapped air. A dry field is essential for such materials. If this is not feasible, an alternative material must be used that is compatible with moisture and saliva. As such, many materials, which are inherently hydrophobic, have components added to them to improve their hydrophilicity and expand their range of uses.

There are instances in which the patient will have mobile soft tissues. This occurs particularly with edentulous patients, who can present with a flabby ridge. If the impression material is very stiff, it may displace such tissues and produce a distorted impression. When this is reproduced in the prosthesis, the soft tissues will need to adapt to the prosthesis rather than the other way around; this will cause discomfort to the patient. Such impression materials are classed as being muco-compressive.

TABLE 2.7.1　Categorization of Impression Materials in Common Use

Elastic Impression Materials

Elastomers	Addition cured silicone, polyether: commonly used
	Condensation-cured silicone, polysulfide: less commonly used
Hydrocolloids	Alginate

Rigid Impression Materials

Plaster

Compo

Zinc-oxide eugenol

TABLE 2.7.3　Requirements of an Impression Material

The Patient	The Clinician
Neutral or pleasant taste and odor	Easily mixed
Short setting time	Short working time
Small/comfortable tray	Easily removed
Easily removed	Good-quality impression
	Low-cost materials
	Easily disinfected

TABLE 2.7.2　Indirect Impression Techniques

Application	Choice of Material	Impression Technique	Choice of Viscosity	Type of Tray
Full dentures	Plaster of Paris	Single stage	–	Stock/special
	Zinc oxide–eugenol	Single stage	–	Special
	Compo/zinc oxide–eugenol	Two stage	–	Stock
	Alginate	Single stage	–	Stock/special
Partial dentures	Alginate	Single	–	Stock/special
	Elastomers	Single	Medium	Special
Crowns, bridges and inlays	Compo	Copper ring	–	–
	Elastomer	Single	Medium	Special tray
		Twin mix	Heavy/light Putty/wash	Special tray Stock tray
		Two stage	Heavy/light Putty/wash	Special tray Stock tray

Impression materials that are sufficiently fluid on placement to prevent displacement of the soft tissues are described as being mucostatic.

Dimensional Accuracy and Stability

Dimensional accuracy is the extent to which the impression accurately reproduces the tissues over the entire area of the impression, whether that is a whole arch or a single tooth. Stability reflects any change in this dimensional accuracy over time. An impression material that shrinks or distorts on setting will have limited dimensional accuracy, and one which changes during storage may have good initial dimensional accuracy but poor stability. In this case the impression must be used to create the model within the limited period during which its dimensional accuracy can be assured.

These two important parameters are dependent on the factors outlined below.

Type of Tray

If the tray is prone to distortion, then the model poured from such a tray will also be distorted. Hence highly flexible trays should be avoided. A good bond between the tray and the impression material is very important. If the impression material comes away from the tray, this will again distort the impression. Manufacturers of impression materials often supply or recommend a suitable adhesive for their material to ensure a good bond. It is important that the manufacturer's instructions are followed to the letter; otherwise, failure of the adhesive bond may result, and care should be taken when mixing manufacturers – using a tray adhesive by one manufacturer with an impression material by another is not necessarily problematic, but compatibility should be checked beforehand. Additional retention may be achieved using perforated trays.

Shrinkage of the Impression Material

Whether the impression material sets by a chemical reaction or some change in physical state, both usually result in some degree of shrinkage of the impression material. Provided the impression material is firmly adhered to the tray, this shrinkage is *away from* the oral tissues and thus increases the space previously occupied by the hard or soft tissues. In the case of a simple crown preparation, the result is a die that is slightly larger than the original tooth preparation (Figure 2.7.1). If the contraction of the impression material is too great, this will result in a loosely fitting crown.

In addition to the changes in dimensions on setting, there is also a slight thermal contraction of the impression material as it cools from mouth to room temperature. Should the balance of this with the setting shrinkage result in a net expansion on setting, then the resultant model will be slightly smaller than the tooth and the crown will not fit. The coefficient of thermal expansion of both the tray and the impression material needs to be small to prevent this from happening. Ideally, an impression material should show a very small contraction ($<1\%$), as this

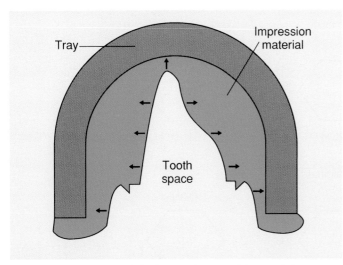

Figure 2.7.1 Shrinkage of the impression material toward the tray resulting in the production of a model which is slightly larger than the original preparation

will result in the production of a crown that is very slightly larger than the situation that it is designed for. This will provide the necessary space for the cement that is to be used.

Plastic or Elastic Behavior Once Set

When an impression is taken of a dentate patient, there will be undercuts due to the bulbous shapes of the tooth crowns. In this case the impression material must be sufficiently flexible to allow removal from the undercut regions without causing distortion; rigid impression materials would therefore be unsuitable. The elastic impression materials must then be used, but, as most are actually viscoelastic materials (see Chapter 1.7), there is a possibility of some permanent deformation.

Storage Stability

There is almost inevitable some delay between the taking of an impression and its arrival in the dental laboratory where the model is poured, and this may be of the order of minutes (when the lab is on site and the technician is ready to receive it) to several days (where the lab is remote and/or the technician has a backlog of tasks to do). It is important that the impression material neither shrinks, nor expands, nor distorts, during this period.

CLINICAL SIGNIFICANCE

Impression materials offer varying degrees of detail reproduction, dimensional accuracy and stability, and also price and ease of use. The clinician must understand the pros and cons of the materials available to make a pragmatic and informed choice.

ELASTIC IMPRESSION MATERIALS

Elastic impression materials are so called because they display elastic behavior once set; that is, the impression can be distorted to some degree, for instance, stretched or bent, and as long as

the stress is not too large or prolonged, it will go on to recover its original shape without permanent deformation.

Most modern elastic impression materials fall into the category of *elastomers* or elastic polymers. The one major exception is *alginate*.

Alginates

Alginate is a *hydrocolloid*. The word colloid is derived from the word *kola*, meaning glue, and *oid*, meaning like. A colloid has a glue-like physical character. The colloidal state represents a highly dispersed phase of fine particles within another phase, somewhere between a solution and a suspension:

- A solution is a homogeneous mixture consisting of a single phase.
- A suspension is a mixture of two distinct phases.
- A colloid is a heterogeneous mixture of two phases, where the two phases are not readily differentiated.

The difference between a colloid and a suspension is that in a colloid the dispersed phase is not readily detectable microscopically. A *hydro*colloid is a colloid where the liquid phase is water. The size of the finely dispersed phase is usually in the range of 1–500 nm. The colloid can exist in the form of a viscous liquid, known as a *sol*, or a solid, described as a *gel*.

The alginates are based on alginic acid, which is derived from algae. The structure of alginic acid is quite complex and is shown in Figure 2.7.2. Some of the hydrogen molecules on the carboxyl groups are replaced by sodium, thus forming a water-soluble salt, with a molecular weight of 20 000–200 000. The setting process in this material is by the creation of cross-links between the polymer chains of the sodium alginate. The composition of a typical alginate impression material is presented in Table 2.7.4.

Setting Reaction

The alginate is supplied as a fine powder (Figure 2.7.3), which is mixed with water. When the powder and water come into contact, a chemical reaction occurs that cross-links the polymer chain, forming a three-dimensional network structure. As these cross-links cannot be broken once formed, this is an irreversible process.

Calcium sulfate dihydrate provides the Ca^{2+} ions for the cross-linking reaction that converts the sol to a gel. The calcium ions are released from calcium sulfate dihydrate, which is partially soluble in the water:

$$(CaSO_4) \cdot 2H_2O \rightarrow 2Ca^{2+} + 2SO_4^{2-} + H_2O$$

The cross-linking mechanism is shown in Figure 2.7.4 and can be described by the general reaction:

$$Na_nAlg + n/2CaSO_4 \rightarrow n/2Na_2SO_4 + Ca_{n/2}Alg$$

| sodium alginate | + | calcium sulphate dihydrate | → | sodium sulphate | + | calcium alginate gel |

The working and setting times are determined by the rate of release of calcium ions and their availability for cross-linking.

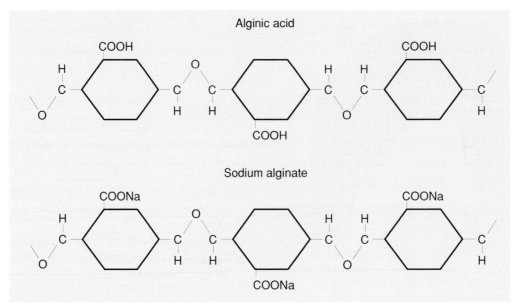

Figure 2.7.2 Structure of sodium alginate with hydrogen ions in alginic acid replaced by sodium ions.

TABLE 2.7.4 Composition of an Alginate Impression Material

Component	Amount (%)	Purpose
Sodium alginate	18	Hydrogel former
Calcium sulfate dihydrate	14	Provides calcium ions
Sodium phosphate	2	Controls working time
Potassium sulfate	10	Setting of model
Fillers (diatomaceous earth)	56	Controls consistency
Sodium silicofluoride	4	Controls pH

Rapid dissolution of the calcium sulfate would give the material an inadequate working time, so to overcome this, sodium phosphate is added to regulate the initial burst of calcium ions. The sodium phosphate acts as a retarder, and the amount included can be varied to produce regular and fast-setting versions of this impression material. Sodium ions are produced by the following reaction:

$$Na_3PO_4 \rightarrow 3Na^+ + PO_4^{3-}$$

The calcium ions will react preferentially with the phosphate ions to form an insoluble calcium phosphate:

$$3Ca^{2+} + 2PO_4^{3-} \rightarrow Ca_3(PO_4)_2$$

Thus the calcium ions that are released initially from the calcium sulfate dihydrate are not available for cross-linking as they react with the phosphate ions. Only when sufficient calcium ions have been released to react with all the sodium phosphate that has been added will the subsequently released calcium ions be free to form cross-links.

There is a considerable pH change on setting, from a pH of 11 to one of about 7. This change in pH has been utilized in some formulations by the incorporation of pH indicators to provide a color change on setting, as a means to assess visually how the setting is progressing.

Properties

These materials are provided as dust-free powders that overcome any potential irritation due to fine dust particles entering the atmosphere and being inhaled. The powder should be mixed thoroughly before use to eliminate the segregation of the components that may occur during storage, and to incorporate the surface layer, which may be contaminated with moisture picked up from the atmosphere. The container must be resealed as soon as the required amount of powder has been removed.

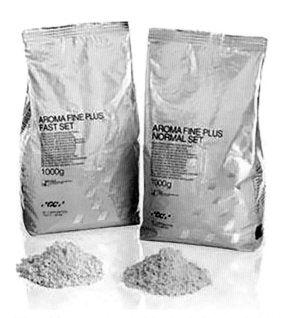

Figure 2.7.3 Alginate powder, which is mixed with water to initiate the setting reaction. Image courtesy of GC Europe.

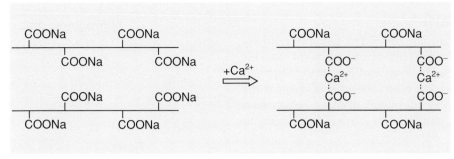

Figure 2.7.4 Cross-linking reaction of sodium alginate in the presence of calcium ions.

The correct proportioning of the powder and water is important, and the manufacturers supply a suitable measuring spoon. Mixing is most easily done in a flexible bowl with a spatula of the type used for mixing plaster and stone, taking care to not introduce bubbles during the mixing.

This material has a well-controlled working time, although this does vary from product to product. The setting reaction is temperature dependent and some clinicians opt to use tepid rather than cold water; this hastens the setting, which is preferable for those patients who find impression taking difficult to tolerate, although care should be taken with this approach; if the water is too warm the alginate may set before it is properly seated in the mouth, and it is rather wasteful, not to say embarrassing, to have to start all over again. Typical values for a regular- and fast-setting alginate impression material are shown in Table 2.7.5. Some clinicians favor – and have access to – automated mixing devices that reduce the time taken for mixing but, of course, these do have an associated cost and space requirement. The clinical setting time can be detected by the loss of tackiness of the surface. The impression should be left in place for 2–3 minutes after the tackiness has gone from the surface.

The surface reproduction with these materials is not as good as that with elastomers, and thus they are not recommended for crown and bridge work, but they are very popular for other applications.

Alginates have poor dimensional stability compared to the elastomers, and the model should generally be poured from the impression as soon as possible after taking the impression, preferably within 10 minutes and, if not, with care to minimize the delay and to store the impression carefully in the meantime. This is because the material is susceptible to:

- Syneresis. This is a process whereby water is forced out onto the surface of the impression as the gel molecules are drawn closer together, with the main driving force being the relief of internal stresses. The water evaporates from the surface and causes the impression material to shrink.
- Imbibition. This is the uptake of water that occurs if the material technique is in too moist/wet an environment. Distortion and swelling of the impression will result if this occurs.

Ideally the model should be poured from the impression straight away, but should this not be possible, the impression material should be kept at a relative humidity of 100% by placing it in a tightly sealed container or bag containing some damp tissue paper nearby (but not in direct contact) to provide a source of water but not to render the impression too wet.

Alginate is highly viscoelastic and a snap-removal technique needs to be employed in order to obtain an elastic response. The amount of compression strain the material may experience on removal from undercuts can be as high as 10%. The permanent deformation in such circumstances may be of the order of 1.5%, which is just about acceptable for the sort of applications in which these materials are used. The permanent deformation can be minimized by ensuring that there are no deep undercuts, as the deeper the undercut, the greater the amount of compression strain. Using a snap removal will ensure that the time for which the material is under compression is as short as possible; this is an advantage because the longer the material is under compression, the greater the amount of permanent deformation due to the viscoelastic nature of the alginates. Some recovery of the deformation will occur once the impression is removed and the compressive load taken off. However, although longer recovery times result in lower permanent sets, this advantage must be offset against the dimensional instability of the material.

The impression must be rinsed after removal from the patient's mouth to remove any saliva, as this will interfere with the setting of the gypsum model. Any surface water should be removed prior to pouring the model, as residual water will dilute the model material and result in a soft surface, which is easily damaged. The alginate should also not be left on the model for too long as it becomes difficult to separate if allowed to dry out. This would result in a poor surface finish, as bits of the alginate are left on the surface of the model. Patient acceptability is generally good with this impression material. The material is cheap but does have a limited shelf life, probably related to water contamination.

TABLE 2.7.5 **A Comparison of Regular- and Fast-Set Alginate**		
	Regular-Set	Fast-Set
Mixing time (minutes)	1	0.75
Working time (minutes)	3–4.5	1.25–2
Setting time (minutes)	1–4.5	1–2

Innovation in Alginates

Although alginate is generally considered a simple, relatively cheap, 'low tech' impression material, it has attracted some innovation that seeks to address some of its shortcomings and expand its range of uses. The most interesting of these are the extended stability, or 'extended-pour', alginates, which have improved dimensional stability, with a reduced propensity to shrink or expand over 5–9 days.

Another quite popular innovation in alginates is 'chromatic' alginates – a rather fanciful name perhaps but it relates to the fact that the setting of the alginate is accompanied by one or more color changes. Products vary according to what the color change(s) signifies but can include an indication of when the material has been appropriately mixed, when it can be placed in the mouth, and/or when it can be removed, indicated by the color of the material at different stages of use, usually triggered by changes in pH.

ELASTOMERIC IMPRESSION MATERIALS

Alginate provides limited reproduction of surface detail and suffers from poor dimensional stability, and this limits its uses. There is a need for an elastic impression material with greater accuracy, a large recoverable deformation, and adequate long-term dimensional stability. These goals can all be met with the elastomeric impression materials.

The elastomeric impression materials are characterized as polymers that are used at a temperature above their glass transition temperature, Tg. The viscosities of these impression materials are governed primarily by the molecular weight of the polymer (i.e. the length of the polymer chains) and by the presence of additives, such as fillers. They are liquid at room temperature, but that can be turned into a solid by binding the long-chain molecules together.

This process of binding the chains to form a three-dimensional network is known as cross-linking (as described in Chapter 1.5) and forms the basis of the liquid-to-solid transition of all the elastomeric impression materials. We will consider two of these in depth: the addition-cured silicones and the polyethers. We will briefly touch on two other elastomeric impression materials: the condensation-cured silicones and the polysulfides. While condensation-cured silicones and polysulfides are still used from time to time, they have become less popular over recent years and have almost – but not quite – been superseded by the addition-cured silicones and polyethers. We will first consider composition, setting, and presentation and will then consider their properties and relative merits.

Polyethers

A simplified version of the polymer structure of a polyether impression material is shown in Figure 2.7.5. The polymer is cured by a reaction with imine end groups. The setting reaction is shown in Figure 2.7.6. There is no by-product associated with this reaction, and therefore the material has fairly good dimensional stability. However, it is inclined to absorb water on storage and must therefore be kept in a dry environment;

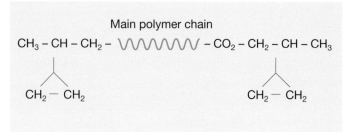

Figure 2.7.5 Structure of a polyether.

certainly, the polymer should never be placed in the same bag as an alginate impression as both will be seriously compromised.

Presentation

The polyethers are supplied as two-paste systems: a base paste (consisting of polyether, a plasticizer such as glycoether or phthalate, and colloidal silica as an inert filler) and an activator paste (consisting of an aromatic sulphonate ester, a plasticizer, and an inert filler). Historically these could only be mixed by hand, but now there are versions that are compatible with automated mixing devices, which brings a degree of convenience, although also at an additional cost. In addition, these materials were previously available only in a single viscosity with an optional thinner to produce a low-viscosity wash, but some manufacturers also now offer different viscosity materials, again adding convenience to this material.

Addition-cured silicones

These materials are based on a polydimethyl siloxane polymer with vinyl terminal groups, as shown in Figure 2.7.7. The setting reaction is via a platinum catalyst and a silanol, as depicted in Figure 2.7.8. An important feature of this setting reaction is the fact that there is no by-product, in contrast to the condensation-cured variety (below).

Presentation

The addition-cured silicones present as a base paste (of polyvinyl siloxane, silanol and a filler) and a catalyst paste (of polyvinyl siloxane, platinum catalyst and a filler). They are commonly supplied in two-barrel cartridges and used with a dispensing 'gun' that extrudes both components into a static mixer or 'tip', a tube with internal filaments that cause very effective mixing (Figure 2.7.9), meaning that the material that comes out of the end is fully mixed with no further mixing required by the clinician. However, since a certain path length is required to achieve this, this is quite a wasteful system, as the material left behind in the tip and the tip itself have to be discarded after each use. Some manufacturers have recently developed shorter path length mixing tips in a bid to reduce waste.

Another common supply method is as two thick pastes that are mixed by hand; this reduces waste but is only suitable for the 'heavy body' and 'putty' options as the lighter body materials are too runny to be handled in this way.

The material is available in a wide range of viscosities, varying from a putty to a heavy-bodied, a medium-bodied, and a light-bodied material. Thus these materials can also be used in a wide range of impression techniques.

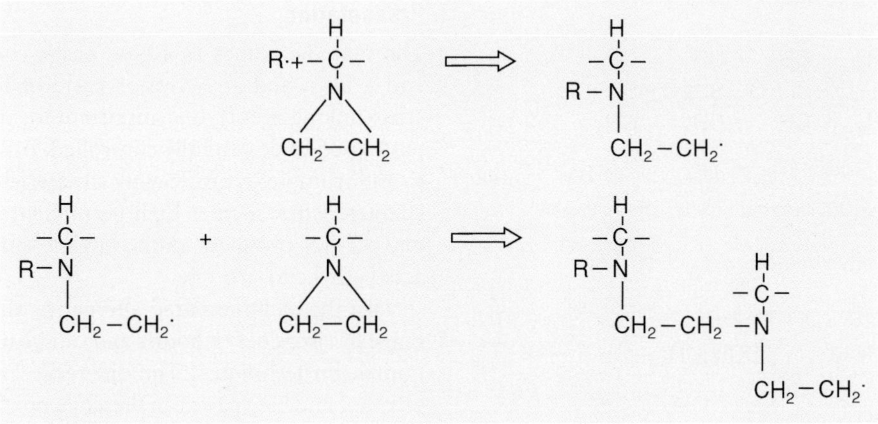

Figure 2.7.6 Cross-linking reaction via the imine pendant groups of a polyether.

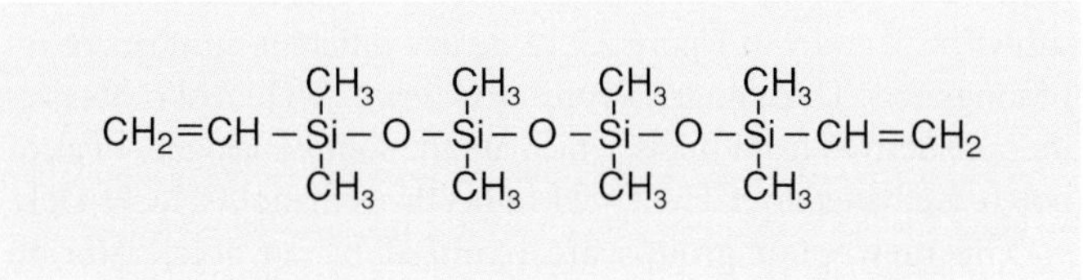

Figure 2.7.7 Polydimethyl siloxane with vinyl end-groups.

If a stock tray is to be used for a single-step impression technique, then there are some addition-cured silicone impression materials, which do not have a tendency to flow when stationary (i.e. when loaded into the tray) but will flow readily under pressure. These are the monophase impression materials.

Relatively recently, an intermediate class of impression material has become available: the polyvinyl ethyl silicone or polyvinyl siloxanether, which combines components of both the polyether and the addition-cured silicone. It has generally been found to have broadly comparable properties to the two parent materials, with (not surprisingly) many parameters falling between the values for the two individual materials, although most data available to date is from laboratory studies. Thus far, there seems scant evidence to significantly differentiate it from either parent material.

Condensation-Cured Silicones

These materials are also based on a polydimethyl siloxane polymer, this time with hydroxyl terminal groups, as shown in

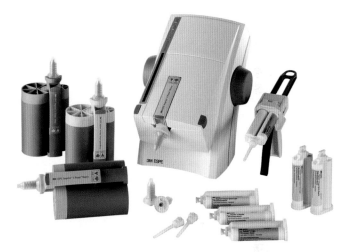

Figure 2.7.9 An example of an addition-cured silicone impression material showing the two-barreled delivery containers and an automated dispensing machine, and a selection of mixing tips of differing lengths. Imprint 4 Family with Pentamix 3 + Garant Dispenser, (2013.02) Courtesy of 3M. © 2023, 3M. All rights reserved.

Figure 2.7.10. Crosslinking is achieved by the use of a tetraethyl silicate (TES), such that as many as three polymer chains can be linked together, as shown in Figure 2.7.11. Three functional groups are needed to form a cross-linking network, as a functionality of two only gives rise to chain lengthening. The by-product of this reaction is an alcohol (R-OH) which has

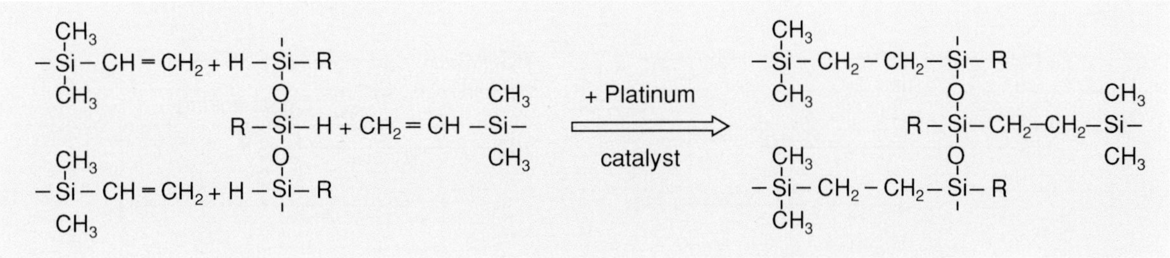

Figure 2.7.8 Cross-linking reaction for an addition-cured silicone impression material.

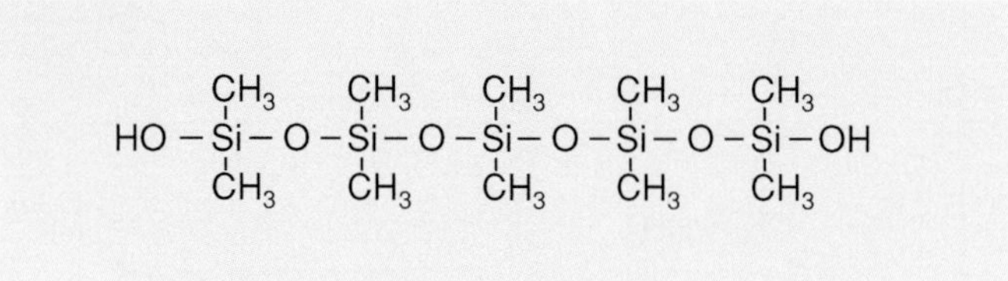

$$HO-\underset{\underset{CH_3}{|}}{\overset{\overset{CH_3}{|}}{Si}}-O-\underset{\underset{CH_3}{|}}{\overset{\overset{CH_3}{|}}{Si}}-O-\underset{\underset{CH_3}{|}}{\overset{\overset{CH_3}{|}}{Si}}-O-\underset{\underset{CH_3}{|}}{\overset{\overset{CH_3}{|}}{Si}}-O-\underset{\underset{CH_3}{|}}{\overset{\overset{CH_3}{|}}{Si}}-OH$$

Figure 2.7.10 Hydroxyl-terminated polydimethyl siloxane.

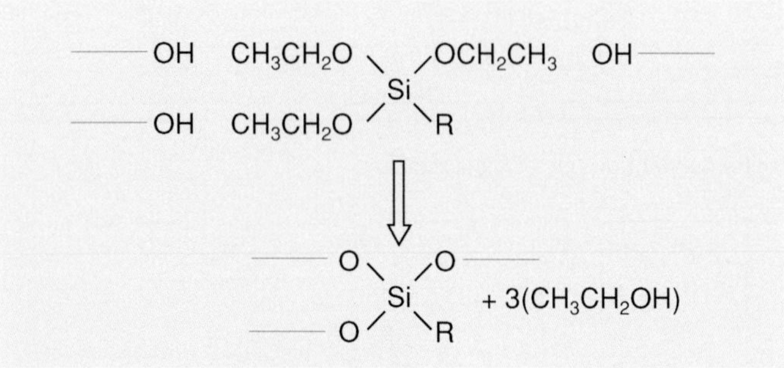

Figure 2.7.11 Cross-linking reaction for a condensation-cured silicone impression material.

unfortunate consequences: the volatile alcohol evaporates under ambient conditions, leading to a shrinkage and warpage of the impression, thus limiting its dimensional stability.

CLINICAL SIGNIFICANCE

The poor dimensional stability of the condensation-cured silicone has meant that clinicians have leaned toward its addition-cured cousin, which does not produce any molecule as a by-product of its setting and thus does not demonstrate this behavior. There are still products that use the condensation-curing method, but these are less common than they once were.

Presentation

The material comes as a base paste, containing silicone fluid and a filler, and an activator paste of tetra-ethyl silicate (the cross-linking agent). It is important for the amount of activator paste used to be carefully controlled. Insufficient TES gives rise to an incomplete cure, leaving a material with poor mechanical characteristics, such as high permanent set. Conversely, an excess of TES also gives an incomplete cure, leaving many unreacted ethyl end-groups.

Like the addition-cured alternative, this material comes in a range of viscosities or bodies and can be used in a wide variety of impression techniques. The difference in viscosity between the activator and base paste can present a problem in that it is difficult to obtain a uniform mix unless a good technique is employed.

Polysulfides

The polysulfide polymer has a molecular weight of 2000–4000, with terminal and pendant mercaptan groups (–SH) (Figure 2.7.12). The subscripts x and y in Figure 2.7.12 denote different numbers of repeating units. These materials are also known as Thiokol rubbers as they are derived from thiols, which are the sulfur analogues of alcohols (e.g. ethanethiol, CH_3CH_2SH, rather than ethanol, CH_3CH_2OH).

The mercaptan groups are oxidized by an accelerator to bring about both chain lengthening and cross-linking, as shown in Figure 2.7.13. This reaction causes a rapid increase in the molecular weight of the polymer, which causes the paste to be converted into a rubber. Water is a by-product of the reaction. The setting reaction is exothermic, with a temperature rise of 3–4°C being typical, although this does depend on the amount of polysulfide used.

Presentation

Polysulfides are presented as a base paste (containing polysulfide and an inert filler, such as titanium dioxide, TiO_2, as 0.3 μm

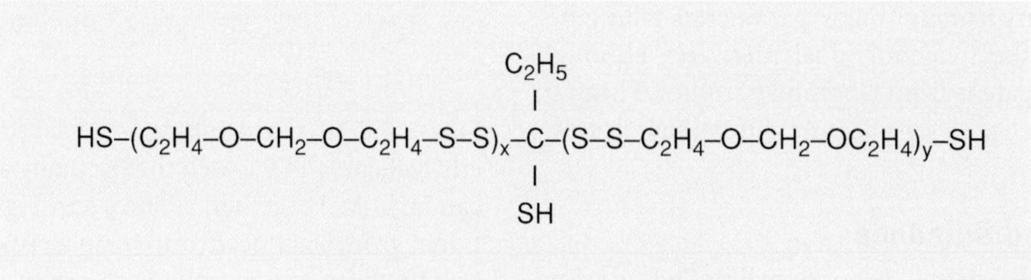

$$HS-(C_2H_4-O-CH_2-O-C_2H_4-S-S)_x-\underset{\underset{SH}{|}}{\overset{\overset{C_2H_5}{|}}{C}}-(S-S-C_2H_4-O-CH_2-OC_2H_4)_y-SH$$

Figure 2.7.12 A typical polysulfide.

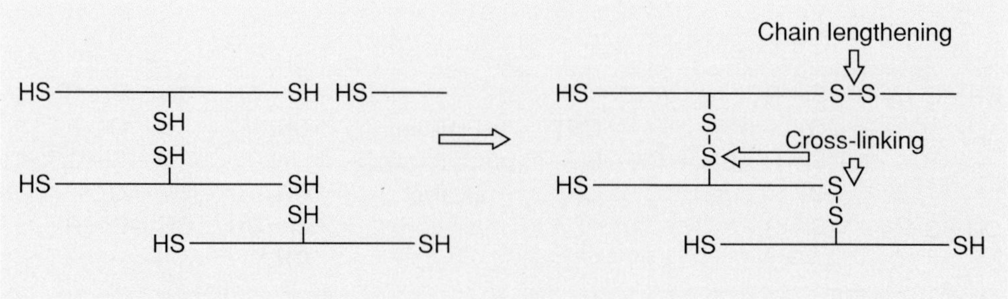

Figure 2.7.13 Cross-linking and chain lengthening of a polysulfide impression material.

particles) and an activator paste (containing lead dioxide, which gives the distinctive brown color, sulfur and dibutyl or dioctyl phthalate). The viscosity of the base paste depends on the amount of filler present, and heavy-, medium- and light-bodied impression paste forms are available. Note that there is no putty version of this impression material, so it must be used with a special tray, using either the medium-bodied material by itself or a combination of the heavy- and light-bodied materials.

The polysulfides have an unpleasant odor due to the mercapto groups. (Small amounts of thiols are added to natural gas to make it easier to detect, and thiols are excreted by the skunk to ward off predators.) The polysulfides are also difficult to clean off clothing if spilled and have certain undesirable mechanical properties such as a high tear strength. When alternative materials are available that do not have these properties, it is not surprising that they have largely fallen out of favor.

> ### CLINICAL SIGNIFICANCE
>
> While polysulfide and condensation-cured silicones are still used from time to time, most clinicians now opt to use either the polyether or addition-cured silicone materials when high precision is required, and alginate when it is not.

RELATIVE MERITS OF THE ELASTOMERIC IMPRESSION MATERIALS

For the reasons described above, polysulfides and condensation-cured silicones will be discussed only to a very limited extent, and we will turn our focus to the addition-cured silicones and polyethers as these now dominate the elastomeric impression materials market.

Handling Characteristics

The setting behavior of the polyether and addition-cured silicone impression materials is generally favorable, with predictable, consistent working and setting times that are provided by the manufacturer. The clinician can choose between regular, fast, and even 'ultra' fast settings to best suit the procedure and patient.

It has been observed that there is an inhibition of the setting of some addition-cured silicone putties when the mixer is wearing latex gloves, probably owing to a sulfur-containing component left on the latex glove as part of the manufacturing process, which interferes with the catalysis that initiates the polymerization of the silicone. The use of nitrile, vinyl, or other gloves overcomes this problem, as does doing the initial mixing with a spatula instead of by hand. The materials are available in a range of working and setting times to suit the particular procedure, patient, and clinician, with typical working times from around 30 seconds to 2–3 minutes, and total setting times ranging from around 2 minutes to over 5 minutes.

The addition-cured silicone impression materials are available in a range of viscosities depending on the amount of filler that is incorporated and include a light-bodied, medium-bodied, and heavy-bodied viscosity and a putty. The mixing of the low-viscosity materials particularly benefits from the use of cartridges combined with dispensing guns, which makes the runny material much easier to handle and avoids the potential for incomplete mixing and the introduction of air bubbles. There are fewer options with the polyethers, although some manufacturers do offer a heavier and lighter body product.

The light-bodied materials are used in the double mix (single-step, two-phase) impression technique in combination with a high-filler-loaded, high-viscosity material (heavy-bodied) in a customized tray. The other use is in the putty/wash (single- or two-step, two-phase) impression technique, where it is used in combination with a very highly filled putty in a stock tray. The medium-bodied material can be used as a single-material, single-step impression technique using a customized tray, or in combination with a light-bodied material in a single-step two-phase technique, again in a customized tray.

Mechanical and Physical Properties
Stiffness

The stiffness of the impression material once it has set can be a major consideration in the ease with which it is removed from undercuts. Earlier high-viscosity impression materials or putties sometimes suffered from excessive stiffness, where removal can be very difficult if the material has been allowed to flow into large interdental spaces. Newer versions of the putties have been introduced that have a lower stiffness once set, the so-called *soft putties*.

Permanent Set

Ideally, when the impression is removed from an undercut, the deformation that results should be totally and immediately recoverable. Elastomeric impression materials are viscoelastic in behavior, so it is important that they are removed from the mouth with a rapid, sharp movement. This will ensure that the impression material is strained for the shortest possible time and that a near-elastic response will be obtained. If the impression is removed slowly, the material will be given the opportunity to flow and not all of the induced strain may be relieved.

The silicones are particularly good at showing virtually no permanent deformation, although polyethers, while they do show more permanent deformation, are generally thought to still lie within acceptable limits.

Tear Strength

The tear strength of the impression material is also important when an impression is taken of the dentate patient. Too low a tear strength, and the impression may break apart while removing it from the mouth, but a high tear strength is not necessarily a good thing, however, as too high a tear strength may give rise to difficulties in removing the impression from the mouth in cases where the impression material has flowed into the interdental spaces. Also, a considerable amount of deformation may occur for materials with a high tear strength before the impression material tears, and this deformation may not be totally recoverable. The tear strength should be sufficient to prevent catastrophic failure, but not so high as to result in excessive deformation or difficulty in removal of the impression.

Accuracy and Reproduction of Detail

It is important that the model of the oral cavity is an accurate three-dimensional replica, since all laboratory work will be based on this model. This is true both at a global scale – the larger dimensions of the tooth or arch – and at a local scale – the fine detail of the tooth surface.

Reproduction of Surface Detail

The elastomeric impression materials reproduce the details of the surface very accurately when a low-viscosity material and the correct technique is employed. The ability to reproduce the surface detail is directly related to the viscosity of the impression material: the lower the viscosity, the better the reproduction. In fact, the reproduction is generally so good that the stone dies are unable to reproduce it.

Factors that give rise to inadequacies in the surface reproduction are generally related to poor technique. For example, great care must be exercised during the mixing of the two pastes to minimize the presence of air bubbles. Air bubbles are not a problem when they are within the bulk of the impression material, but they will present difficulties when close to or at the surface, as detail will be lost. Another problem that may manifest itself is the occurrence of areas where the impression material has not set properly and retains a tacky feel. This is usually due to improper mixing resulting in a non-homogeneous mix.

An impression material's ability to adapt to the surface of the hard and soft tissues is affected by its hydrophilicity: the extent to which it can tolerate a wet surface. Polyethers are not excessively hydrophobic, but silicones are inherently hydrophobic materials, and early versions of these impression materials typically had rather high water contact angles (Chapter 1.9), signifying that they would not adapt well to a surface that wasn't thoroughly dried. The other favorable properties of addition-cured silicones meant that there was ample motivation for researchers and manufacturers to put their minds to this problem, however, and modern silicone impression materials have surfactants added to them to reduce the contact angle to be closer to that of the polyether impression materials.

Dimensional Stability and Accuracy

Besides the problems of distortion, there are also the dangers of expansion and contraction of the impression. While some impression materials have limited dimensional stability (such as the condensation-cured silicones and alginates) and some limited accuracy (such as alginates again, although it is adequate for many applications), with the current versions of the addition-cured silicones and the polyethers, impression materials are most probably as accurate as they will ever need to be. The principal innovation in recent years has been in making their handling and storage more convenient, and some manufacturers are becoming increasingly mindful of the waste associated with impression materials and are trying to address this.

Setting Shrinkage and Thermal Contraction

In general, the setting shrinkage of polyether and addition-cured silicone impression materials is very low. The cross-linking process results in considerably less shrinkage than is usually associated with polymers, as it merely involves a process of linking the pre-existing polymer chains to each other; there is no polymerization shrinkage because there is no polymerization. As mentioned above, the condensation-cured silicones had a significantly higher degree of contraction soon after setting due to the evaporation of the alcohol by-product, and this was a major factor in their being largely replaced by addition-cured silicones.

The thermal contraction of the material is important, as the impression sets at mouth temperature but is handled at room temperature, and any contraction that occurs as a result of that change in temperature must be taken into account. The polyethers have a somewhat higher thermal contraction (320 ppm $°C^{-1}$) than the silicones (200 ppm $°C^{-1}$). Both the setting shrinkage and the thermal contraction are also affected by the amount of filler present, in that the higher the filler loading, the smaller the contraction, and this affects the light-bodied materials the most, as these have the lowest filler loading.

> **CLINICAL SIGNIFICANCE**
>
> The amount of light-bodied material used should always be kept to a minimum, as it exhibits more setting and thermal contraction than the heavy-bodied materials.

Stability on Longer-Term Storage

The polyethers are very stable in storage as long as they are kept dry; if they are placed in a high-humidity environment, they will absorb water and expand. If this occurs, the resultant model is going to be smaller than the original tooth, and a crown produced on such a model will not fit under any circumstances. The addition-cured silicone materials exhibit excellent long-term stability and do not shrink or expand significantly on storage.

> **CLINICAL SIGNIFICANCE**
>
> The addition-cured silicones are extremely stable once set and show virtually no dimensional change on storage. Thus these materials are particularly good to use in situations where duplicate stone dies are needed. Polyethers also show excellent stability but do require dry storage conditions.

IMPRESSION TECHNIQUE

The wide variety of presentations of the addition-cured silicone impression materials provides an opportunity to use various impression-taking techniques. While there are differences in the specific technique, the general principle is that a first impression is taken with a more viscous, putty material which represents the overall anatomy, and this impression is used in conjunction with a less viscous wash material to take a further impression that captures the finer details (Figure 2.7.14). The most popular are putty/wash procedures, which allow the use of a stock tray.

Twin-Mix Technique

In this technique the low-viscosity wash is mixed and placed in a syringe and, while the impression material is placed around

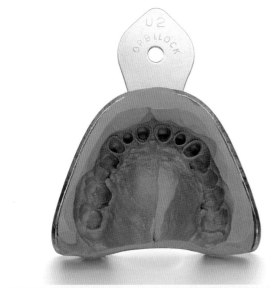

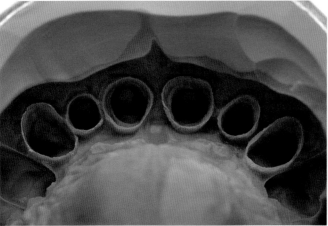

Figure 2.7.14 An example of a two-stage impression showing the viscous putty supporting the less viscous wash material, permitting the capture of the finer details of the tissues of interest. Courtesy of 3M. © 3M 2023. All rights reserved.

those teeth for which an accurate impression is needed, the putty is mixed and placed in the stock tray. The loaded tray is then inserted in the patient's mouth, and the two impression materials are allowed to set simultaneously. There will be some deformation of the impression material on removal, most of which is recovered immediately by a recoil action.

> **CLINICAL SIGNIFICANCE**
>
> The permanent set is a measure of the ability for elastic recovery; the larger the permanent set, the greater the potential for distortion on removal of the impression from the mouth.

If the model is poured virtually immediately, little or no shrinkage (due to cooling and storage contraction) will have taken place, and the resultant model will be only slightly bigger than the tooth. Due to storage contraction (in the case of the condensation-cured silicone), the longer the delay before pouring the model, the larger the model will be. As the addition-cured

silicones are extremely stable on storage, the model will be of the same size no matter when it is poured.

The potential problems with this technique are related to the removal of the addition-cured silicones. Although there are now some softer putties, removal can be difficult if the putty has flowed into the interdental spaces; the larger these are, the more difficult it will be to remove the impression. Another problem that may arise is that the putty may displace the wash in areas where surface accuracy is desirable.

Two-Stage With Spacer Technique

This technique effectively involves the production of a special tray by using the putty first. A primary impression is taken either directly from the oral surfaces or sometimes with a thin cellophane sheet laid over the putty. In the former situation the poor-quality impression of the teeth is then cut out, creating a channel for the wash material. After this, a second impression is produced using the low-viscosity wash, which provides the necessary surface detail. When this method is used with the addition-cured silicones, it avoids the need to remove a stiff putty material from undercuts.

Two-Stage Without Spacer Technique

In this technique the first impression is taken with the putty. Subsequently, the wash is placed around the teeth and in the tray containing the set putty and is reseated in the mouth. The process of reseating in itself can be quite problematic. As a certain amount of space is required by the wash, there will be some compression of the putty to accommodate this.

The excellent recovery of the silicone impression materials means that, immediately after the material has set and is removed from the mouth, there will be a recoil action as the pressure on the putty is relieved. If a model is poured virtually immediately, then for both impression materials the model is likely to be slightly smaller than the tooth. For the condensation-cured silicones, the shrinkage on storage will ensure that, after a delay of 24 hours, this situation will have reversed. However, the addition-cured silicones are so dimensionally stable that the model will always be too small.

Compatibility With Model Materials

The hydrophobicity of some silicone impression materials can make them susceptible to poor wetting by the aqueous slurries of the gypsum-based products used to pour models or dies, which can lead to air bubbles and voids. While this problem has been addressed to some degree by the inclusion of surfactants in the impression material, it has not completely disappeared. One way in which the occurrence of air bubbles and voids can possibly be minimized is by the application of a surfactant to the surface of the impression after it has been disinfected and before pouring the model.

COST AND SUSTAINABILITY OF ELASTIC IMPRESSION MATERIALS

The elastomers are considerably more expensive than alginate, and most clinicians therefore only use them when necessary,

Table 2.7.6 Advantages and Disadvantages of Addition-Cured Silicone and Polyether Impression Materials

Advantages	Disadvantages
Polyethers	
Hydrophilic	High permanent deformation
Good surface detail	Swells in disinfectants or moist environments
Good dimensional accuracy	Difficult to remove
Good resistance to deformation	Low tear strength
Highly acceptable to patient	Care needed when disinfecting
Addition-Cured Silicones	
Good surface detail (dry surfaces)	Hydrophobic (unless surfactant added)
Good dimensional accuracy	Low tear strength
Good storage stability	
Low permanent deformation	
Wide range of viscosities	
Easy to disinfect	
Highly acceptable to patient	

opting for a cheaper option when it will fulfill their clinical needs adequately. The relative merits of the two most commonly used elastomeric impression materials are summarized in Table 2.7.6.

From a sustainability point of view, impression materials differ from most restorative materials in that their use is fleeting: once the impression is taken, the mold poured and used, stored, or scanned, the impression is no longer usually required. As such, there is both the sourcing of the material and the disposal of the finished impression to consider. Alginate is one of the more sustainable dental materials, as algae is a renewable raw material and the end product (the impression) is biodegradable. It has been suggested that it may be possible to recycle alginate impressions for use as a crop fertilizer, and proof of principle has been achieved in research studies, although this has yet to be widely adopted. Silicones, on the other hand, do not have as positive a sustainability profile. For one thing, the mixing tips commonly used lead to a lot of waste – both the single-use tip itself and the material that is lodged within the tip and cannot be used. At least silicones are made primarily from silica, or sand; less of a concern than materials sourced mostly from petrochemicals, although recycling would be challenging and as yet would not appear to be under serious consideration. Little work seems to have been done to develop sustainable and/ or recyclable polyethers for dentistry, although this is gaining attention in other industries and may yet find its way to the dental clinic.

CLINICAL SIGNIFICANCE

From a sustainability point of view, the profile of dental impression materials is not favorable, and researchers, manufacturers, and clinicians will all have their part to play in developing more environmentally sound solutions.

DISINFECTION OF IMPRESSION MATERIALS

The dental team is continually exposed to microorganisms that can cause infections such as the common cold, pneumonia, tuberculosis, herpes, and hepatitis. Cross-infection may occur from the patient to the dentist or hygienist, to the dental surgery assistant, and eventually to the laboratory technician. Thus the whole dental team is at risk, and stringent infection control is paramount.

Dental laboratories will not accept impressions unless there is assurance from the clinician that they have been disinfected. This adds yet another requirement for the successful impression: that the disinfection process must be effective yet not compromise the accuracy or stability of the impression. All the care and attention paid to the taking of a good-quality impression could be totally undermined if the impression should distort during the disinfecting procedure. It is up to the clinician to choose the most appropriate impression material and the associated disinfection procedure.

Disinfectants

Sterilization of impressions is rarely possible using an autoclave because of the high temperature and time needed. There are some brands that are now autoclavable as long as the temperature and duration are controlled, but these are in the minority, and the clinician must always check very carefully if this is the case for a specific material. Much more commonly, disinfection is the method of choice for infection control. The most effective means of disinfecting impressions is to immerse them in disinfectant solution for up to 30 minutes. When disinfection of impressions cannot be carried out by immersion, a disinfectant spray may be used. There are a variety of solutions which may be used for spray or immersion disinfection of impression materials. Historically some rather unpleasant chemicals were used for this purpose, which tended to have strong, unpleasant odors and could irritate the skin and eyes and damage surfaces that they came into contact with. These included bleach, aldehydes, and phenols. Nowadays, the most common active ingredients in products used to disinfect impressions are alcohols (propanol and ethanol being the most common), quaternary ammonium salts (common broad-spectrum antiseptics), and sodium percarbonate (a chlorine-free bleach alternative).

Effects of Disinfectants on the Accuracy of Impression Materials

It is important that the disinfection protocol does not adversely affect the accuracy or dimensional stability of the impression.

Alginate is by far the most vulnerable in this regard. It is a hydrophilic material and will readily take up water from its surroundings. For this reason, immersion in a disinfectant solution causes it to swell, even if the immersion is only for a short period. For alginate impressions, a spray disinfectant is preferred, and for the shortest acceptable time that still has been shown to give suitable killing of the infectious agents that might potentially be found on the impression's surface. Different alginate-disinfectant combinations give subtly different specifications, and the 'extended pour' alginates tend to fare a little better in this regard, but typically the spray must not be left on the surface for more than 15 minutes to ensure that the impression is not distorted.

Polyether impression materials are known to expand when exposed to moisture. It is not surprising then that immersion in a variety of disinfectants causes excessive swelling in some disinfectant solutions after as little as 10 minutes. Spray disinfectants are acceptable, although some polyethers are compatible with short immersions in particular disinfectant solutions. Following the instructions specific to both the impression material and the specific disinfectant product is very important to avoid a lot of time wasted down the line.

The addition-cured silicones offer a more convenient option in this specific regard. Many studies have been undertaken on the effects of disinfectants on the dimensional stability of addition-cured silicones, and these conclude that no adverse effects result from even an extended exposure (up to 18 hours) of addition-cured silicones to all varieties of disinfectant.

FAILURES OF IMPRESSION-TAKING

As the quality of the prosthesis is directly dependent on the quality of the impression, it is important that a poor-quality impression is identified readily and is not passed to the dental laboratory for processing.

In many instances the need for retakes can be avoided by being aware of the kinds of problems that might arise and how these may be avoided. The main failures are associated with poor reproduction of surface detail and poor fit of the prosthesis.

Poor Reproduction of Surface Detail

Factors that give rise to poor reproduction of surface detail are:
* *Rough or uneven surface on impression.* This may be due to incomplete setting (usually associated with premature removal), improper mixing, or the presence of surface contaminants. A set that is too rapid will also give a poor surface reproduction and may be due to the wrong temperature, humidity, or mix.
* *Bubbles.* These usually arise if the material is allowed to set too quickly or if bubbles have been introduced during the mixing process.
* *Irregular-shaped voids.* These will appear due to moisture or debris on the surface.

Poor Fit of Prosthesis

Factors that give rise to poor fit are:
* *Distortion.* The use of excessively flexible trays will result in distortion of the impression as the tray is distorted during seating. If the working time of the impression material is exceeded, the material will not flow properly and there is a temptation to use more pressure when taking the impression, causing distortion of the tray and permanent set of the impression material. Movement of the tray while the impression material is setting will also cause distortion. Adhesive failure between the tray and the impression material can occur if there is insufficient adhesive, if the wrong adhesive is used, or if insufficient time is allowed for the adhesive to become ef-

fective. An inappropriate disinfecting procedure will also give rise to distortion.
* *Castings too big or too small.* Although it would be difficult to distinguish between prostheses that fit poorly due to being the wrong size or being distorted, the most common causes of the wrong-sized castings are: the use of inappropriate impression techniques, pouring the model at the wrong time, or the impression having been stored under unsuitable conditions of temperature and humidity.

RIGID IMPRESSION MATERIALS

These are the materials that, once set, are rigid; in contrast to the elastic impression materials, they display no elastic behavior and if stressed (i.e. stretched, pulled, or bent) are likely to break. They must therefore not be used when a patient has any undercuts, as to remove the impression would require either the impression to break or the tooth to come out with it!

Impression Compound (Compo)

Impression compound is a thermoplastic material with a glass transition temperature of about 55–60°C. Above its glass transition temperature it becomes soft and will take up a new form. On cooling to mouth temperature, it hardens and can be removed, retaining an impression of the oral cavity. Thus no chemical reaction is involved in the use of this material.

Composition

The composition of impression compounds tends to vary from product to product but typically consists of a combination of resins and waxes, plasticizers, and fillers, each having a specific function:
* *Resins and waxes.* Resins are amorphous organic substances that are insoluble in water. Typical naturally occurring resins used in impression compound include rosin and shellac, although some products use synthetic resins to give greater control and consistency of the composition. Waxes are straight-chain hydrocarbons of the general formula $CH_3(CH_2)_n CH_3$, where n is between 15 and 42. They are characteristically tasteless, odorless, colorless, and greasy to the touch. Waxes used in impression compound include beeswax and colophony.
* *Plasticizers.* The waxes and resin, if used on their own, would tend to produce a brittle material with a tendency toward tackiness. The brittleness is overcome by the addition of plasticizers, such as gutta percha and now, more commonly, stearic acid.
* *Fillers.* To overcome the tackiness, control the degree of flow, and minimize shrinkage due to thermal contraction, a filler is added. Commonly used fillers are calcium carbonate and limestone. The fillers also improve the rigidity of this impression material.

Properties

Impression compound is muco-compressive, as it is the most viscous of the impression materials used. This can present particular problems in those patients who have a flabby mandibular ridge.

Table 2.7.7 Coefficient of Thermal Expansion of Waxes

Source	Name	Temperature Range (°C)	Coefficient of Expansion (ppm °C⁻¹)
Mineral	Paraffin	20–28	307
		28–34	1631
Plant	Carnauba	22–52	156
Insect	Beeswax	22–41	344
		41–50	1048

Compo is rigid once cooled and therefore cannot be used to record undercuts. It has a high viscosity, so reproduction of surface detail is not very good. However, the reproduction can be improved by reheating the surface of the impression material after taking the first impression and then reseating it in the patient's mouth. Even then, the surface detail is not as good as can be achieved with virtually all of the other impression materials. It is therefore better to use compo as a simple and quick means of producing a special tray and then use a wash of zinc oxide–eugenol to provide the surface detail.

The coefficient of thermal expansion of resins and waxes is very high, as indicated in Table 2.7.7, and is highly non-linear within the temperature range of dental interest (Figure 2.7.15). Shrinkage is in the order of 1.5% and is due to the thermal contraction from mouth to room temperature.

The material has poor dimensional stability, and the model must be poured as soon as possible after the impression is taken; this should take place within 1 hour.

The thermal conductivity of impression compound is very low, meaning that, on softening, the outside will always soften first. This can give the impression that the material is ready for use when the inside might still be quite hard. Differential expansion gives rise to internal strains, which relieve themselves in due course by distortion of the impression. Thus the material must be placed in the water bath to allow sufficient time for it

to achieve a uniform temperature. Even then, internal strains will inevitably build up during cooling and will eventually give rise to distortion, which is why the model must be poured as soon as possible.

Application

Its main application is for recording preliminary impressions of edentulous arches. This gives a model on which a special tray can be constructed and which can subsequently be used with a low-viscosity impression material (such as zinc oxide–eugenol) for recording the fine surface detail (see below). The material is used relatively little these days, as other impression materials are found more convenient, although it does still have its adherents.

Zinc Oxide–Eugenol Paste

Whereas there are many zinc oxide–eugenol products that are presented as powder–liquid systems, the impression material is in the form of two pastes. There is typically a *base paste* consisting of zinc oxide, olive oil, linseed oil, zinc acetate, and a trace of water and a *reactor paste* consisting of eugenol and fillers, such as kaolin and talc.

Zinc oxide and eugenol are the reactive components that take part in the setting reaction (see Chapter 2.4). The water initiates the setting reaction, and the zinc acetate is present to speed up the setting process. The oils and fillers are inert substances, which allow the material to be used in a paste–paste formulation, and help to provide the appropriate handling characteristics.

Properties

The liquid is very fluid, that is, mucostatic, and, being a water-based system, readily adapts to the soft tissues. It therefore provides a detailed reproduction of the soft tissues without causing displacement of the soft tissues but is rigid once set and is thus unable to record undercuts. This limits its application to the edentulous mouth, where it is used with a special tray.

It has the advantage of being dimensionally stable and shows little shrinkage on setting. However, as it is used with a special tray, the tray may impose limitations on the dimensional stability of the whole impression.

Although the material is non-toxic, eugenol can cause a tingling, burning sensation in the patient's mouth and leave a persistent taste that the patient may find unpleasant. The paste tends to adhere to skin, so the skin around the lips should be protected with petroleum jelly.

Impression Plaster
Presentation and Composition

Impression plaster consists of a powder to which water is added to produce a smooth paste. The composition of the powder is similar to that of the model materials discussed in more detail in Chapter 3.1, as is the setting process. The impression material consists typically of calcium sulfate β-hemihydrate $(CaSO_4)_2 \cdot H_2O$, potassium sulfate to reduce the expansion, borax to reduce the rate of setting, and starch to help disintegration of the impression on separation from the plaster/stone model.

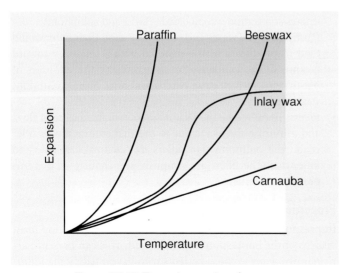

Figure 2.7.15 Thermal expansion of waxes.

Properties

The impression plaster is easy to mix, but great care must be taken to avoid trapping air bubbles, as these will give rise to surface inaccuracies. The material has well-controlled working and setting characteristics, which are governed by the relative amounts of borax and potassium sulfate.

The amount of potassium sulfate is generally more than would be found in model plaster, as for impressions, the expansion must be kept to a minimum. Since the potassium sulfate also acts as an accelerator of the set, borax is needed to counteract it. The working time is of the order of 2–3 minutes, as is the setting time.

The mixed material has a very low viscosity and so is mucostatic. It is hydrophilic and thus adapts readily to the soft tissues, recording their surface detail with great accuracy. The material is best used in a special tray, made of acrylic or shellac, to a thickness of 1.0–1.5 mm. Alternatively, it can be used as a wash with a compo special tray.

The dimensional stability of impression plaster is very good, so a time delay in pouring the model is of no consequence, although extremes of temperature should be avoided. A separating medium (usually a solution of sodium alginate) must be used between the model plaster and the impression plaster.

The material is rigid once set and thus unable to record undercuts. This limits its application to the edentulous patient.

From the patient's point of view, it is not an unpleasant material, although it tends to leave a sensation of dryness in the mouth for some time after the impression has been taken.

DIGITAL IMPRESSIONING

Intraoral digital impression systems are rapidly coming to the forefront of dentistry. The first serious application of the intraoral impressioning system was developed for the chair-side computer-aided design–computer-aided manufacture (CAD–CAM) system from Sirona (CEREC™). In order to be able to produce a CAD–CAM-processed restoration at the chair side, it is necessary to have a digital image of the oral anatomy. The imaging system is based around an infrared (840 nm) or blue light-emitting diode (LED; 470 nm) scanner. A process known as triangulation is used to determine the position of the laser dot. In most cases a laser stripe, instead of a single laser dot, is swept across the object to speed up the acquisition process. One drawback of the early models is that the surfaces of the teeth needed to be covered with a white powder (titanium dioxide) to prevent unwanted reflections and thus aid the data collection, although this has now become quite unusual with more recent instruments not requiring this step. Once the intraoral data have been captured, they can be used to produce a milled definitive restoration in a single visit. The advantage is that the digital impression can be reviewed on screen for accuracy and it is easy to ensure that the margins of the prepared teeth are readily identified.

CEREC™ is a fully integrated system, and not all dentists are able or willing to devote the extra time and effort needed to learn the various stages of designing, milling, and characterization of the restorations. A number of manufacturers, including 3Shape (Trios4™), 3M/ESPE (LAVA COS™), and Cadent (iTero™), have invested heavily in free-standing chair-side intraoral scanners. The LAVA COS™ system, for example, captures three-dimensional data in a video sequence that is able to record approximately 20 three-dimensional data sets per second, or close to 2400 data sets per arch, for an accurate and high-speed scan. The most impressive achievement is the ability of the system to model those data in real time at the chair side, which is due to the increased processing power of the latest computers. This has made it possible to display on the monitor the three-dimensional image that is being taken in the mouth as it is being captured. As with the CEREC™ system, the dentist can confidently and immediately assess whether enough information has been captured for a completed digital impression. These free-standing intraoral scanners are intended to capture the digital data, which are then transferred to a facility that can either proceed directly to the manufacture of the restoration or convert the data into a highly accurate model; this, in turn, can be sent to the laboratory of the dentist's choice for more conventional processing.

The potential benefits of these systems are enormous, as they replace the tray-and-putty method of impressing patients with a highly detailed digital scan of the tooth preparation area. This approach has a number of benefits, as it:

- eliminates the imprecision synonymous with conventional impressions
- improves patient interaction
- improves patient comfort, as no bulky tray is needed and there is no waiting while the impression material sets
- improves communication between the dental laboratory and the dentist
- increases productivity
- reduces the need for retakes.

At present, the systems are only able to take accurate impressions of the hard tissues, so the type of restoration that can be made from digital impressions from the various systems include inlays, onlays, crowns, fixed bridges and mouthguards, occlusal guards, and orthodontic appliances. There are at least a dozen systems on the market, and as they are a costly investment, it is important that one chooses the best intraoral scanner to meet one's needs. Factors that should be taken into account are speed of data capture, the size of the scanner (the more bulky, the less comfortable for the patient), ease of use, and the quality of the data capture. Most of the intraoral scanners are now powderless (by employing a polarizing filter), and some also have the ability to capture the data in color. This is a remarkably rapidly changing field, especially as the demands on the system that will optimize its use become clearer with increasing use in the dental clinic.

FURTHER READING

Heuttig, F., Klink, A., Kohler, A., Mutschler, M., Rupp, F., 2021. Flowability, tear strength, and hydrophilicity of current elastomers for dental impressions. Materials (Basel) 14 (11), 2994.

Nassar, U., Aziz, T., Flores-Mir, C., 2011. Dimensional stability of irreversible hydrocolloid impression materials as a function of pouring time: a systematic review. Journal of Prosthetic Dentistry 106 (2), 126–133.

Seraq, M., Nassar, T.A., Avondoglio, D., Weiner, S., 2018. A comparative study of the accuracy of dies made from digital intraoral scanning vs. elastic impressions: an in vitro study. Journal of Prosthodontics 27 (1), 88–93.

Stober, T., Johnson, G.H., Schmitter, M., 2010. Accuracy of the newly formulated vinyl siloxanether elastomeric impression material. Journal of Prosthetic Dentistry 103 (4), 228–239.

Takeuchi, Y., Koizumi, H., Furuchi, M., Sato, Y., Ohkubo, C., Matsumura, H., 2018. Use of digital impression systems with intraoral scanners for fabricating restorations and fixed dental prostheses. Journal of Oral Science 60 (1), 1–7.

Punj, A., Bompolaki, D., Garaicoa, J., 2017. Dental impression materials and techniques. Dental Clinics of North America 61 (4), 779–796.

Laboratory and Related Dental Materials

Models, Dies, and Refractories: Traditional and CAD/CAM Techniques and Materials

INTRODUCTION

A *model* is a replica of the fitting surfaces of the oral cavity; it is poured from an impression of the oral anatomy and is then used to construct an appliance, such as a full or a partial denture. A *mold* is used for the construction of a denture. *Dies* are replicas of individual teeth and are generally used in the construction of crowns and bridges. A *refractory investment* is a high-temperature-resistant material that uses gypsum or phosphates as a binder and is used as a mold material for lost wax casting of dental casting alloys and a mold or support structure for the construction of ceramic restorations such as veneers, crowns, and inlays using sintering or hot pressing. In this chapter we will focus on the chemistry and properties of these materials.

MODELS AND DIES

The basic ingredient for models and dies is gypsum, more commonly known as plaster of Paris.

Chemistry of Gypsum
Composition
Gypsum is calcium sulfate dihydrate, $CaSO_4 \cdot 2H_2O$. When this substance is calcined – that is, heated to a temperature sufficiently high to drive off some of the water – it is converted into calcium sulfate hemihydrate $(CaSO_4)_2 \cdot H_2O$, and at higher temperatures still the anhydrite is formed as shown below:

Gypsum	$CaSO_4 \cdot 2H_2O$
$\downarrow$ Up to 130°C	
Hemihydrate	$(CaSO_4)_2 \cdot H_2O$
$\downarrow$ Up to 200°C	
Anhydrite	$CaSO_4$

The production of calcium sulfate hemihydrate can be undertaken in one of three ways, producing versions of gypsum with different properties and hence different applications. These are plaster, dental stone, and densite (improved stone). It should be noted that the three versions are chemically identical, differing only in form and structural detail.

Plaster. Calcium sulfate dihydrate is heated in an open vessel. Water is driven off, and the dihydrate is converted into hemihydrate, known as calcined calcium sulfate or β-hemihydrate. The resultant material consists of large irregular porous particles, and these particles do not pack together very tightly.

The powder needs to be mixed with a large amount of water to obtain a mix satisfactory for dental use, as much of the water is absorbed into the pores between the particles. The usual mix is 50 mL of water to 100 g of powder.

Dental stone. If the dihydrate is heated in an autoclave, the hemihydrate that is produced consists of small, regular-shaped particles which are relatively non-porous. This autoclaved calcium sulfate is known as α-hemihydrate. Due to the non-porous and regular structure of the particles, they can be packed more tightly together using less water. The mix is 20 mL water to 100 g of powder.

Densite (improved stone). In the production of this form of calcium sulfate hemihydrate, the dihydrate is boiled in the presence of calcium chloride and magnesium chloride. These two chlorides act as deflocculants, helping separate the individual particles that would otherwise tend to agglomerate. The hemihydrate particles that are produced are yet more compact and smoother than those of the dental stone. The densite is mixed in the ratio of 100 g of powder to 20 mL of water.

Applications of Gypsum Materials
Plaster is used as a general-purpose material, mainly for bases and models, as it is cheap and easy to use and shape. The setting expansion (see below) is not of great importance for these applications. A similar composition is used for plaster impression material (see Chapter 2.7) and for gypsum-bonded refractory investments, although for these applications, the working and setting times and the setting expansion are carefully controlled by the incorporation of various additives (see below).

The dental stone is used for models of the mouth, while the denser, improved stone is used for individual tooth models, called dies. The latter are used for the shaping of wax patterns from which castings are produced.

Setting Process
Heating the hydrate to drive off some of the water produces a substance that is effectively dehydrated. As a consequence of this, the hemihydrate is able to react with water and revert back to calcium sulfate dihydrate as follows:

$$\left(CaSO_4\right)_2 \cdot H_2O + 3H_2O \rightarrow 2CaSO_4 \cdot 2H_2O$$

The setting process for gypsum products is believed to occur in the following sequence:
- Some calcium sulfate hemihydrate dissolves in the water.
- The dissolved calcium sulfate hemihydrate reacts with the water and forms calcium sulfate dihydrate.

- The solubility of calcium sulfate dihydrate is very low, and a supersaturated solution is formed.
- This supersaturated solution is unstable, and calcium sulfate dihydrate precipitates out as stable crystals.
- As the stable calcium sulfate dihydrate crystals precipitate out of the solution, more calcium sulfate hemihydrate is dissolved, and this continues until all the hemihydrate has dissolved.

Working and Setting Times

The material must be mixed and poured before it reaches the end of its working time. The working times vary from product to product and are chosen to suit the particular application.

For impression plaster, the working time is only 2–3 minutes, whereas it approaches 8 minutes for a gypsum-bonded refractory investment. Short working times give rise to short setting times, as both are controlled by the speed of the reaction. Hence, for an impression plaster, the setting time is typically 2–3 minutes, whereas the setting time can vary from 20 to 45 minutes for gypsum-bonded refractory investments.

The model materials have working times similar to those of impression plaster, but their setting times are somewhat longer. For plaster, the setting time is 5–10 minutes, while for stone it can be up to 20 minutes.

The handling characteristics are controlled by the inclusion of various additives. Additives that speed up the setting process are gypsum ($\leq 20\%$), potassium sulfate, and sodium chloride ($\leq 20\%$). These act as nucleating sites for the growth of dihydrate crystals. Those that slow down the setting rate are sodium chloride ($\geq 20\%$), potassium citrate, and borax, which interfere with dihydrate crystal formation. These additives also affect the dimensional change on setting, as discussed later.

The manipulation of the powder–liquid system will also affect the setting characteristics. The operator can change the powder-to-liquid ratio, and, by adding more water, the setting time is extended, because it takes longer for the solution to become saturated and thus for the dihydrate crystals to begin to precipitate out. Increasing the spatulation time will result in a reduction of the setting time, as it has the effect of breaking up the crystals as they form, hence increasing the number of sites for crystallization.

CLINICAL SIGNIFICANCE

Longer spatulation times will tend to reduce the setting time and increase the setting expansion, as it modifies the way in which the material crystallizes.

An increase in temperature has only a minimal effect, since the increased rate of dissolution of the hemihydrate is offset by the higher solubility of the calcium sulfate dihydrate in the water.

Dimensional Changes on Setting

On setting, the crystals that are formed are spherulitic in appearance (Figure 3.1.1), not unlike snowflakes. These crystals impinge on one another as they grow and push each other apart. The result of this action is that there is a dimensional expansion on setting. The material in fact does shrink, in the sense that its molar volume is less by 7.1 vol. %, as shown in Table 3.1.1. However, large, empty spaces form between the

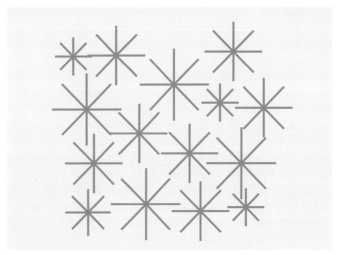

Figure 3.1.1 Spherulitic structure of calcium sulfate dihydrate

TABLE 3.1.1 **Change in Molar Volume That Occurs as Calcium Sulfate Hemihydrate Is Rehydrated**			
	$(CaSO_4)_2 \cdot H_2O$	$+ 3H_2O \rightarrow$	$2CaSO_4 \cdot 2H_2O$
Molecular weight	290	54	344
Density	2.75	1.0	2.32
Molar volume	105	54	148
Change in volume = $(148 - 159)/159 \times 100 = -7.1\%$			

crystals, leading to a high porosity. It is this that accounts for the observed net dimensional expansion of 0.6 vol. %.

This ability to expand on setting is a very important feature of this material, and it is the factor that makes it so useful for a large number of dental applications. In particular, there is a school of thought that models and dies are best produced slightly larger than the oral anatomy. This is to ensure that crowns, bridges, and dentures are not too tight a fit when placed in the mouth. The expansion is also made use of in investments, as it helps compensate for the shrinkage of metallic casting on cooling from the melting temperature.

Although it is desirable generally that models produced from plaster or stone are slightly on the big side, the unchecked expansion of this material would be excessive.

CLINICAL SIGNIFICANCE

There are various additives in gypsum products that are used to control the degree of expansion, which in the case of plaster is 0.2–0.3 vol. % and for stones and dies is in the region of 0.05–0.10 vol. %.

Sodium chloride. Sodium chloride provides additional sites for crystal formation. The higher density of crystals limits the growth of the crystals and hence reduces their ability to push each other apart. This results in a reduction of the observed expansion. The increased number of sites for nucleation of the dihydrate crystals has the effect of increasing the rate of setting of the material. The hemihydrate also dissolves more rapidly, which again increases the rate of reaction.

If present in high concentrations ($\geq 20\%$), the sodium chloride will deposit onto the surface of the crystal and prevent further growth. This reduces the reaction rate, rather than increasing it.

Potassium sulfate. Potassium sulfate (K_2SO_4) reacts with the water and calcium sulfate hemihydrate to produce $K_2(CaSO_4)_2 \cdot H_2O$. This compound crystallizes very rapidly and encourages the growth of more crystals. This has the effect of reducing the overall expansion and accelerating the setting reaction. When present as a 2% solution in water, it will reduce the setting time from approximately 10 minutes to 4 minutes.

Calcium sulfate dihydrate. The addition of a small amount of calcium sulfate dihydrate will provide additional sites for nucleation and act as an accelerator; it will reduce both the working and the setting times.

Borax. The addition of borax ($Na_2B_4O_7 \cdot 10H_2O$) is important because it counteracts the increased rate of setting due to the inclusion of the above additives. It is a *retarder* of the setting process. The addition of borax leads to the formation of calcium tetraborate, which deposits on the dihydrate crystals and prevents further growth.

Potassium citrate. Potassium citrate acts as a retarder and is sometimes added in addition to borax.

Thus, by carefully regulating the amount of the above additives, gypsum-based products can be produced with the required control over degree of expansion and working and setting times, making the materials appropriate for a range of applications. The typical setting expansions for gypsum products are as shown in Table 3.1.2.

CLINICAL SIGNIFICANCE

The low setting expansion of stone and densite makes these materials ideal for the production of dies and models for both metal and ceramic work.

Hygroscopic Expansion

The setting expansion can be increased substantially by immersing the material in water while it is setting. When it is in air, the surface tension of the free water tends to draw the crystals together, and this limits the ability of the crystals to grow.

However, when the crystals are immersed in water, they can grow more freely, resulting in a greater degree of expansion. This process is called *hygroscopic expansion* and is sometimes used with gypsum-bonded refractory investments for the casting of alloys that have a high coefficient of thermal expansion (CTE) or a high contraction on solidification.

Gypsum and Sustainability

Gypsum is increasingly under the spotlight from the point of view of sustainability and environmental pollution. If gypsum models and investments are disposed of in such a way as the material comes into contact with biodegradable waste, this results in the production of hydrogen sulfide gas, which is highly toxic and can cause both acute and chronic health problems for those exposed to it. Gypsum must be disposed of via a specialist waste disposal contractor to ensure this does not occur, but sadly this is not always done, and for this reason the use of gypsum in dentistry can contribute to pollution.

Properties

Dimensional Stability

Once the material has set, there is little or no dimensional change. The storage stability is excellent, although the material *is* slightly soluble in water. For this reason, washing the surface with hot water should be avoided.

Compressive Strength

The compressive strength is the mechanical property most commonly used for assessing the strength of gypsum products. These values are typically as shown in Table 3.1.3.

The compressive strength is affected considerably by the powder-to-liquid ratio that is used. It is clear from the above data that the reduction in the amount of water that is required to produce an acceptable mix gives a significant improvement in the compressive strength. Thus the compressive strength of the set product is affected by straying from the recommended powder-to-liquid ratio. The use of an excessive amount of water has the advantage that a smooth mix, which can be readily poured, is obtained. The air that is incorporated during the mixing process is more readily removed from such a mix for stone and densite by vibration, but the compressive strength after setting will be inferior. On the other hand, using less water than is recommended results in a thick mix from which incorporated air is more difficult to remove, leading to an increased porosity and a significantly reduced strength. There is also a danger that insufficient water will be present for the full reaction to take place.

Thus using less water has the potential of increasing the compressive strength, but inferior properties are obtained if too little is used.

There is a marked difference in the wet and dry strength of plaster products. In general, the dry strength is about twice the wet strength.

Tensile Strength

The wet tensile strength of plaster is very low (approximately 2 MPa). This is due to the porosity and brittle nature of the material, which has the disadvantage that teeth and margins on the model can be easily damaged if handled roughly. Dental stone has a tensile strength about twice that of plaster and is therefore preferred for the production of crown and bridge models and dies.

TABLE 3.1.2 Setting Expansions of Some Gypsum Products	
Plaster	0.20–0.30%
Stone	0.08–0.10%
Densite	0.05–0.07%

TABLE 3.1.3 Compressive Strengths of Some Gypsum Products	
Plaster	12 MPa
Stone	30 MPa
Densite	38 MPa

Hardness and Abrasion Resistance

The surface hardness of gypsum products is very low, so the material is highly susceptible to scratching and loss through abrasion. The epoxy resins have been explored as alternative die materials, since these exhibit much better detail reproduction, abrasion resistance, and transverse strength than the gypsum materials but are subject to polymerization shrinkage.

CLINICAL SIGNIFICANCE

The contraction of epoxy resins during setting can compromise the fit of castings unless this is taken into account in the processing.

Reproduction of surface detail

In the American National Standards Institute/American Dental Association specification no. 19, compatibility of impression materials with dental stones is assessed by the presence of a 20-μm-wide line reproduced on an unmodified calcium sulfate dihydrate cast. As the surface of gypsum products is slightly porous, minute surface details that are less than 20 μm are not readily reproduced. However, macroscopic surface details are very accurately reproduced, although air bubbles (trapped between the plaster and the impression, for example) can contribute to the loss of surface details.

When a mold is being waxed up for casting, the die has to be kept moist. Since the gypsum is, to some degree, soluble in water, some surface loss of material will occur and therefore repeated drying and wetting should be avoided.

CLINICAL SIGNIFICANCE

Whenever a die needs to be rewetted, this should be done with a saturated solution of calcium sulfate dihydrate in water.

Summary

The advantages and disadvantages of the use of plaster for the production of models can be summarized as shown in Table 3.1.4.

REFRACTORIES

As mentioned previously, refractories are materials that can withstand high temperatures of up to 1500°C. They are used to construct molds used in the lost wax casting technique for the fabrication of metal restorations and the hot pressing of

TABLE 3.1.4 Advantages and Disadvantages of Plaster for Model Making

Advantages	Disadvantages
Dimensionally accurate and stable	Low tensile strength, brittle, poor abrasion resistance
Cheap	Poor surface detail
Good color contrast	Poor wetting of rubber impression materials

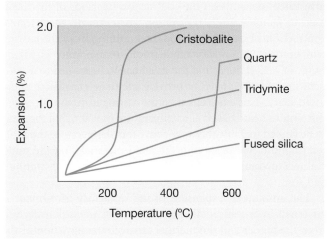

Figure 3.1.2 Thermal expansion behavior of three silica allotropes.

ceramic restorations and are also used as a base in the sintering process for the production of ceramic restorations such as veneers, crowns, and inlays.

In 1929, Coleman and Weinstein invented a gypsum-bonded cristobalite investment to replace the plaster of Paris, eliminating most of the shrinkage and distortion problems that had plagued the production of gold castings up to that point. Cristobalite is one of the three allotropic forms of silica, the others being quartz and tridymite, and it has thermal expansion qualities that make it especially suitable as an investment material for gold casting (Figure 3.1.2). The term investment originated from the solid mold process, in which a material like plaster of Paris is poured or 'invested' into a container that holds the wax pattern that is identical to the gold casting to be produced. After the plaster has set, the mold is heated up to a temperature of 900–1000°C so that the wax pattern is burnt out and a high degree of thermal expansion is achieved, leaving a hollow cavity into which the molten metal is poured. However, the addition of cristobalite to plaster of Paris to create a gypsum-bonded investment did not immediately produce perfect gold alloy castings, and it was not until the 1940s that cristobalite investment materials were formulated that compensated for all of the distortions encountered in the original lost wax technique.

Refractories for lost wax casting of dental alloys

The basic principles of lost wax casting are described in Chapter 3.3. The most important feature of a dental refractory investment is the amount it will expand on heating without distorting or disintegrating. The concept is that the mold cavity will expand by an amount sufficient to compensate for the shrinkage of the wax pattern due to the change in temperature at which the wax pattern is prepared and subsequently invested, and the shrinkage of the metal as it cools down from its casting temperature.

wax shrinkage + metal shrinkage =
setting expansion + hygroscopic expansion + thermal expansion

The aim is to produce a restoration that will be a perfect fit. Naturally, the degree of expansion required from the refractory investment depends on the contraction behavior of the metal used to manufacture a restoration. For example, the effective contraction of dental gold alloys on cooling from the casting temperature (1100–1300°C) to room temperature is in the range of 1.25–1.80%, and the mold has to be heated to a temperature of 900–1000°C to provide adequate expansion of the mold space. This contrasts with the casting of titanium, where the mold is heat-soaked at a temperature of 900°C but then has to be cooled to 350°C because above this temperature the molten titanium will react with the mold materials. Yet the mold still has to compensate for a thermal contraction of titanium of 1.6%.

The amount of expansion of the refractory investment is governed by a combination of the setting expansion derived from the binder and the thermal expansion/contraction of the binder and filler.

The type of refractory and its properties depend on the particular application, but there are currently two types of refractory materials that are still widely used, namely gypsum-bonded and phosphate-bonded refractories. The gypsum-bonded investments are used primarily for casting with low-melting-temperature gold alloys, while the phosphate-bonded investments are used with base metal alloys and with high-melting-temperature gold and precious metal alloys, and for the casting, hot pressing and sintering of dental glasses and glass–ceramics.

Gypsum-Bonded Refractory Investments

Gypsum-bonded dental refractory investments are used primarily in conjunction with relatively low-melting-temperature gold alloys and silver/palladium alloys, which are typically melted in the range of 1100–1300°C. Gypsum-bonded dental refractory investments consist of some 70% silica, typically a mixture of quartz and cristobalite, and 30% binder (calcium sulfate hemihydrate).

The setting expansion is governed by the composition of the binder and will clearly be a function of the relative amounts of plaster and stone and all the other ingredients that are incorporated to control the expansion and the setting time, as explained in detail above when considering models and dies. The setting expansion can be enhanced by placing the mold in water or adding water to the surface of the mold during the initial setting process. The hygroscopic expansion that this gives rise to is caused by the capillary action of the water, which is attracted into the spaces between the dihydrate crystals as they form and pushes the crystals further apart. It is important to appreciate that, when hygroscopic expansion is used, the mold temperature at casting may need to be some 200°C lower. Along with the addition of sodium chloride and/or potassium sulfate, the setting expansion can vary from 0.25 to 0.80%. However, much of this is lost when the investment is heated, when the gypsum binder will shrink as it loses water and it converts from calcium sulfate dihydrate, through calcium sulfate hemihydrate to anhydrite ($CaSO_4$).

The thermal expansion of most refractory materials would be insufficient to provide enough expansion to compensate for the contraction of a dental casting alloy. To overcome this problem, cristobalite is used as a major ingredient in dental refractory investments along with the binder. Cristobalite undergoes a rapid expansion at 220°C due to an inversion from cubic high cristobalite to tetragonal low cristobalite, resulting in a less dense crystal structure. At the same time, the room-temperature form of quartz, α-quartz, undergoes a reversible change in crystal structure at 573°C to form β-quartz, and this is accompanied by a linear expansion of 0.45%. The thermal expansion of a gypsum-bonded investment can be carefully controlled by selecting appropriate amounts of each ingredient and is typically in the range of 1.20–1.50%.

Phosphate-Bonded Refractory Investments

Gypsum-bonded refractory investments are not suitable for use with many high-melting-temperature gold alloys used to construct metal–ceramic restorations and most base metal alloys such as Ni–Cr and Co–Cr alloys. For such alloys, which typically are cast at temperatures between 1400°C and 1550°C, a phosphate-bonded investment is required, since the gypsum-bonded investment would disintegrate on contact with the molten metal. Also, as a consequence of the high casting temperature, the thermal contraction for such alloys is typically around 2.0–2.3% and the gypsum-bonded investments are not able to compensate for this degree of contraction.

A phosphate-bonded investment consists of a powder containing ammonium diacid phosphate ($NH_4 \cdot H_2 \cdot PO_4$), calcined magnesia (MgO), and silica (quartz and cristobalite). The powder is mixed with a liquid consisting of water, colloidal silica, surfactant, deflocculant, glycerine, and defoaming agent. On mixing, a reaction takes place between the phosphate, magnesia, and water as follows:

$$NH_4 \cdot H_2 \cdot PO_4 + MgO + 5H_2O \rightarrow Mg \cdot NH_4 \cdot PO_4 \cdot 6H_2O$$

The crystalline solid that forms as a result of this setting reaction binds the silica particles together. As with the plaster of Paris, the crystals push each other apart and this results in a small setting expansion, but again most of this is lost when the mold is heated. When the temperature reaches approximately 300°C, ammonia and water are released:

$$2(Mg \cdot NH_4 \cdot PO_4 \cdot 6H_2O) \rightarrow Mg_2 \cdot P_2O_7 + 2NH_3 + 13H_2O$$

On further heating, any remaining $NH_4 \cdot H_2 \cdot PO_4$ reacts with the colloidal silica to form a silicophosphate, which helps increase the strength of the investment at high temperatures.

The release of ammonia on heating the refractory investment is a potential environmental hazard but there are now phosphate-bonded investments that do not release ammonia. This has been achieved by substituting the ammonium diacid phosphate ($NH_4 \cdot H_2PO_4$) with $Mg(H_2PO_4)_2$.

When considering the use of a phosphate-bonded refractory investment as a mold for hot pressing or support for the construction of ceramic restorations, there is, in fact, very little literature on the subject. During the laboratory construction stage of, for example, a veneer, careful consideration must be given to the dimensional changes that may take place within the variety of refractory and ceramic materials available. When the ceramic is fired on a refractory mold, it is important that there is no differential contraction, as this may cause distortion or even cracking of the restoration. Generally speaking, matched refractory investment and ceramic systems have a closely matched CTE, but huge discrepancies, by as much as a factor of 2, can arise with the injudicious selection of a refractory/ceramic combination. Some veneering ceramics, such as those based on a feldspathic glass, will have a CTE of 6–7 ppm $°C^{-1}$ and the phosphate-bonded refractory investments can have a CTE of up to 13 ppm $°C^{-1}$.

> ### CLINICAL SIGNIFICANCE
>
> By carefully controlling the composition of the binder and the refractory investment, the setting and thermal expansion can be controlled and, in turn, it is possible to compensate for the contraction of the metal or the ceramic such that the restoration will have a clinically acceptable quality of fit on the tooth.

DIGITAL MANUFACTURING OF MODELS AND DIES

New digital technologies are significantly changing practices in dental laboratories, in particular computer-aided design and computer-aided manufacture (CAD/CAM) and 3D printing. Many of the traditional ways of producing dental prostheses are being replaced by digital manufacturing routes. A major distinction between CAD/CAM and 3D printing is that CAD/CAM is a subtractive manufacturing process (material is removed from a block or disc), while 3D printing is an additive process (the material is built up in layers to create the precise shape required), resulting in minimal waste of material.

Computer-Aided Design and Computer-Aided Manufacture: CAD/CAM

CAD/CAM began its dental life in 1970s when Duret and Preston began to explore its applications in dentistry. This was followed by the work of Moermann in the 1980s, which was instrumental in developing the CEREC® system. CAD/CAM has now become a well-accepted technology in many modern dental laboratories as well as for dental clinicians who use it at the chairside. Its use has increased considerably in the last few decades, partly driven by the increased use of digital imaging systems such as intraoral scanners, which in the early days were somewhat cumbersome but have since become better, smaller, faster, and easier to use, providing the digital data needed to input into the design. The software used to design the prostheses has also become much more user-friendly, and many of the processing steps are now automated. Alongside the technological innovation, developments in biomaterials science have allowed an ever-increasing range of materials to be available for use in dental CAD/CAM applications.

CAD/CAM is based on three elements, namely (1) data acquisition, (2) data processing, and (3) manufacturing. The extraordinary increases in the processing speed and memory of microchips over recent years have resulted in major advances in all of these areas, one example being the wide range of intraoral scanners on the market. It is now possible to create a digitized 3D model of the oral cavity directly with such a system, and consequently there is no need to take an impression or pour a model.

The digital model is used to design the restoration using one of the numerous software packages available for the design of dental restorations such as models, dies, crowns, bridges, partial denture frameworks, and denture bases. At the end of the design process, a digital file is created of the component to be manufactured. This file can then be transferred to a milling unit or 3D printing machine for the production of the final prosthesis.

A significant development in the CAD/CAM technologies used in dentistry has been the transition from closed to open-access systems. The first systems were designed to be closed systems but now the technology is being opened up and the component parts of a CAD/CAM system can be purchased separately. This allows for greater flexibility as data can be acquired from a multitude of sources (intraoral scanner, contact or laser model digitizer, CT, MRI) and appropriate design software can be matched to the object to be manufactured (e.g. crown and bridge frameworks, partial denture frameworks, customized implant and implant abutments). Another advantage of open systems is that this widens access to a much greater range of manufacturing methods such that the most appropriate manufacturing processes and associated materials can be selected. The competition also helps to drive down the price.

The CAM part of CAD/CAM in dentistry is based on the process of subtractive manufacturing. Using computer numerically controlled machining, power-driven machine tools such as saws, lathes, milling machines, and drill presses are used to remove material from a block or disc in order to achieve the desired geometry. Thus one starts out with a block or disc of the material and the machine cuts away the bits that are not wanted. These technologies are now so advanced that they are able to produce highly complex models, which would otherwise be difficult and sometimes impossible to make by the conventional dental processes. CAD/CAM milling of crown copings and bridge frameworks is now widely used by dental laboratories, gradually replacing the role of the highly skilled dental technician sitting at the bench.

3D Printing

3D printing, also referred to as additive manufacturing or rapid prototyping (RP), is a disruptive technology that is having a profound effect on the manufacturing, engineering, and retail sectors. The aerospace and automotive industries use expensive materials and if it is possible to reduce the cost of materials used by reducing the amount of waste, this can result in significant cost savings. Subtractive manufacturing is inherently wasteful as only a small amount of the block of material one starts with is used in the final component. The advantage with additive manufacturing is that there is little or no waste material created.

What Is Additive Manufacturing?

Additive manufacturing is defined by the American Society for Testing and Materials (ASTM) as:

The process of joining materials to make objects from 3D model data, usually layer upon layer, as opposed to subtractive manufacturing methodologies.

In principle, the process works by taking a 3D computer file and creating a series of cross-sectional slices. Each slice is then printed one on top of the other to create the 3D object. One attractive feature of this process is that there is no waste. Additive manufacturing processes first started to be used in the 1980s to manufacture prototypes, models, and casting patterns, then referred to as rapid prototyping (RP). A feature of additive manufacturing is that it is a remarkably rapidly changing field with a huge investment in developing enhanced manufacturing technologies, which is changing the way we make things. Additive manufacturing has changed from only RP models to manufacturing functional parts for use as final products. As it becomes more widely used, costs are coming down compared to traditional manufacturing techniques in terms of price, speed, reliability, and cost of use. As with CAD/CAM, the increased ability for 3D data capture using laser scanners, CT and MRI, and developments in software encourages greater and greater use of the technology.

An added benefit is that the number of materials that the industry uses has increased dramatically and modern machines can utilize a broad array of polymers, metals, and ceramics. This becomes all the more necessary as the industry makes the transition from prototypes to functional devices, where the materials used need to have the appropriate properties for their desired function. When a prototype is produced, it is sufficient for it to look good, but for functional objects such as customized implants and oral prostheses, the materials and their properties have to be suitable for clinical use.

Additive manufacturing is in fact ideally suited to dentistry, which has a tradition of producing customized parts made to fit the patient and not the other way around. There are a number of additive manufacturing technologies that we can use, including:

- Stereolithography (SLA)
- Direct light processing (DLP)
- Fused deposition modeling (FDM)
- Selective electron beam melting (SEBM)
- Laser powder forming
- Inkjet printing

This list is by no means exhaustive and further technologies are added to this list frequently. 3D printing is reshaping the way dentists approach personalized care. One of the earliest applications of 3D printing was the production of models of the human skeleton using SLA to aid in the design and placement of customized implants (Figure 3.1.3).

This was made possible with the developments in 3D imaging systems such as CT and MRI and software that allowed 3D reconstruction of the hard and soft tissues. The introduction of intra-oral scanners, producing a 3D model of the oral anatomy, means that 3D printing is now being used in the production of drill guides for dental implants, the production of physical models for prosthodontics, orthodontics and surgery, the manufacture of dental, craniomaxillofacial and orthopedic implants, and the fabrication of copings and frameworks for implant and dental restorations.

CLINICAL SIGNIFICANCE

With the improvements in the speed, reliability, and accuracy of the hardware, additive manufacturing will seriously compete with traditional labor- and skill-intensive manufacturing methods.

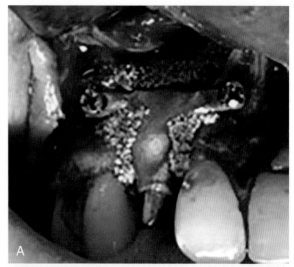
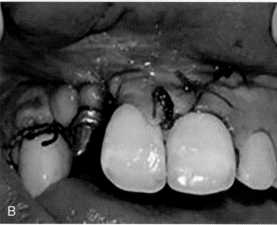

Figure 3.1.3 Customized transmucosal titanium implant for a cleft palate patient. Images courtesy of and copyright Dr Shirin Shahr Baf and Dr Behnam Mirzakouchaki, Sheffield, UK.

For the dental materials scientific community, these technologies provide the opportunity to develop and use a whole new range of materials. The materials first used in additive manufacturing were chosen primarily to suit the aerospace and automotive industries and not the medical industries. However, many new materials are now being explored specifically for the dental market.

Models and Dies Produced Using CAD/CAM

Whereas the original driving force for the development of dental CAD/CAM systems was for the production of ceramic restorations, the flexibility of CAD/CAM means that, given the right tools, nearly anything can be produced. There are milling units that use blocks or discs in a wide range of materials. A number of companies now produce discs that can be fitted into a milling unit that are of sufficient size to produce models and dies.

The material most commonly used for the production of models is still PMMA, but now it is also used to produce models from blocks made from polyurethane. In the case of prefabricated PMMA the advantage is that there is no residual monomer, and for the polyurethane it is claimed to be very hard wearing. For the production of dies, a range of wax discs in a variety of contrasting colors (to differentiate from the model) are available.

3D Printing of Models and Dies

Essentially the printing of models and dies works by building up items by depositing ultraviolet (UV) or visible light–activated resins layer by layer. Using this new technology, it is possible to produce dental models and dies in a range of polymeric materials. Thus the models and dies are made from resins, not plaster or stone. The original data of the oral anatomy can be acquired either by the use of an intraoral scanner or by digitizing the impression.

There are a number of systems that are widely used in dental laboratories to produce models using 3D printing, the most common of which are SLA and DLP. In SLA a vat of liquid photopolymer resin is cured by a UV laser to solidify the pattern layer by layer to create a solid 3D model (Figure 3.1.4). Each layer is traced out by the laser on the surface of the liquid resin, at which point a 'build platform' descends, and another layer of resin is wiped over the surface, and the process is repeated.

Desktop SLA 3D printers contain a resin tank with a transparent base and non-stick surface, which serves as a substrate for the liquid resin to cure against, allowing for the gentle detachment of newly formed layers. The printing process starts as the build platform descends into a resin tank, leaving space equal to the layer height in between the build platform, or the last completed layer, and the bottom of the tank. A laser points at two mirror galvanometers, which direct the light to the correct coordinates on a series of mirrors, focusing the light upward through the bottom of the tank and curing a layer of resin. The cured layer then gets separated from the bottom of the tank and the build platform moves up to let fresh resin flow beneath. The process repeats until the print is complete.

Just like their SLA counterparts, desktop DLP 3D printers are built around a resin tank with transparent bottom and a build platform that descends into a resin tank to create parts upside down, layer by layer. The difference is the light source.

TABLE 3.1.5 **Model Composition (EvoDent) for DLP (%w/w)**	
Polyurethane acrylate	20–40
N/A Dipropylene glycol diacrylate	60–80
2,4,6-trimethylbenzoyldiphenyl phosphine oxide	2–6
Pigment	0.2–1

DLP 3D printers use a digital projector screen to flash an image of a layer across the entire platform, curing all points simultaneously. This has the benefit of significantly speeding up the printing process.

Most SLA and DLP printers are now very user-friendly, with easily replaceable build platforms and resin tanks. Some systems come with a cartridge system that automatically refills the tank with liquid resin, which requires less attention and allows printing overnight. The resins come in a wide range of formulation configurations: materials can be soft or hard, and heavily filled with secondary materials like glass and ceramic. A wide variety of UV light–cured acrylate-based resins can be used with these printers, and the composition of an example of such a resin is described in Table 3.1.5. One drawback is that models printed with either SLA or DLP technologies require post-processing after printing. First, the parts need to be washed in a solvent to remove excess resin, followed by a post-curing cycle to ensure the resin model is fully cured. The advantages of 3D printing models are numerous in that the resin models are accurate and durable. The cost keeps coming down as the equipment is able to print multiple models in a single print run. 3D printing can improve the efficiency of the dental laboratory by freeing up staff as they no longer have to make the molds by hand so that they can instead focus their efforts elsewhere.

For the production of dies for the lost wax casting process using 3D printing, still the most popular material used is wax. The 3D printing process uses technologies known as fused deposition modeling (FDP) and jetting. In both instances droplets of the wax are deposited onto a build platform. In FDM two materials are deposited, one being the wax die material and the other being a water-soluble support material. Once printed, the support material is dissolved away, leaving only the required die ready for lost wax casting.

FURTHER READING

Chan, T.K., Darvell, B.W., 2001. Effect of storage conditions on calcium sulphate hemihydrate-containing products. Dental Materials 17, 134.

Dawood, A., Marti, B., Sauret-Jackso, V., Darwood, A., 2015. 3D printing in dentistry. British Dental Journal 19 (11), 521–529.

Derrien, G., Le Menn, G., 1995. Evaluation of detail reproduction for three die materials by using scanning electron microscopy and two-dimensional profilometry. Journal of Prosthetic Dentistry 74, 1.

Duke, P., Moore, B.K., Haug, S.P., 2000. Study of the physical properties of type IV gypsum, resin-containing, and epoxy die materials. Journal of Prosthetic Dentistry 83, 466.

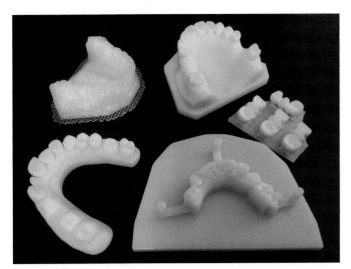

Figure 3.1.4 Stereolithography printed models in resin. Permission from Envisiontec pending.

Ireland, A.J., McNamara, C., Clover, M.J., House, K., Wenger, N., Barbour, M.E., et al., 2008. 3D surface imaging in dentistry: what we are looking at. British Dental Journal 205, 387.

Miyazaki, T., Hotta, Y., Kunii, J., Kuriyama, S., Tamaki, Y., 2009. A review of dental CAD/CAM: current status and future perspectives from 20 years of experience. Dental Materials Journal 28 (1), 44–56.

Mörmann, W.H., Bindl, A., 1997. The new creativity in ceramic restorations: dental CAD–CAM. Quintessence International 27, 821.

Oberoi, G., Nitsch, S., Edelmayer, M., Janjić, K., Müller, A.S., Agis, H., 2018. 3D printing – Encompassing the facets of dentistry. Frontiers in Bioengineering and Biotechnology 6, 172.

van Noort, R., 2012. The future of dental devices is digital. Dental Materials 28, 3–12.

Whyte, M.P., Brockhurst, P.J., 1996. The effect of steam sterilization on the properties of set dental gypsum models. Australian Dental Journal 41, 128.

Wildgoose, D.G., Winstanley, R.B., van Noort, R., 1997. The laboratory construction and teaching of ceramic veneers: a survey. Journal of Dentistry 25 (2), 119–123.

Denture Base Resins

INTRODUCTION

The world's population is aging. In 2019, 1 in 11 people were over the age of 65; by 2050, this is predicted to rise to 1 in 6 (The United Nations Department of Economic and Social Affairs, 2019). Although improvements in oral health have been seen across many countries, and alternative means of replacing missing teeth such as implants have developed significantly, it is nevertheless probable that with this increase in older people, there will be a continued demand for full or partial dentures to replace missing teeth. Market research predicts a 6% Compound Annual Growth Rate (CAGR) in denture products. In the United Kingdom's most recent Adult Dental Health Survey it was found that 1 in 5 adults wore removable dentures, split approximately 1:2, with one-third of these edentate and two-thirds partially dentate. It is important that current and future denture patients can be provided with an aesthetically pleasing, comfortable, highly functional denture, and it is likely that a substantial number will find this option preferable to dental implants.

In this section we will consider the materials used to create *non*-metallic dentures. A consideration of the alloys used for metallic-framed denture creation can be found in Chapter 3.3.

The construction of a denture involves many steps. The first step is taking an impression, which is then followed by the various laboratory stages. These include producing a model, setting the teeth, preparing a waxed model, investing in a denture flask, and boiling out the wax, which then leaves a space to be filled by the denture base material.

Various materials have been used historically to construct dentures, including cellulose products, phenol-formaldehyde, vinyl resins, and vulcanite, although each had its limitations that have led to them falling out of favor:

- Cellulose products suffered from warpage in the mouth, and from a taste of camphor due to its use as a plasticizer. This camphor leached out of the denture, causing blistering and staining with loss of color within a few months.
- Phenol-formaldehyde (Bakelite) proved to be too difficult to process and also lost its color in the mouth.
- Vinyl resins were found to have a low resistance to fracture, and failures were common, possibly due to fatigue.
- Vulcanite was the first material to be used for the mass production of dentures, but its aesthetic qualities are not very good and it has now been replaced by acrylic resins.

Polymethylmethacrylate (PMMA), more commonly called acrylic resin, is the material of choice for non-metallic dentures; it has the required aesthetic quality, being available in colors and translucencies that provide a good representation of the dental soft tissues, and is cheap and easy to process. Even so, it is not ideal in all respects. The ideal properties of a denture base material are shown in Table 3.2.1.

Acrylic resins are popular because they meet many of the criteria set out in Table 3.2.1. In particular, dentures made from acrylic resin are easy to process using inexpensive techniques and are aesthetically pleasing. Besides its use in the construction of full dentures, the material is also used for a wide range of other applications such as the construction of customized trays for impression taking, the soft-tissue replication on cast metal frameworks, denture repairs, soft liners, and denture teeth.

COMPOSITION AND STRUCTURE OF ACRYLIC RESIN

An acrylic resin denture is made by the process of free radical addition polymerization to form PMMA. The monomer is methyl methacrylate (MMA):

$$
\begin{array}{cc}
H & Me \\
| & | \\
C & = C \\
| & | \\
H & C = O \\
 & | \\
 & O \\
 & | \\
 & Me
\end{array}
$$

TABLE 3.2.1 Criteria for an Ideal Denture Base Material

Natural appearance
High strength, stiffness, hardness and toughness
Dimensional stability
Absence of odor, taste or toxic products
Resistance to absorption of oral fluids
Good retention to polymers, porcelain and metals
Ease of repair
Good shelf life
Ease of manipulation
Low density
Accurate reproduction of surface detail
Resistance to bacterial growth
Good thermal conductivity
Radiopacity
Ease of cleaning
Inexpensiveness to use

TABLE 3.2.2   **Constituents of a Heat-Cured Resin**
Powder
Beads or granules of poly methyl methacrylate
Initiator – benzoyl peroxide
Pigments/dyes
Opacifiers – titanium/zinc oxides
Plasticizer – dibutyl phthalate
Synthetic fibers – nylon/acrylic
Liquid
Methyl methacrylate monomer
Inhibitor – hydroquinone
Cross-linking agent – ethylene glycol dimethacrylate

where Me stands for CH_3. The conversion of the monomer into a polymer involves the normal sequence of activation, initiation, propagation, and termination, as described in Chapter 1.5. The resins are available in either heat-cured or cold-cured forms.

Heat-Cured Resins

These materials consist of a powder and a liquid, which, on mixing and subsequent heating, form a rigid solid. The constituents of the powder and liquid are shown in Table 3.2.2.

The reasons for the particular formulation of a powder–liquid system are threefold:
- Processing is possible by the dough technique.
- Polymerization shrinkage is minimized.
- The heat of the reaction is reduced.

The dough technique helps to make the processing of dentures a relatively straightforward process. A flask containing the teeth set in plaster is packed with the dough and then closed under pressure such that the excess dough is squeezed out. In addition, by adapting the dough to the model and trimming off any excess, cold-cure varieties of the acrylics are easily manipulated (when in the doughy stage) to produce special trays. Granules dissolve more readily in the monomer than beads and hence reduce the time taken to reach the doughy stage.

The polymerization shrinkage is reduced when compared to using a monomer because most of the material that is being used (i.e., the beads or granules) has already been polymerized.

The polymerization reaction is highly exothermic, as a considerable amount of heat energy (80 kJ mol^{-1}) is released in reducing the C=C to –C–C– bonds. Since a large proportion of the mixture is already in the form of a polymer, the potential for

overheating is reduced. As the maximum temperature reached will be less, the extent of thermal contraction will also be reduced.

The monomer is extremely volatile and highly flammable, so the container must be kept sealed at all times and must be kept away from naked flames. The container is a dark glass bottle, which extends the shelf life of the monomer by avoiding spontaneous polymerization from the action of light. Hydroquinone also extends the shelf life of the monomer by reacting rapidly with any free radicals that may form spontaneously within the liquid and producing forms of stabilized free radicals that are not able to initiate the polymerization process. Contamination with the polymer beads or granules must be avoided, as these carry the benzoyl peroxide on their surface and only a tiny amount of the polymer is needed to start the polymerization reaction.

The polymer powder is very stable and has a virtually indefinite shelf life. A cross-linking agent such as diethylene glycol dimethacrylate is included in order to improve the mechanical properties (Figure 3.2.1a). These are incorporated at various points along the methyl methacrylate polymer chain and form cross-links with adjacent chains by virtue of their two double-bond sites (Figure 3.2.1b). Thus, although the PMMA is a thermoplastic resin, the inclusion of the cross-linking agent prevents post-processing.

Cold-Cure Resins

The chemistry of these resins is identical to that of the heat-cured resins, except that the cure is initiated by a tertiary amine (e.g., dimethyl-P-toluidine or sulfinic acid) rather than heat.

This method of curing is not as efficient as the heat curing process and tends to result in a lower-molecular-weight material. This has an adverse effect on the strength properties of the material and also raises the amount of uncured residual monomer in the resin. The color stability is not as good as for the heat-cured material, and the cold-cured resins are more prone to yellowing.

The size of the polymer beads is somewhat smaller than in the heat-cured resin (which has a bead size of 150 μm) to ease dissolution in the monomer to produce a dough. The doughy stage has to be reached before the addition curing reaction begins to affect the viscosity of the mix and prevents the adaptation of the mix to the mold walls.

The lower molecular weight also results in a lowering of the glass transition temperature, with Tg being typically 75–80°C. While one might think that this makes the material more inclined to warpage, this is not so. As no external heat source is

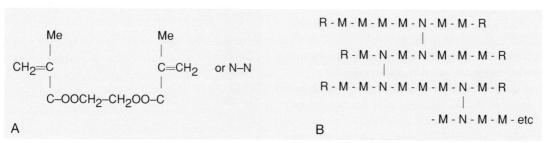

Figure 3.2.1 Diethylene glycol dimethacrylate (a) and its formation of cross-links (b).

used to cure the resin, there is less build-up of internal strain. Nevertheless, the material is highly susceptible to creep, and this can contribute significantly to the eventual distortion of the denture when in use.

ASPECTS OF MANIPULATION

Powder-to-Liquid Ratio

It is important to use the correct powder-to-liquid ratio (2.0/1.0 wt %; 1.6/1.0 vol. %). Too much powder could result in inadequate filling by the monomer of the free space between the powder particles, resulting in a weak material as a consequence of porosity in the final product. Too much monomer will produce excessive polymerization shrinkage and a loss of quality of fit to the denture-bearing surface.

The additives tend to settle out at the bottom of the container, and it is important that the container is shaken before use to ensure an even distribution of the powder ingredients.

Control of Color

The coloring pigment is usually incorporated in the polymer powder, but in some cases it may simply be on the surface of the polymer beads and may be washed off by too rapid a contact with the monomer. In this case the polymer should be added to the monomer slowly. Too little powder will produce too light a shade.

Mold Lining

There is a danger that the resin may penetrate the relatively rough surface of the plaster mold and adhere to it. To prevent this, a separating medium must be employed. Nowadays, the separating medium is usually a solution of sodium alginate, although some still recommend the use of tin foil.

Processing

There are two problems in particular to watch out for in the processing of acrylics for dentures: one is their porosity and another is the presence of processing strains.

Porosity

The problem one is most likely to experience with acrylic resin dentures is the occurrence of porosity during the processing stage. There are two major causes of porosity: polymerization shrinkage-associated *contraction porosity* and volatilization of the monomer, termed *gaseous porosity*.

Contraction porosity. Contraction porosity occurs because the monomer contracts by some 20% of its volume during processing. By using the powder–liquid system, this contraction is minimized and should be in the region of 5–8%. However, this is not translated into a high linear shrinkage, which, on the basis of the volumetric shrinkage, should be of the order of 1.5–2% but is in fact somewhere in the region of 0.2–0.5%. It is believed that this is because the observed contraction is due in large part to the thermal contraction as a result of the change from curing temperature to room temperature rather than due to the polymerization contraction. In order to activate the polymerization process, the temperature in the flask has to be raised to more than 60°C, such that the benzoyl peroxide breaks down and forms free radicals (see Chapter 1.5). Once the reaction has been initiated, it continues to generate heat of its own due to the exothermic reaction. This can push up the temperature of the acrylic to well above 100°C.

At the processing temperature, the resin is able to flow into the spaces created by the curing contraction. The driving force for this flow is provided by pressure that is exerted during the processing; packing a slight excess of denture base material into the mold ensures that the material is under pressure when the mold is closed. This pressure is maintained throughout the processing cycle.

The resin only becomes rigid once it gets below its glass transition temperature, at which point the curing contraction will have been completed. From this point on, it is the thermal contraction that contributes to the observed changes in dimensions of the denture base. Cold-cured resins should give a better fit for the denture, as the processing temperature is considerably lower (around 60°C, compared to 100°C for the heat-cured resin). However, the fit is normally compromised due to the increased likelihood of creep at the lower Tg.

It is therefore important that sufficient dough is packed in the mold to ensure that the material is constantly under pressure during processing. This will cause any voids present in the mix to collapse and should also help to compensate for the curing contraction. Thus the packing of the mold should only be carried out when the mix has reached the doughy stage, as, prior to this, the high flow causes a rapid loss of pressure.

If there is evidence of localized porosity, this may be due to poor mixing of the components or to packing the mold before the doughy stage is reached. The associated differential contraction can lead to distortion of the denture.

Gaseous porosity. As noted above, on polymerization, there is an exothermic reaction. This could cause the temperature of the resin to rise above 100°C, which is just above its boiling temperature. If this temperature is exceeded before the polymerization process is completed, gaseous monomer will be formed, which is the cause of gaseous porosity. The amount of heat generated depends on the volume of resin present, the proportion of monomer, and the rapidity with which the external heat reaches the resin. The occurrence of gaseous porosity can be avoided by allowing the temperature to be raised in a slow and controlled fashion.

> ### CLINICAL SIGNIFICANCE
> Polymerization must be carried out *slowly* (to prevent gaseous porosity) and *under pressure* (to avoid contraction porosity), such that the temperature of the denture acrylic never exceeds 100°C.

Processing Strains

The restriction imposed on the dimensional change of the resin will inevitably give rise to internal strains. If such strains were allowed to relax, the result would be warpage, crazing, or distortion of the denture base. Although many of the strains generated during the curing contraction can be relieved by the flow

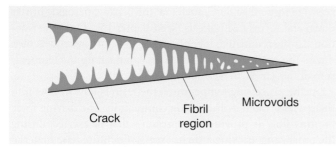

Figure 3.2.2 Crack formation resulting from a craze

that occurs above the glass transition temperature, some strain that is due to thermal contraction will remain. The level of the internal strain can be minimized by using acrylic rather than porcelain teeth (so that there is no differential shrinkage on cooling) and by allowing the flask to cool slowly.

The relief of internal strain can produce tiny surface defects in the resin. These are known as *crazes* and can be identified by a hazy or foggy appearance to the surface of the denture base. A craze is a localized region of high plastic deformation of the polymer, which may be filled with tiny voids. At this stage, it is not yet a crack since, unlike a crack, the crazed region can still support stress. However, crazing can lead to brittle fracture of the polymer. As the voids in the crazed region grow, these become separated only by thin fibrils of polymer until eventually the fibrils fail and a crack is formed (Figure 3.2.2). This crack will grow under an externally applied load such that it will reach a size at which it will continue to grow spontaneously and cause the denture to fracture.

The crazes may be formed in response to heat (due to polishing, for example), differential contraction around porcelain teeth, or attack by solvents such as alcohol.

CLINICAL SIGNIFICANCE

The introduction of cross-links in the polymer chains by the addition of diethylene glycol dimethacrylate has been found to reduce the potential for craze formation.

PROPERTIES

Dimensional Stability and Accuracy

Given that the denture is placed on an adaptable cushion of soft tissues, one may wonder why it is so important that the denture does not change its shape. In fact, it is a matter of great concern to the *retention* of the denture, where retention can be defined as the resistance to forces that tend to displace the denture in an occlusal direction. This is distinct from *stability*, which is the resistance to movement in a horizontal direction.

The factors that determine the retention of dentures in the mouth are essentially physical in nature. Anatomical factors such as undercuts are a nuisance rather than an advantage, as the denture is rigid and cannot engage them. In some instances pre-prosthetic surgery may be required to remove the undercut.

The most appropriate explanation of the factors that govern the retention of a denture is the viscous flow model (as discussed in Chapter 1.9), which is based on the relationship

$$F = 3\pi\eta R^4 / 2h^3\delta t$$

for a disc with radius R, and a thickness of saliva h.

Adhesion of the denture to the mucosa is provided by saliva, and the greater the surface area, the better the adhesive bond (i.e., R should be as large as possible). At the same time, it is important that the cohesion of the saliva film is not destroyed, and this is best guarded against by having as thin a film of saliva between the mucosa and denture as is possible (i.e., h should be small), so the denture should fit as accurately as possible.

The establishment of a peripheral seal around the edge of the denture is very important for retention. The tighter the seal, the more difficult it is for additional saliva to enter the space between the denture and the mucosa, and this means that more force needs to be applied to separate the denture from the mucosa. Anything that may upset the peripheral seal, such as over-extension, interferences (e.g. a frenal notch), and occlusal imbalance, will impair the retention of the denture.

As patients get older, the rate of production and the consistency of their saliva may change. The saliva becomes less adhesive to the denture, due to poor wetting of the surface by an inadequate supply of saliva, and it also becomes less viscous. Denture retention can then become a particular problem, and denture fixatives may have to be employed.

CLINICAL SIGNIFICANCE

For a denture to have the optimum retention, it should (1) cover the maximum area of mucosa compatible with the functional muscular activity and (2) be a close fit, so as to minimize the thickness of the saliva film and retain a good peripheral seal.

Mechanical properties

The tensile strength of acrylic resins is typically no more than 50 MPa. The elastic modulus is low, with the flexural modulus being in the region of 2200–2500 MPa. When this is combined with a lack of fracture toughness, it is perhaps not surprising that dentures are prone to fracture. Some 30% of denture repairs carried out by dental laboratories involve midline fractures, which are most prevalent among upper dentures.

Most fractures are associated with some traumatic incident to the denture, although this may not be easily recognized. If dropped on the floor, a denture does not necessarily break instantly, but the chances are that a crack will have formed that will continue to grow unnoticed until the denture fails suddenly and catastrophically. Thus eventual failure of the denture occurs due to flexural fatigue.

Some fractures may be associated with poor-quality processing. Lack of bonding between the resin and the acrylic teeth is such a possibility and gives rise to a weak interface from which a fracture is likely to be initiated. The formation of crazes due to processing faults or exposure to solvents is another possibility.

For those patients who fracture their dentures on a regular basis, it is possible to consider a high-impact-resistant denture base resin. These resins are formulated with a rubber toughening agent, such as a fine dispersion of butadiene styrene. The rubbery inclusions stop cracks from developing, showing a higher degree of resistance to fracture as a consequence. However, they also cause a lowering of the flexural modulus, and long-term fatigue failure due to excessive flexure can be a problem.

An alternative approach to the strengthening of acrylic dentures is the incorporation of fibers so as to produce a fiber-reinforced composite. Many different fibers have been explored in this regard; those that show the best properties in clinical use are ultra-high-molecular-weight polyethylene (UHMWPE), which are neutral in color, have low density and known biocompatibility, and can be surface-treated to enhance bonding to the resin and are available as a fiber weave that has been treated to improve adhesion to PMMA, although this remains somewhat limited, and glass fibers, which can be either incorporated in the resin as short fibers or embedded in cloth or loose form and are usually pre-treated with silane to improve the coupling to the acrylic resin in a similar way to the coupling between filler particles and resin in a resin-based composite.

CLINICAL SIGNIFICANCE

The lack of strength and toughness of acrylic resin dentures is a serious problem and can result in fractures of up to 10% of dentures within 3 years of use.

Creep is a problem with acrylic resins (particularly the cold-cured resins), as they are viscoelastic materials. The addition of a cross-linking agent reduces the amount of creep, but it cannot be totally eliminated.

Physical Properties
Thermal Conductivity
The thermal conductivity of PMMA is approximately 6×10^{-4} cal·g^{-1}·cm^{-2}. This is very low and can present problems during denture processing, as the heat produced cannot escape, leading to a temperature rise.

From the patient's point of view, the problem with a low coefficient of thermal conductivity is that the denture isolates the oral soft tissues from any sensation of temperature. This can lead to a patient consuming a drink that is far too hot without realizing it, which may lead to the back of the throat and possibly even the esophagus being scalded.

Coefficient of Thermal Expansion
The coefficient of thermal expansion is approximately 80 ppm °C^{-1}. This is quite high, as one might expect from a resin. In general, this does not present a problem, except that there is a possibility that porcelain teeth set in denture base resin may gradually loosen and be lost due to the differential expansion and contraction.

Water Sorption and Solubility
Due to the polar nature of the resin molecules, PMMA will absorb water. This water sorption is typically of the order of 1.0–2.0% by weight.

In practice, this helps to compensate for the slight processing shrinkage. However, given the low rate of diffusion of water through the resin, it would take the denture some weeks of continuous immersion in water to reach a stable weight.

Although PMMA is soluble in most solvents (e.g., chloroform), as it is only lightly cross-linked, it is virtually insoluble in most of the fluids that it may come into contact with in the mouth. However, some weight loss *will* occur, due to the leaching of the monomer in particular, and possibly some of the pigments and dyes.

Biocompatibility
In general, PMMA is highly biocompatible and patients suffer few problems. Nevertheless, some patients will show an allergic reaction. This is most probably associated with the various leachable components in the denture, such as any residual monomer or benzoic acid.

The allergic reaction tends to be virtually immediate and is more likely to occur with cold-cured resin dentures because of their higher residual monomer content. Sometimes it may be possible to overcome this problem by subjecting the denture to an additional curing cycle, but there is a danger that this will cause the denture to distort as internal processing stresses are relieved.

When a patient has a confirmed delayed hypersensitivity to methacrylate resins, then an alternative denture base material may have to be considered.

Alternative Denture Base Materials
Nylon was first considered for dentures in the 1950s, but in the early days deterioration of the color, excessive water sorption, and a high flexibility due to the low elasticity limited the material's success in this application. While they remain something of a niche material, their elastic properties do make them useful when the patient has severe soft and/or hard tissue undercuts, as their flexibility allows them to engage these undercuts. They still have a significant list of limitations, however, including the need for a thicker base, porosity, which leads to plaque accumulation and discoloration, a greater risk of alveolar resorption, and poor repair prospects. As such, nylon dentures find rather sparse use, limited to those patients with severe undercuts, few missing teeth, and where the denture does not experience significant loading.

Other polymers used for denture bases, as alternatives to PMMA and/or the cobalt chrome alloy used for metal-framed dentures, include acetal resin (polyoxymethylene), chemically related to nylon with lower porosity, polyacryletherketones which have found applications in medicine but are still rather new to dentistry and thus little is known about their long term suitability and limitations, and aryl ketone polymers, which are again somewhat new to market so have limited data available, but early observations would appear to indicate properties that make them a suitable substitute for cobalt chrome frameworks.

Summary
The advantages of the use of poly methyl methacrylate are that it:
- has excellent aesthetics
- is easy and cheap to process
- has a low density.
  The disadvantages are that the material:
- has barely adequate strength characteristics
- is susceptible to distortion
- has a low thermal conductivity
- is radiolucent.

DIGITAL MANUFACTURING OF DENTURES

CAD–CAM-Produced Denture Bases

While the conventional technique of making a denture base is via the dough molding technique using a plaster model in a flask, it is now also possible to use CAD–CAM. An important feature of this development was the production of software that included a virtual articulator. Examples of the software are 'Formlabs', 'The Ivoclar Digital Denture' software, and 'Dentca Design'. Interestingly, the latter is a web-based denture design software package, which is made possible by the availability of high-speed internet connections. All these systems have demonstration videos that are available on YouTube. The digital denture workflow involves the following steps:

1. **Scan:** both the fully articulated model and the wax-rim are scanned in a desktop model scanner. Alternatively with some denture CAD–CAM systems, the scanning is of the impression, or of the oral cavity itself, removing the need for impression-taking altogether. For further information on this, see Chapter 2.7 on digital impressions.
2. **Design:** the scanned date is imported into the denture CAD software and the denture is designed digitally.
3. **CAM:** the designs are sent to the milling unit for machining from an acrylic disc/block.
4. **Post-processing:** the printed parts are washed and the supports are removed.
5. **Assemble:** the teeth are bonded to the denture base and post-cured.
6. **Finish:** the full denture is polished.

Thus the denture base and the teeth are designed as two separate STL files, machined separately, and then the teeth are bonded to the base. For the denture base, a block of pink PMMA is used as the source material, which is available in a variety of shades. Similarly blocks of PMMA in various tooth shades are available to machine the teeth. Being prefabricated, this significantly reduces the presence of residual monomer. Remakes are simplified and faster as the original designs are always available and the digital denture is completely patient specific.

3D-Printed Denture Bases

For 3D printing, the data capture and design processes are essentially the same as for CAD–CAM. STL files are created of the denture base and the teeth and these are then 3D printed. A direct light printer (DLP) system is preferred as it is faster than stereolithography. The 3D printing denture and teeth materials are UV light–cured acrylic resins (e.g., NextDent Denture 3D+ or Dentca) and have the same properties as conventional acrylic with the convenience of curing with UV light instead of temperature.

> **CLINICAL SIGNIFICANCE**
>
> With the development of these new technologies, patients will spend less time in the clinic and make fewer visits. For the dental technician, these techniques have the advantage that the dentures are fabricated without the need for casts, flasking, or other processing methods.

> **CLINICAL SIGNIFICANCE**
>
> CAD–CAM and 3D printing open up the possibility of using reinforced acrylics or materials other than PMMA with potentially far superior properties, which cannot be processed using the more conventional techniques.

DENTURE-LINING MATERIALS

The denture-lining materials fall essentially into three groups, namely:

- permanent hard reline materials
- semi-permanent soft liners
- tissue conditioners/temporary soft liners.

Hard Reline Materials

Although the expected mean life of a complete denture may be 4–5 years, the actual life will depend on the rate of resorption of the alveolar bone. If the fitting surface of a denture needs to be replaced to improve the fit of the denture, a *hard reline* material can be employed. Relining a complete denture may be required due to soft-tissue changes arising from bone resorption. This tends to be more of a problem with mandibular than maxillary dentures. The criteria for relining are:

- poor retention or stability
- collapse of the vertical dimension of the occlusion
- degradation of the denture base
- lack of denture extension into mucobuccal fold areas
- in a patient for whom habituation to a new denture may be difficult or impossible, perhaps owing to cognitive decline or contributory health factors.

Either the reline can be achieved with a cold-cure acrylic resin at the chair side, or the denture is sent to a dental laboratory for relining with a heat-cured acrylic.

The heat-cured acrylics used by laboratories are identical to those used for the construction of dentures.

The cold-cured resins come in two types, with constituents as listed in Table 3.2.3. The reason for the second type of reline material is that MMA can be very irritant to soft tissues and can sensitize the patient. The poly ethyl methacrylate (PEMA) and butyl methacrylate are less irritant to the patient but have the disadvantage that they cause a reduction in the Tg, and this increases the possibility of dimensional instability.

One of the most serious drawbacks with attempting a chairside reline is that there is little control over the amount of denture material removed and the thickness of the reline material that replaces it. Other problems include high exothermic reactions, unacceptable taste, and poor color stability over time.

TABLE 3.2.3 Two Types of Cold-Cured Resin

	Type I	Type II
Powder	Poly methyl methacrylate	Poly ethyl methacrylate
	Benzoyl peroxide	Benzoyl peroxide
	Pigments	Pigments
Liquid	Methyl methacrylate	Butyl methacrylate
	Di-*n*-butylphthalate	Amine
	Amine	

Semi-Permanent Soft Liners

Occasionally, a patient will complain of persistent pain and discomfort from a denture, even though the denture would appear satisfactory in all other respects. This problem is seen most commonly in the lower jaw, where there is a smaller surface area over which to distribute the load, and where patients may have a sharp, thin, or heavily resorbed alveolar ridge. In such cases, the patient has difficulty tolerating a hard denture. If the pain persists when all possible measures have been taken to minimize the occlusal load and redistribute the load over as large an area as possible, the denture may be made more comfortable by the use of a soft liner. This provides a means of absorbing some of the energy involved in mastication, by interposing a highly resilient material between the denture and the mucosa.

Polymers with a glass transition temperature just above the temperature in the mouth will have a rubbery behavior and are highly resilient. Some polymers have a naturally low glass transition temperature (e.g. silicone polymers) and others (e.g., PMMA) can be modified by the inclusion of plasticizers to reduce their glass transition temperature (Table 3.2.4). The plasticizer acts as a lubricant for the polymer chains, making it easier for them to slide past one another, allowing the material to deform more easily and giving it a lower elastic modulus. In fact, soft liners are usually constructed from one or the other of these two materials.

Silicone Rubber

Silicone rubber materials consist of a poly dimethyl siloxane polymer to which filler is added to give it the correct consistency. The material solidifies by a cross-linking process rather than by a polymerization process, as the material is already a polymer. This cross-linking can be achieved either by heat, using benzoyl peroxide, or at room temperature, using tetraethylsilicate (see Chapter 2.7).

Silicone does not bond readily to the acrylic resin of the denture, so an adhesive needs to be employed. This adhesion can be achieved using silicone polymer dissolved in a solvent, or by the use of an alkyl-silane coupling agent. In both cases the bond is very weak and usually fails due to delamination within a relatively short time owing to the stresses that form at the interface between liner and denture when the silicone absorbs water from the saliva and swells. Another drawback is that this material tends to support the growth of *Candida albicans,* which leads to

denture stomatitis. They do, however, retain their softness better than acrylic soft liners as this is an intrinsic property rather than the result of an additive, which can itself leach out.

Acrylic Soft Liners

Acrylic soft liners have the advantage that they bond relatively well to the PMMA denture, although these can sometimes delaminate from the denture base and become more susceptible to the retention of *Candida*. These materials can be subdivided into those containing leachable plasticizers and those containing polymerizable plasticizers.

Leachable Plasticizer Systems

PEMA has a glass transition temperature of only 66°C, compared with 100°C for PMMA. A combination of these two polymers, with a small amount of plasticizer (such as dibutylphthalate) is highly resilient. Thus the powder is a mixture of PEMA and PMMA, and the liquid is MMA, containing 25–50% plasticizer.

Unfortunately, the plasticizer gradually leaches out and the liner becomes stiff as it loses its resilience. How rapidly this transition takes place depends to some extent on the patient's regime for cleaning the denture. In general, high temperatures and strong bleaching agents should be avoided.

Polymerizable Plasticizer Systems

Plasticizers have been developed that polymerize, and thus resist dissolution, but which maintain their lubricating effect.

Exact formulations of this new material are not known, but some use alkyl-maleate or alkylitaconate, while for one experimental system, the liquid component is known to be a mixture of tridecyl methacrylate, 2-diethylhexyl maleate, and ethylene glycol dimethacrylate. The liquid is mixed with either PEMA or copolymers of n-butyl and ethyl methacrylate.

The material is fairly hard at room temperature, which makes it easy to finish, and softens when taken up to mouth temperature.

Relative Merits of Soft Liners

The relative merits of the silicone and acrylic soft liners are outlined in Table 3.2.5. Although the use of soft liners is perceived as a long-term solution to poor load distribution, their clinical life is generally no more than 6 months due to the problems described above. Hence they are described as semi-permanent soft liners.

TABLE 3.2.4 Glass Transition Temperatures for Polymethacrylate Esters

Group	Transition Temperature (°C)
Methyl	125
Ethyl	65
Propyl	38
Butyl	33

TABLE 3.2.5 Relative Merits of Soft Liners

Silicone Rubber	Acrylic
Highly resilient	Less resilient
Retain softness	Go hard with time
Requires bonding agent	Self-adhesive
Susceptible to growth of *Candida albicans*	More resistant to bacteria
Weak bond	Permanent bond
Poor tear strength	Acceptable tear strength
No permanent deformation	Susceptible to creep

Tissue Conditioners/Temporary Soft Liners

In some instances the denture can give rise to inflammation or ulceration of the load-bearing soft tissues. A simple solution would be for the patient to stop wearing the denture until the inflammation has subsided. This is generally not acceptable to the patient, and a tissue conditioner can be employed to overcome the problem.

A tissue conditioner is a soft material that is applied temporarily to the fitting surface of the denture for the purpose of allowing a more even stress distribution. This permits the mucosal tissue to return to its normal shape and to resolve any inflammation of the denture-bearing tissues. Once the inflammation has receded and the tissue has recovered, an impression can be taken for a new denture.

Such a material must be exceptionally soft, yet not so soft as to squeeze out from between the denture and the mucosa. These materials typically consist of a powder such as PEMA, which, when mixed with a solvent such as ethyl alcohol and an aromatic ester such as a plasticizer (e.g., butyl phthalylbutylglycolate), produces a gel-like substance. Its consistency will depend on the initial powder-to-liquid ratio and the relative amounts of each of the components. When the powder and liquid are mixed together, the solvent readily penetrates the polymer beads, and this allows the plasticizer to enter the polymer very rapidly so as to create a gel structure.

The alcohol and plasticizer will leach out quickly, and therefore the tissue conditioner needs to be replaced *every few days* if the traumatized tissue is to revert to a healthy state as soon as possible. For some patients, the tissue conditioner may be maintained for up to 3 weeks; hence the frequently used term 'temporary soft liner'.

One suggestion to improve the short lifespan of the tissue conditioners is to coat them with a thin surface layer of semi-set methyl methacrylate resin so as to reduce the rate at which the solvent and plasticizer leach out.

FURTHER READING

Chow, C.K., Matear, D.W., Lawrence, H.P., 1999. Efficacy of antifungal agents in tissue conditioners in treating candidiasis. Gerodontology 16, 110.

Diaz-Arnold, A.M., Vargas, M.A., Shaull, K.L., 2008. Flexural and fatigue strengths of denture base resin. Journal of Prosthetic Dentistry 100 (1), 47–51.

Garcia, L.T., Jones, J.D., 2004. Soft liners. Dental Clinics of North America 48, 709.

Goiato, M.C., Freitas, E., dos Santos, D., de Medeiros, R., Sonego, M., 2015. Acrylic resin cytotoxicity for denture base – Literature review. Advances in Clinical and Experimental Medicine 24 (4), 679–686.

Gray, D., Barraclough, O., Ali, Z., Nattress, B., 2021. An update on indirect prosthodontic materials and their manufacturing techniques. Dental Update 48 (4), 699–705.

Hamanaka, I., Takahashi, Y., Shimizu, H., 2011. Mechanical properties of injection-molded thermoplastic denture base resins. Acta Odontologica Scandinavica 69 (2), 75–79.

Lee, S., Hong, S.-J., Paek, J., Pae, A., Kwon, K.-R., Noh, K., 2019. Comparing accuracy of denture bases fabricated by injection molding, CAD/CAM milling, and rapid prototyping method. Journal of Advanced Prosthodontics 11, 55–64.

Parvizi, A., Lindquist, T., Schneider, R., 2004. Comparison of the dimensional accuracy of injection-molded denture base materials to that of conventional pressure-pack acrylic resin. Journal of Prosthodontics 13, 83.

Pronych, G.J., Sutow, E.J., Sykora, O., 2003. Dimensional stability and dehydration of a thermoplastic polycarbonate-based and two PMMA-based denture resins. Journal of Oral Rehabilitation 30, 1157.

Rickman, L.J., Padipatvuthikul, P., Satterthwaite, J.D., 2012. Contemporary denture base resins. Dental Update 39 (1) Part 1, 25–30, and Part 2, 176–187.

Shim, J.S., Watts, D.C., 2000. An examination of the stress distribution in a soft-lined acrylic resin mandibular complete denture by finite element analysis. International Journal of Prosthodontics 13, 19.

Takahashi, T., Gonda, T., Mizuno, Y., Fujinami, Y., Maeda, Y., 2017. Reinforcement in removable prosthodontics: a literature review. Journal of Oral Rehabilitation 44 (2), 133–143.

The United Nations Department of Economic and Social Affairs. World Population Ageing 2019. https://www.un.org/en/global-issues/ageing.

Wimmer, T., Gallus, K., Eichberger, M., Stawarczyk, B., 2016. Complete denture fabrication supported by CAD/CAM. Journal of Prosthetic Dentistry 115 (5), 541–546.

Yunus, N., Rashid, A.A., Azmi, L.L., 2005. Some flexural properties of a nylon denture base polymer. Journal of Oral Rehabilitation 32, 65.

Alloys for Metallic Restorations

INTRODUCTION

The production of metallic restorations such as crowns, bridges, inlays, cast posts and cores, and partial dentures is commonly carried out in the dental laboratory by the *lost wax* casting technique. This method of casting has been around for a considerable time, with the earliest known example of an object created using the lost-wax technique being a 6000-year-old amulet from Mehrgarh in Pakistan. The technique is used to this day in many industries, particularly those where small, complex shapes are required such as in jewelry and ornament making. It was first used in dentistry in the 1890s.

The basic principles are simple. A wax model is produced of the desired shape, and this model is embedded or *invested* in a material resistant to high temperatures. The wax is then removed by melting and burning, leaving behind a cavity of the desired shape. This void can now be filled with molten metal so that the metal assumes the shape of the original wax carving. The stages in the production of a dental casting are therefore as follows:

- preparation of the dentition
- production of an impression
- pouring of a model
- waxing of the desired shape
- investing the wax pattern
- burn-out and heating
- melting and casting the alloy
- finishing and polishing
- heat treatments.

Thus it can be seen that many different materials are involved in the production of a metal casting. These include impression materials, model and die materials, waxes, investment materials, and casting alloys. Some of these have already been discussed in previous sections.

A detailed account of the various practical stages involved in the production of a metal casting will not be provided here, as this process is the prerogative of the dental technician. Instead, attention will be focused on the alloys that are used and the requirements that are placed on them for their applications in restorative dentistry.

When the lost wax casting technique was first developed for application in dentistry by Taggart in the early 1900s, the alloys of choice were gold alloys. For the construction of removable partial dentures, the gold alloys were gradually replaced by cobalt–chromium (Co–Cr) alloys during the 1950s and, to a lesser extent, Co–Cr–Ni alloys. In the latter part of the 20th century titanium made its appearance as a fixed and removable partial denture-casting alloy.

It is the responsibility of the dentist to request the most suitable alloy for a particular application when instructing a dental laboratory to produce a prosthesis. This choice should not be left to the dental technician. After all, it is the dentist who will be placing these materials in the patient's mouth.

CLINICAL SIGNIFICANCE

It is the dentist's responsibility to know what metals they are providing for their patients. This requires a knowledge of the types of alloys available, and their composition and properties.

DESIRABLE PROPERTIES

The choice of alloy is governed by several factors. *Cost* is a serious consideration due to the volatile prices of many metals. Other considerations are the *biocompatibility* of the alloy and its resistance to *corrosion* and *tarnish*. These requirements apply to all applications in dentistry and limit the range of alloys that can be used; further considerations specific to the use then allow us to narrow down that range even further.

Suitability for a specific application, be it a low-stress-bearing inlay or an item subject to much greater stresses such as a posterior bridge, is determined primarily by the *mechanical properties* of the alloy, such as its stiffness, strength, ductility, and hardness. Stiffness is a consequence of both the design of the prosthesis – the shape – and the inherent properties of the alloy itself such as the elastic modulus. The higher the elastic modulus, the stiffer the structure will be for a given shape. This is an important consideration, especially for long-span bridges, cast posts, partial dentures, and denture clasps, which are likely to be subjected to fairly high loads and therefore need to have not only a suitable stiffness but also to be resistant to permanent deformation. This requires the alloy to have a high yield stress or proof stress. However, for such things as clasps, high strength needs to be balanced against ductility, since it is important that the alloy is not so brittle as to fracture when small adjustments are made.

In the case of inlays, where marginal adaptation is usually improved by burnishing, ductility is even more important. Alloys for these applications need to be very ductile and soft if they are not to fracture during this procedure.

The *ease of casting* of the alloy is an important consideration for the dental laboratory technician. The dental technician will want to know what the melting range and casting temperature are for the alloy as, in general, the higher these are, the more problems the alloy presents in handling. Another important consideration in this context is the quality of fit of the restoration, which is a function of the casting shrinkage and cooling contraction of the alloy. These have to be accounted for if the casting is not to be too small. The higher the shrinkage, the more of a problem this becomes.

The *density* of the alloy is also important. Most castings are carried out in a centrifugal force-casting machine, and the higher the density of the alloy, the easier it is to force the air out of the mold space and to fill the space completely with alloy.

Thus alloys with a wide range of properties are needed to satisfy these varied requirements. As we find often in biomaterials science, it is necessary to consider the specific needs and priorities and select the material that best meets the demands of the application overall while accepting that no single material has the 'perfect' profile of properties and attributes. The main alloys that are employed in dentistry are noble and precious metal alloys and various base-metal alloys such as Co–Cr alloys. Titanium is unusual in that it is one of the very few metals that may be used in its pure form in dentistry, although titanium alloys are also sometimes encountered.

CLINICAL SIGNIFICANCE

It is important for the dentist to have a close working relationship with the dental laboratory, and to take into account their views when choosing an alloy.

NOBLE AND PRECIOUS METAL ALLOYS

The noble and precious metals consist of eight elements that have some features in common. They are very resistant to corrosion (noble) and expensive (precious). The noble metals are considered to be gold, platinum, rhodium, ruthenium, iridium, and osmium, whereas silver and palladium are generally referred to as the precious metals.

High-Gold Alloys

This is a group of alloys that have been around for some considerable time and that can be distinguished from other alloys used in dentistry by their high precious metal content, which must not be less than 75%, with a gold content in excess of 60%. The precious metal content is usually made up of gold, silver, platinum, and palladium. These alloys can be classified into four distinct groups, as indicated in Table 3.3.1.

The amount of gold in an alloy is defined in one of two ways:
- *Carat.* Pure gold has a carat value of 24, and an alloy's carat is expressed in terms of the number of 24th parts of gold

within it. Thus an alloy with 50% gold would be designated as a 12-carat gold alloy. Much jewelry is 9-carat gold (37.5%) or 18-carat gold (75%).
- *Fineness.* Pure gold has a fineness rating of 1000, so 18-carat gold is 750 fine, and 9-carat gold is 375 fine.

Thus the dental gold alloys in Table 3.3.1 vary from 21.6 to 14.4 carat, or 900 to 600 fine.

Alloying Elements in Dental Gold Alloys

The largest fraction by far of these alloys is gold, with lower amounts of silver and copper. Some formulations also contain very small amounts of platinum, palladium, and zinc.

The silver has a slight strengthening effect and counteracts the reddish tint of the copper.

The copper is a very important component, as it increases the strength, particularly of type III and IV gold alloys, and reduces the melting temperature. The limit to the amount of copper that can be added is 16%, as amounts in excess of this tend to cause the alloy to tarnish.

Platinum and palladium increase both the strength and the melting temperature.

Zinc acts as a *scavenger* during casting, preventing oxidation, and improves the castability.

A variety of other elements, such as iridium, ruthenium, and rhenium ($<0.5\%$), may be present. These have very high melting temperatures and act as nucleating sites during solidification, thus helping to produce a fine grain size.

Strengthening Mechanisms

Although all of the alloying elements give rise to some increase in the yield strength of the gold alloy by forming a solid solution, the most effective strengthening mechanism is the addition of copper, in what is known as *order hardening*.

This hardening heat treatment is carried out after the homogenizing anneal at approximately 700°C, which is performed to ensure a uniform composition throughout the casting. It involves reheating the alloy to 400°C and holding it at that temperature for approximately 30 minutes. Rather than being randomly distributed, the copper atoms arrange themselves in little ordered clusters.

This ordered structure prevents slippage of the atomic layers, which has the effect of raising the yield stress and the hardness of the alloy. There must be at least 11% copper in the gold alloy for order hardening to occur, so it cannot occur in type I and type II gold alloys. Type III gold alloys have just enough copper, and a small improvement in strength is observed. For type IV gold alloys, the improvement in strength is quite significant.

TABLE 3.3.1	Composition of High-Gold Alloys						
Type	Description	Au%	Ag%	Cu%	Pt%	Pd%	Zn%
I	Soft	80–90	3–12	2–5	–	–	–
II	Medium	75–78	12–15	7–10	0–1	1–4	0–1
III	Hard	62–78	8–26	8–11	0–3	2–4	0–1
IV	Extra hard	60–70	4–20	11–16	0–4	0–5	1–2

TABLE 3.3.2 Range of Mechanical Properties of High-Gold Alloys

Type	Condition	σ_y (MPa)	UTS (MPa)	Elongation (%)	VHN
I	As cast	60–140	200–310	20–35	40–70
II	As cast	140–250	310–380	20–35	70–100
III	As cast	180–260	330–390	20–25	90–130
	Hardened	280–350	410–560	6–20	115–170
IV	As cast	300–390	410–520	4–25	130–160
	Hardened	550–680	690–830	1–6	200–240

UTS, Ultimate tensile strength; VHN, Vickers hardness number.

The effect of this strengthening process is shown in Table 3.3.2. The addition of copper, combined with the hardening heat treatment, can result in a 10-fold increase in the yield strength. The importance of the hardening heat treatment for the type III and IV gold alloys is also indicated. However, there is a price to pay in terms of a reduction in the ductility of the alloy, as shown by the lower percentage elongation at which failure occurs. Thus excessive bending may give rise to brittle fracture, a problem that may arise when producing partial denture clasp arms out of a type IV gold alloy.

For some alloys, the hardening process is to allow the alloy to cool slowly on the bench rather than quenching it immediately on casting. This technique is commonly known as *self-hardening*. The disadvantage with this approach is that it is not as well controlled as when the alloy is first given a homogenizing anneal and then a hardening heat treatment. It is important that the dentist stipulates to the dental technician that a hardening heat treatment is to be carried out if a type III or IV gold alloy is chosen. If a self-hardening alloy has been selected, then it should be allowed to cool slowly on the bench and should not be quenched.

Other features

As the alloying elements form a solid solution readily with the gold, the difference between the liquidus and the solidus is small. This makes these alloys relatively easy to cast and produces a reasonably homogeneous result. The addition of platinum and palladium gives a larger gap between the liquidus and the solidus. The larger this gap, the more compositional segregation occurs on solidification, making a homogenizing anneal more desirable for the type III and IV gold alloys.

Due to their low casting temperature, the casting shrinkage (~1.4%) is readily compensated for by the use of a gypsum-bonded investment.

The low Vickers hardness numbers (VHNs) make these alloys easy to polish to a smooth surface finish, although, in the case of the heat-hardening alloys this is better done in the as-cast condition.

In general, it can be said that the use of these alloys does not present a major problem to the dental technician, and good-quality, well-fitting castings can be produced. Their corrosion and tarnish resistance is excellent, as is their biocompatibility.

Applications

Given their different mechanical properties, the recommended applications for the use of these alloys are as follows.

Type I alloys. These are best used for single-surface inlays in low-stress situations. As they are relatively soft and easily deformed, they need plenty of support to prevent deformation under occlusal loading. The low yield stress of these alloys allows the margins to be burnished easily. Given the high ductility, they are unlikely to fracture.

Type II alloys. These can be used for most inlays. However, those with thin sections should be avoided, as deformation is still a possibility.

Type III alloys. These can be used for all inlays, onlays, full-coverage crowns and short-span bridges, and cast posts and cores because of their greater strength compared with type I and type II alloys. However, they will be more difficult to burnish and have a higher potential for localized fracture if they are burnished excessively.

Type IV alloys. These are used for cast posts and cores, long-span bridges, and, in partial denture construction, particularly clasp arms. Clasp arms can be adjusted in the as-cast state and then heat-hardened. Of course, this will not be possible when using a self-hardening alloy. The low elastic modulus and high yield strength of the gold alloy provide a high degree of flexibility to clasp arms, which allows them to be withdrawn over quite severe undercuts without danger of permanent deformation. These alloys cannot be burnished in their hardened state and are therefore unsuitable for inlays.

Medium- and Low-Gold Alloys

The high prices of gold and other noble metals stimulated manufacturers to produce alternative alloys with reduced gold contents. Compositions of a few representative examples are presented in Table 3.3.3.

Some of these may be classed as *medium-gold alloys*, with the gold content varying from 40 to 60%. The palladium and silver contents are increased to compensate for the reduced gold content, while the copper content is in the range of 10–15%. Palladium is added to counteract the tendency of silver to tarnish.

The palladium, silver, and copper readily form substitutional solid solutions, with the gold producing a single-phase structure throughout the entire compositional range. The presence of copper allows order hardening, just as with the type III and IV gold alloys.

TABLE 3.3.3	Composition of Medium- and Low-Gold Alloys							
Alloy	Type	Color	Au%	Pd%	Ag%	Cu%	In%
Solaro 3 (Metalor)	Medium-gold	Yellow	56	5	25	11.8	–
Stabilor G (Degussa)	Medium-gold	Yellow	58	5.5	23.3	12.0	–
Mattident E (Johnson Matthey)	Medium-gold	Yellow	55	8.0	24.0	11.5	–
Palaginor 2 (Metalor)	Low-gold	White	12.5	18.9	53.7	14.2	–
Palliag MJ (Degussa)	Low-gold	White	12.5	20.9	55.0	8.5	–
Mattident B (Johnson Matthey)	Low-gold	White	11.0	20.0	54.5	12.5	–
Realor (Degussa)	Low-gold copper-free	Yellow	20.0	20.0	39.0	–	16.0
Selector 3 (Metalor)	Low-gold copper-free	Yellow	20.0	21.0	38.7	–	16.5
Mattieco J (Johnson Matthey)	Low-gold copper-free	Yellow	20.0	20.0	40.1	–	17.8

There are also a number of *low-gold alloys*, which have gold contents typically of the order of 10–20%. The other elements are silver (40–60%) and palladium (up to 40%); these alloys could thus be described as Ag–Pd alloys, but we will leave that description for those alloys containing minor amounts of gold (<2%) or no gold at all.

Due to the reduced gold content, these alloys are white in appearance; they may be less attractive to those patients who prefer the appearance of the yellow gold alloys. In order to overcome this disadvantage, there are also a number of copper-free low-gold alloys, which contain high levels of indium. These have a two-phase structure consisting of a face-centered cubic (FCC) matrix with islands of a body-centered cubic (BCC) phase due to the high indium content. The matrix phase is essentially an Ag–Au solid solution with minor additions of palladium, indium, and zinc. The BCC phase consists of Pd–In with substantial amounts of gold, silver, and zinc, giving the alloy its yellow color. Thus the color seems to be related to the presence of the indium rather than the absence of copper.

Properties and Applications

Some of the properties of these alloys are compared in Table 3.3.4. The medium-gold alloys are recommended for the same applications as type III and IV gold alloys. Their ductility tends to be lower than that of the type IV gold alloys, and their high yield stress makes them difficult to burnish. There is even a danger of fracture on burnishing, due to the localized work hardening that occurs and further reduces their ductility. However, they are very suitable for long-span prostheses and may be used for implant-supported prostheses and posts and cores.

The low-gold content alloys tend to have poorer mechanical properties than the medium-gold alloys and are recommended as an alternative to type III gold alloys. However, their white color makes them less popular than they might otherwise be. These alloys are extensively used for posts and cores, where the white color does not present a problem, as the casting will be covered with another material.

The removal of the copper and the addition of the indium again produce alloys with properties similar to those of the type III gold alloys but with the advantage of the yellow color. However, the gap between the solidus and the liquidus is greater, which can result in a less homogeneous structure, and their melting temperature is considerably higher, making the casting process more difficult.

Although, in general, the medium-gold alloys are a suitable alternative to the type IV gold alloys, and the low-gold alloys to

TABLE 3.3.4	Comparison of Some Properties of Medium- and Low-Gold Casting Alloys Compared to a Type IV Gold Alloy*						
Alloy	Type	VHN	Elastic Modulus (GPa)	0.2% Proof Stress (MPa)	Elongation (%)	Solidus–Liquidus Temperature (°C)	Casting Temperature (°C)
Aurofluid 3	Type IV	255	80	480	10	885–920	1070
Solaro 3	Medium-gold	285	90.5	600	10	870–920	1070
Stabilor G	Medium-gold	275	–	830	6	–	1000–1100
Mattident E	Medium-gold	269	–	685	7	885–945	1045–1145
Palaginor 2	Low-gold	170	82	340	12	875–970	1200
Palliag MJ	Low-gold	265	–	630	4	940–1010	1100–1200
Mattident B	Low-gold	256	–	645	3.5	945–1000	1100–1200
Realor	Low-gold Cu-free	185	–	405	6	860–1035	1200
Selector 3	Low-gold Cu-free	180	75	370	8	875–1035	1200
Mattieco J	Low-gold Cu-free	200	–	740	5	870–940	1080–1150

*Data taken from manufacturers' data sheets.

type III gold alloys, one problem with these alloys is that their properties are more variable from alloy to alloy than for each of the four types of high-gold alloys (see Table 3.3.4).

The biocompatibility of these alloys appears to be excellent, and corrosion does not seem to be a problem, even with the two-phase, low-gold, copper-free alloys.

CLINICAL SIGNIFICANCE

The dentist must understand the properties of each alloy and, if necessary, seek advice from the manufacturer or dental laboratory in order to determine the suitability of an alloy for a particular clinical application.

Silver–Palladium Alloys

As the name implies, Ag–Pd alloys contain predominantly silver with significant amounts of palladium.

The palladium improves the resistance to corrosion and helps prevent tarnish, which is usually associated with the silver. These alloys were introduced in the 1960s as an alternative to the high-gold alloys and are commonly called 'white golds'.

The composition and the properties of some representative alloys after their heat-hardening treatment are presented in Table 3.3.5. Although there is some self-hardening with these alloys if they are left to bench-cool, the properties are generally inferior when compared to a carefully controlled hardening heat treatment.

There are two notable features of the data presented in Table 3.3.5. First, there is the wide range of properties in the different alloys, which again highlights the need to select the alloy for the application in mind very carefully. The low strength and hardness and the high ductility of one of the alloys shown (Palliag W) suggest that this alloy is suitable only for low-stress-bearing inlays. The other alloy with a similar composition (Mattieco 25) has superior mechanical properties, being more comparable to a type III gold alloy, and could be used for crowns, short-span bridges, and post and cores.

However, those alloys with reduced silver content and increased palladium content have properties similar to those of the type IV gold alloys. Nevertheless, their use for long-span prostheses is generally contraindicated. This may be associated

with the high casting temperatures for these alloys, which is the second most notable feature of these materials.

These high casting temperatures require the use of phosphate-bonded investments and high-temperature casting techniques, and it is well recognized that accurate casting at high temperatures is a problem for the dental technician.

The alloys have a tendency to work-harden rapidly, which precludes excessive adjustment and any burnishing. Although they are highly biocompatible, tarnishing does occur with these alloys. These disadvantages have resulted in this group of alloys being considerably less popular than the medium- and low-gold alloys.

BASE METAL ALLOYS

Cobalt–Chromium Alloys

Co–Cr alloys were first introduced to the dental profession in the 1930s and, since then, have effectively replaced the type IV gold alloys for the construction of partial denture frameworks, primarily due to their relatively low cost, which is a significant factor with these large castings.

Composition

The alloy consists of cobalt (55–65%) with up to 30% chromium. Other major alloying elements are molybdenum (4–5%) and, in at least one case, titanium (5%) (Table 3.3.6).

The cobalt and chromium form a solid solution for up to 30% chromium, which is the limit of solubility of chromium in cobalt; additional chromium would produce a highly brittle second phase.

In general, the higher the chromium content, the better the corrosion resistance of the alloy. Therefore the manufacturers try to maximize the amount of chromium without introducing the brittle second phase. Molybdenum is present in order to refine the grain size by providing more sites for crystal nucleation during the solidification process. It has the added benefit that it produces a significant solid solution hardening effect, an effect shared by the addition of iron. Nevertheless, the grains are very large, although grain boundaries are difficult to identify due to the coarse dendritic structure of the alloy.

TABLE 3.3.5 Composition and Properties of Silver/Palladium Alloys*

Alloy	Ag%	Pd%	Cu%	Zn%	VHN	0.2% Proof Stress (MPa)	Elongation (%)	Solidus–Liquidus Temperature (°C)	Casting Temperature (°C)
Palliag W (Degussa)	70.0	27.5	–	–	55	80	33	1080–1180	–
Mattieco 25 (Johnson Matthey)	68.5	25.0		3.0	199	500	31	1050–1110	1210–1290
Palliag M (Degussa)	58.5	27.4	10.5	–	310	940	3	950–1040	1100–1200
Palliag NF IV (Degussa)	52.0	39.9	–	4.0	270	595	6	1070–1145	1200–1250
Mattident P (Johnson Matthey)	46.6	33.4	19.0	–	290	780	3	1005–1040	1140–1240

*Data taken from manufacturers' data sheets.

TABLE 3.3.6 **Properties of Some Co–Cr Alloys***

Alloy	Co%	Cr%	Mo%	VHN	0.2% Proof Stress (MPa)	Elongation (%)	Solidus–Liquidus Temperature (°C)	Casting Temperature (°C)
Biosil H (Degussa)	65.7	28.5	4.5	360	600	8	1320–1380	1500
Vitallium (Nobelpharma)	60.6	31.5	6.0	428	616	3	1300–1370	1550
Wisil (Krupp)	65	28	5.0	390	580	7	1355–1375	1535

*Data taken from manufacturers' data sheets.

Carbon, which is present only in small quantities, is nevertheless an extremely important constituent of the alloy, as small changes in the carbon content can significantly alter the strength, hardness, and ductility of the alloy. Carbon can combine with any of the other alloying elements to form carbides. The fine precipitation of these can dramatically raise the strength and hardness of the alloy. However, too much carbon will result in excessive brittleness. This presents a problem for the dental technician, who needs to ensure that no excess carbon is absorbed by the alloy during melting and casting.

The distribution of the carbides also depends on the casting temperature and the cooling rate, with discontinuous carbide formation at the grain boundaries being preferable to continuous carbide formation.

Properties

For the dental technician, these alloys are considerably more difficult to handle than the gold alloys because they must be heated to high temperatures before they can be cast. Casting temperatures are in the region of 1300–1400°C and the associated casting shrinkage is ~2.0%.

This problem has largely been overcome with the introduction of induction casting equipment and high-temperature-resistant phosphate-bonded refractory investments. Accuracy is compromised at these high temperatures, which effectively limits the use of these alloys to partial dentures.

The high hardness of these alloys makes them difficult to polish mechanically. Electrolytic polishing is used for the fitting surfaces, so as not to compromise the quality of fit, but non-fitting surfaces are still mechanically polished. The benefit is that the highly polished surface is retained for a very long time, which is a distinct advantage with a removable prosthesis.

The lack of ductility so easily exacerbated by carbon contamination *does* present problems, especially as these alloys are also prone to casting porosity. These limitations combine to give rise to a common problem with partial dentures: clasp fractures. This problem becomes even more pronounced when an attempt is made to adjust a clasp arm, and excessive or frequent adjustments will invariably lead to a clasp-arm fracture.

Nevertheless, there are some features of these alloys that make them ideally suited to the construction of partial denture frameworks. The modulus of elasticity of a Co–Cr alloy is typically 250 GPa, whereas, for the alloys previously discussed, the modulus is in the range of 70–100 GPa. This high modulus of elasticity has the advantage that the denture, and particularly the clasp arms, can be made thinner in cross-section while maintaining adequate rigidity. This, combined with a density of about half that of the gold alloys, means that the castings are considerably lighter. This is of great benefit to the comfort of the patient.

The addition of chromium makes this a highly corrosion-resistant alloy, as can be emphasized by the fact that the alloy also forms the basis of many surgically implanted prostheses, such as hip and knee joints. It can be said therefore that these alloys have an excellent history of biocompatibility.

Some of the commercially available alloys also contain nickel, which is added by the manufacturer in order to increase the ductility and reduce the hardness. However, nickel is a well-known allergen, and its use in the mouth may trigger an allergic reaction. Therefore, for patients known to have a propensity for allergic reactions, it is advisable to use a nickel-free Co–Cr alloy.

Titanium Alloys

The interest in titanium-based castings for removable and fixed prosthodontics came about at approximately the same time as the development of titanium dental implants. Titanium has several attractive features, such as high strength with low density and excellent biocompatibility. In addition, however, there were concerns that, if a metal different from the titanium used in dental implants were used to produce the crowns and bridges, this might lead to galvanic effects.

The discovery of the element titanium has been attributed to the Reverend William Gregor in 1790, but it was not until 1910 that the first pure form of titanium was produced and, even now, titanium is still very expensive compared with, for example, stainless steel. Pure titanium is produced via the Kroll process, which involves heating titanium ore (e.g. rutile) in the presence of carbon and chlorine. The resultant $TiCl_4$ is reduced with molten sodium to produce a titanium sponge, which is subsequently fused under vacuum or in an argon atmosphere to produce an ingot of the metal.

Composition

Clinically, two forms of titanium have received the most interest. One is the commercially pure form of titanium (cpTi) and the other is an alloy of titanium–6% aluminum–4% vanadium.

Commercially pure titanium. Titanium is allotropic, with a hexagonal close-packed (HCP) structure (α) at low temperatures and a BCC structure (β) above 882°C. Commercially pure titanium (cpTi) is, in fact, an alloy of titanium with up to 0.5% oxygen. The oxygen is in solution, so the metal is single-phase. Elements such as oxygen, nitrogen, and carbon have a greater solubility in the HCP structure of the α-phase than in the cubic form of the β-phase. These elements form interstitial solid solutions with titanium and help to stabilize the α-phase. Transition elements, such as molybdenum, niobium, and vanadium, act as β-stabilizers.

Titanium–6% aluminum–4% vanadium. When aluminum and vanadium are added to titanium in only small quantities, the strength of the alloy is much increased over that of cpTi. Aluminum is considered to be an α-stabilizer, with vanadium acting as a β-stabilizer. When these are added to titanium, the temperature at which the α–β transition occurs is depressed, such that both the α and β forms can exist at room temperature. Thus Ti–6% Al–4% V has a two-phase structure of α and β grains.

Properties

Pure titanium is a white, lustrous metal, which has the attraction of low density, good strength, and an excellent corrosion resistance. It is ductile and constitutes an important alloying element with many other metals. Alloys of titanium are widely used in the aircraft industry and military applications because of its low density, high-tensile strength (~500 MPa), and ability to withstand high temperatures. The elastic modulus of cpTi is 110 GPa, which is half that of stainless steel or Co–Cr alloy.

The tensile properties of cpTi depend significantly on the oxygen content and, although the ultimate tensile strength, proof stress, and hardness increase with increased oxygen concentration, this is at the expense of the ductility.

By alloying titanium with aluminum and vanadium, a wide range of mechanical properties superior to the cpTi are possible. Such alloys of titanium are a mixture of the α- and β-phase, where the α-phase is relatively soft and ductile while the β-phase is harder and stronger but also less ductile. Thus by changing the relative proportions of α and β, a wide variety of mechanical properties can be achieved.

For the Ti–6% Al–4% V alloy, considerably higher tensile properties (~1030 MPa) are achievable than for pure titanium, which makes it attractive for use in high-stress-bearing situations such as partial dentures.

An important feature of these materials is the fatigue resistance of titanium alloys. Both cpTi and Ti–6% Al–4% V have a well-defined fatigue limit, with the S–N curve leveling out after 10^7–10^8 cycles of stress reversal at a tensile strength reduced by 45–50%. Thus cpTi should not be used in situations where the tensile stress may exceed 175 MPa. In contrast, for the Ti–6% Al–4% V, the fatigue limit is approximately 450 MPa.

Corrosion of alloys can be a serious problem, both in terms of degradation of the prosthesis and the release of potentially toxic or allergenic compounds. Titanium has become popular because it is exceptionally corrosion-resistant and this applies equally to the alloys. Although titanium is a highly reactive metal, this is also one of its strengths because the oxide formed on the surface (TiO_2) is extremely stable and this has a passivating effect on the metal. The potential for corrosion of titanium in the biological environment has been studied and has confirmed its excellent corrosion resistance.

Castability does present a serious problem with these alloys. Titanium has a high melting point (~1670°C), which creates problems with regard to the compensation of the cooling

TABLE 3.3.7 Comparison of Some Properties of Base Metal Casting Alloys

Property	Co–Cr alloy	Titanium	Ti–6% Al–4% V
Density (g cm^{-3})	8.9	4.5	4.5
Casting temperature (°C)	~1500	~1700	~1700
Casting shrinkage (%)	2.3	3.5	3.5
Tensile strength (MPa)	850	520	1000
Proportional limit (MPa)	550–650	350	920
Elastic modulus (GPa)	190–230	110	85–115
Hardness (Vickers)	360–430	200	–
Ductility (%)	2–8	20	14

contraction. Because the metal is very reactive, all castings need to be carried out in a vacuum or an inert atmosphere, which requires special casting equipment. Thus only a few dental laboratories will be set up for the casting of titanium alloys. The other problem is that the molten alloy has a propensity to react with the refractory investment mold, leaving behind a surface scale, which can compromise the quality of fit of the restoration. When constructed for implant-supported superstructures, very tight tolerances are required in order to achieve a passive fit on the implants. If this is not the case, the retention of the implant in the bone may be compromised. Internal porosity is also often observed with titanium castings. Hence other forms of processing titanium for dental prostheses are also used, such as milling by computer-aided design–computer-aided manufacture (CAD–CAM) or electrical discharge machining.

Some of the properties of the base metal alloys discussed above are presented in Table 3.3.7 for comparison.

SUMMARY

A growing variety of casting alloys are used in dentistry. In order to make a rational choice from the current spectrum of high-gold alloys and their alternatives, the dentist needs to have more knowledge about their appearances and their physical and mechanical properties than ever before.

Although the cost of the alloy is an important consideration, one generally finds that the cost savings on the prostheses are lower than might be expected. This is because the lower cost of the alloy is often offset by the increased cost of production. Also, in general, it can be said that the higher the gold content of the alloy, the better the quality of fit of the restoration.

When the dentist wishes to use alternative alloys to the precious metal alloys, it is important to liaise closely with the dental laboratory and find out what alloys are regularly used there, and what the laboratory's recommendations are, because of the wide range of properties obtainable.

CLINICAL SIGNIFICANCE

The ultimate responsibility for the materials used in the patient's mouth rests with the dentist, and not the dental technician.

CAD–CAM and 3D Printing of Metal Frameworks

Multi-axis CAD–CAM milling allows the production of metal frameworks with a high degree of precision. However, the method is slow and wasteful of material and the complexity of the design is limited. In contrast, no such limitations in the complexity of the design exist when 3D printing, which means that nowadays, this is the preferred route for digital manufacturing of metal frameworks. 3D printing is ideally suited to the production of highly accurate, one-off parts in metals. A number of 3D printing technologies are able to print metal objects and these include electron beam melting (EBM) and metal powder bed fusion technology, also referred to as selective laser melting (SLM). It is the latter technology that has become the preferred method in dentistry. 3D printers developed specifically for the dental industry produce millions of metal 3D-printed dental parts each year (Figure 3.3.1).

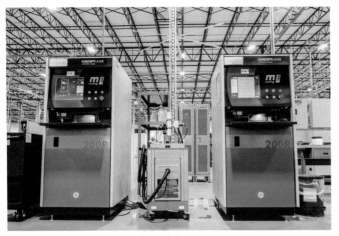

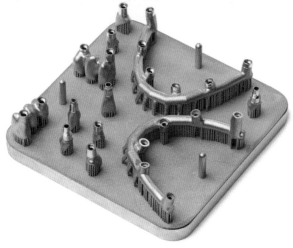

Figure 3.3.1 3D printers and the printed crown bridge and denture parts in Co-Cr alloy. Images courtesy of and copyright GE Additive, with thanks.

Metal 3D printing is well suited to dentistry because

- each patient is unique and each restoration has to be designed to suit that patient
- dental prostheses are small and complex, ideally suited to the small build envelope of the 3D printers
- dental prostheses are small but high in value, which helps to offset the high cost of the metal 3D printers
- metal 3D printing can significantly reduce the length and complexity of the manufacturing process when compared with lost-wax casting.

The digital approach can significantly reduce the number of steps involved in the manufacturing process as well as eliminate a number of materials. For example, it could be as simple as:

- Take an intraoral scan (no impression material and no casting of plaster models)
- Import the scanned data into the design software and produce a CAD model (no wax-up)
- Send the file of the model to the 3D metal printer and print the part (no refractory die etc.)
- Finish the part and return to the clinic

Not only can this be achieved in a matter of days, but because the metal 3D printer can print numerous prostheses in one go, the cost of each prosthesis is also much reduced, and all this without compromising the accuracy. Since the impression is stored digitally, replacement prostheses can also be produced easily. At present, the majority of metal parts fabricated are produced in Co-Cr alloy but other options in gold alloys or titanium alloys are becoming available.

FURTHER READING

Au, A.R., Lechner, S.K., Thomas, C.J., 2000. Titanium for removable partial dentures (III): 2-year clinical follow-up in an undergraduate programme. Journal of Oral Rehabilitation 27, 978.

Cruickshank-Boyd, D.W., 1981. Alternatives to gold 1: non-porcelain alloys. Dental Update 8, 17.

Laverty, D.P., Thomas, M.B.M., Clark, P., Addy, L.D., 2016. The use of 3D metal printing (direct laser metal sintering) in removable prosthodontics. Dental Update 43 (9), 826–828.

Leinfelder, K.F., 1997. An evaluation of casting alloys used for restorative procedures. Journal of the American Dental Association 128, 37.

Revilla-Leon, M., Meyer, M.J., Ozcan, M., 2019. Metal additive manufacturing technologies: literature review of current status and prosthodontics applications. International Journal of Computerized Dentistry 22 (1), 55–67.

Watanabe, I., Kiyosue, S., Ohkubo, C., 2002. Machinability of cast commercial titanium alloys. Journal of Biomedical Materials Research 63, 760–764.

Traditional Dental Ceramics

INTRODUCTION

Ceramic restorations are indicated where aesthetics is paramount and when the size or shape of the preparation exceeds the limit for the use of direct composite resins. The uses of ceramic include the construction of crown and bridgework, veneers, inlays and onlays, and sometimes artificial teeth for dentures. The construction of such restorations is usually undertaken in dental laboratories by technicians skilled in the art of fusing ceramics. In recent years the advent of computer-aided design–computer-aided manufacture (CAD–CAM) in dentistry has opened up opportunities to use new materials and the potential to extend the use of ceramics.

As people retain their teeth for much longer than in the past, the need for aesthetically acceptable restorations has increased and is likely to continue doing so. This is reflected in the growing use of ceramics in restorative procedures. Ceramics have developed a great deal over the last few decades, and there are many different materials available, sometimes dressed up with confusing or unhelpful terminology. In an attempt to demystify and clarify this important family of materials, the coverage of ceramics in this book has been changed compared to in earlier editions and is divided into two chapters: *Traditional dental ceramics*, which provides the historical context and describes those ceramics that have been in use relatively unchanged for some considerable time; and *Contemporary dental ceramics*, which describes those more recent developments including technologies that have found popularity or are gaining traction.

The reader should not be tempted to neglect study of traditional ceramics; these are very far from obsolete and are still in widespread use. The science that underpins them is of direct relevance to the modern ceramics and is also important to understand in what ways the modern ceramics differ from the materials that preceded them. Furthermore, the more traditional materials have *themselves* been the subject of innovation and development such as reinforcement, and their use in CAD–CAM, so the distinction between traditional and contemporary is a loose one with a good degree of overlap.

HISTORICAL PERSPECTIVE

Pottery in Europe up to CE 1700

The achievement of making usable pottery was a considerable feat and involved many trials and tribulations for the early potters. The raw material used for pottery is clay, and this presented the potter with two major problems.

The first problem was how to convert the clay into a form that provided the best consistency for manipulation and firing. Clay is usually too sticky to handle when simply mixed with water, and this problem was overcome by the addition of sand and ground seashells. In addition, clay shrinks as it dries out and hardens. If this shrinkage is non-uniform, either in rate or in overall magnitude, the pots will crack even before they have been fired. Again, the addition of a coarse-grained filler went some way toward overcoming this problem.

It was during the firing of the pots that the problems really began to be serious. Gases present in the mixture, whether air bubbles or gases formed during heating (such as water vapor and CO_2), created voids in the clay and even sometimes caused it to fracture during firing. Early potters overcame this problem by beating the clay prior to molding to get rid of the air (*wedging* is the term often used by artisans to describe this process). Another development was the technique of raising the temperature very gradually during the firing process, as then, the steam and gases could diffuse out of the clay slowly, rather than bursting out and causing the pot to crack.

The most serious obstacle during this phase in the development of ceramic technology was the temperature at which the pottery could be fired. The conversion of clay from a mass of individual particles loosely held together by a water binder to a coherent solid relies on a process known as *sintering*. In this process the points at which the individual particles are in contact fuse at sufficiently high temperatures (Figure 3.4.1).

The process relies on diffusion, which is greatly accelerated by elevated temperatures. The demand for high uniform temperatures could not be met by the traditional open fires, and this led to the invention of the *kiln*. The earliest of these was the *up-draught kiln*, in which higher temperatures and greater uniformity of temperature were obtained by drawing air through the fire and putting the pots in the rising hot gases.

Early kilns were able to reach temperatures of up to 900°C, and pottery fired at this temperature is called *earthenware*. The resultant pottery is porous, as the sintering process has only just managed to fuse the particles of clay where they touch. Such pots were suitable for the storage of solid foods but could not hold any liquids. This problem was overcome eventually by fusing a thin layer of a glassy material, that is, a glaze, over the surface of the pot. This technology was used as far back as 5500 BCE in various places, including Turkey.

Gradual progress was made toward higher kiln temperatures so that many more clays could be partially melted. The liquid phase would invariably solidify as a glass, resulting in impervious

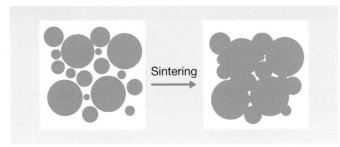

Figure 3.4.1 Sintering of ceramic particles.

pottery that is generally known as *stoneware*. Stoneware appeared in Europe in the CE 15–16th centuries.

Chinese Porcelain

In contrast to what was happening in Europe, stoneware had been produced in China by 100 BCE, and by the CE 10th century, ceramic technology in China had advanced to such a stage that Chinese artisans were able to produce:

A ceramic so white that it was comparable only to snow, so strong that vessels needed walls only 2–3 mm thick and consequently light could shine through it. So continuous was the internal structure that a dish, if lightly struck, would ring like a bell. This is porcelain!

As trade with East Asia grew, this infinitely superior material came to Europe from China during the 17th century. Until then, there had been a distinct lack of interest in tableware. The majority of the population ate off wooden plates, and the nobility were satisfied with metal ones. For special occasions, gold and silver tableware would be used by the very wealthy.

This all changed with the introduction of Chinese porcelain, which stimulated demand for high-quality ceramic tableware. There was no way in which the trade could possibly satisfy this demand, so strenuous efforts were made by the European pottery industry to imitate Chinese porcelain.

Passable imitations were made by using tin oxide as a glaze (producing the white appearance of porcelain), but this method did not reproduce the translucency of Chinese porcelain. For example, Meissen in Germany in 1708 managed to produce what they called "white porcelain," but their product more closely resembled northern Chinese stoneware. Many other manufacturers, now well-established names, were unable to produce genuine porcelain but still made a name for themselves with high-quality stoneware, such as Majolica from Italy, Wedgwood from England, and Delft's Blue from Holland.

In the up-draught kiln the technology existed to produce high temperatures, although the Chinese down-draught kiln was somewhat superior at controlling the temperature. The problem of reproducing Chinese porcelain was essentially one of selecting the material and the method of processing. Many, such as John Dwight of Fulham, who was granted a patent by Charles II in 1671, claimed to have discovered the secret of Chinese porcelain but really only managed to make white stoneware.

In order to produce porcelain, the material has to remain or to become white on firing and must be so strong that vessels with walls less than 3 mm thick can be produced. If the product needs to be made with walls thicker than 3 mm, even porcelain appears opaque. So the major differences between stoneware and porcelain are that porcelain is white and can be made in such thin sections that it appears translucent. Stoneware could be made to look white but had to be used in such a thickness that it was invariably opaque.

This situation prevailed for some time until, in 1717, the secret was leaked from China by a Jesuit missionary, Father d'Entrecolles. He performed his missionary work in a place called King-te-Tching, which, at that time, was the porcelain center of China. Going among the people in their place of work, he managed to acquire samples of the materials used. He sent the samples to a French friend of his, together with a detailed account of how the porcelain was manufactured. The samples and the description were passed on to M. de Réaumur, a scientist, who was able to identify the components used by the Chinese, such as kaolin, silica, and feldspar.

Kaolin, known as china clay, is a hydrated alumino-silicate. The silica is in the form of quartz and remains as a fine dispersion after firing; the feldspar is a mixture of sodium and potassium–aluminum silicates. These were mixed in proportions of 25–30% feldspar, 20–25% quartz, and 50% kaolin. It should be said that by the early 1700s, the Meissen factory in Dresden was already producing a very passable porcelain based on kaolin, silica, and alabaster.

In a way, it is a little surprising that it took so long before the composition of Chinese porcelain was unraveled. The art of making porcelain involves no complex chemistry, since the process is one of taking three rather common minerals (kaolin, feldspar, and flint) and firing them at high temperatures. Once the mystery had been solved, however, it did not take long for new porcelains to be developed in Europe. Soon it was possible to make it in any shade or tint, and its translucency gave such a depth of color that it was not long before the dental potential of this material was recognized.

The dental application of porcelain dates back to 1774, when a French apothecary named Alexis Duchateau considered the possibility of replacing his ivory dentures with porcelain. Ivory, being porous, soaks up oral fluids and eventually becomes badly stained, as well as being highly unhygienic. Duchateau, with the assistance of porcelain manufacturers at the Guerhard factory in Saint Germain-en-Laye, succeeded in making himself the first porcelain denture. This was quite a feat, since the porcelain shrinks considerably on firing. This shrinkage had to be taken into account if the denture was going to fit at all well in the mouth. Since then, other materials such as vulcanite and, more recently, poly methyl methacrylate have helped replace porcelain for denture applications.

Porcelain teeth, in conjunction with an acrylic denture base, are still used. However, the most important application of dental porcelain is in the construction of veneers, inlays, crowns, and bridges, where the aesthetic qualities of the porcelain are still superior to that of any other substitute for enamel and dentine.

Porcelains were the first materials used in the construction of the porcelain jacket crown (PJC). Many new materials have appeared on the market over recent years that are described as porcelains but are, in fact, very different forms of ceramic when compared with the early porcelains.

One of the most serious drawbacks with the early dental porcelains described above was their lack of strength and toughness, which seriously limited their use. As early as 1903, Land described, in an issue of *Dental Cosmos*, how to make porcelain crowns but came up against the problem that the crowns would break too easily. Similarly, Pincus described the concept of the ceramic veneer in an article in the *Californian Dental Association Journal* of 1938 but was also frustrated by the lack of strength of the porcelains available at the time. This has changed considerably beginning in the 1960s with the introduction of a raft of innovations such that now we have a wide range of dental ceramics at our disposal.

CLINICAL SIGNIFICANCE

It is now more appropriate to use the more general description of *dental ceramics*, as this encompasses a wider range of materials than the term *porcelain*.

CLASSIFICATION OF DENTAL CERAMICS

When seeking to classify dental ceramics, there are several approaches that can be adopted. One of the earliest classifications was based on the fusion temperatures of the ceramic powders: the dental ceramics were classified as either high-fusing, medium-fusing, or low-fusing materials. This was fine when the only manufacturing route was by the process of sintering. However, nowadays, there are multiple manufacturing routes that can be used besides sintering that include hot pressing, casting, and CAD–CAM. There is even ongoing research to develop 3D printing methods for dental ceramics. All of this means that the convention of classifying dental ceramics by their fusion temperatures is no longer suitable, as it doesn't encompass the full range of ceramics that we encounter. Another option is to classify dental ceramics according to the processing routes used. The drawback with this approach is that in some instances the same ceramic can be used in different processing routes giving rise to duplication and a good deal of confusion. Yet another approach is to classify dental ceramics according to their application, such as veneers, cemented high-strength core and monolithic ceramics, and resin-bonded ceramics, but again some dental ceramics would overlap, leading to duplication.

The classification adopted in this book is based on the microstructure of the dental ceramics and is as follows:
1. Glasses, including particulate-filled glasses and reinforced glasses, for example, feldspar, leucite-containing-feldspar, alumina-reinforced feldspar, and glass-infiltrated ceramics.
2. Glass-ceramics, for example, leucite, lithium disilicate, and apatite glass-ceramics.
3. Crystalline ceramics, for example, alumina and zirconia.
4. Resin matrix ceramics, for example, resin composites and interpenetrating networks.

The range of dental applications of these ceramics is shown in Table 3.4.1. The methods of processing include powder/liquid sintering, slip casting, hot-ceramic pressing, and

TABLE 3.4.1 Applications of Dental Ceramics

Description	Application
Feldspathic glass	Veneers for porcelain jacket crowns and resin-bonded laminate veneers
Alumina-reinforced feldspathic glass	Core of the porcelain jacket crown
Leucite containing feldspathic glass	Veneer for metal and zirconia substructures and resin-bonded laminate veneers
Leucite glass-ceramics	Resin-bonded laminate veneer, anterior crowns and posterior inlays
Lithium disilicate glass-ceramics	Resin-bonded anterior and posterior crowns and bridges
Fluorapatite glass-ceramics	Veneer for lithium disilicate cores for crowns and bridges
Glass infiltrated spinel	Core for anterior crowns and bridges
Glass infiltrated alumina	Core for anterior crowns and bridges and posterior crowns
Glass infiltrated alumina/zirconia	Core for anterior and posterior crowns and bridges
Crystalline ceramic: alumina	Core for anterior and posterior crowns and bridges
Crystalline ceramic: zirconia	Core for anterior and posterior crowns and bridges and monolithic posterior crowns and bridges
Resin matrix ceramics	Veneers, inlays, onlays, anterior and posterior crowns, implant-supported crowns

CAD–CAM. The ceramics described in 1 are considered traditional dental ceramics, including the use of these in metal–ceramic devices; those in 2-4 are discussed in the following chapter under the heading of contemporary dental ceramics.

DENTAL GLASSES AND REINFORCED DENTAL GLASSES

The fundamental building block of dental glasses is a glassy material called feldspar. Feldspar was critical in the development of dental porcelains, as discussed above. Thus it is of interest first to take a closer look at the development of dental porcelains.

DENTAL PORCELAIN

The earliest dental porcelains were mixtures of kaolin, feldspar, and quartz, and were quite different from earthenware, stoneware, and domestic porcelain, as indicated in Figure 3.4.2.

This shift away from the composition of Chinese porcelain was driven by the need to enhance the aesthetics of the dental porcelain. It was not until 1838 that Elias Wildman produced dental porcelain with a translucency and shades that reasonably matched those of the natural teeth. The compositions of domestic and dental porcelain are shown in Table 3.4.2.

Kaolin is a hydrated aluminum silicate ($Al_2O \cdot 2SiO_2 \cdot 2H_2O$) and acts as a binder, making the unfired porcelain easier to mold. It is opaque, however, and its presence, even in very small

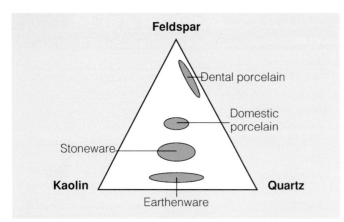

Figure 3.4.2 Relative composition of ceramic products based on feldspar, kaolin, and quartz.

TABLE 3.4.3 Typical Oxide Composition of a Dental Porcelain

Material	Wt %
Silica	63
Alumina	17
Boric oxide	7
Potash (K_2O)	7
Soda (Na_2O)	4
Other oxides	2

TABLE 3.4.2 Composition of Household and Dental Porcelains

Porcelain	% Kaolin	% Quartz	% Feldspar
Household	50	20–25	25–30
Dental	0	25	65

quantities, meant that the earliest dental porcelains lacked adequate translucency. Thus, for dental porcelains, the kaolin was omitted and they could thus be considered to be a feldspathic glass with crystalline inclusions of silica.

The quartz remains unchanged during the firing process and acts as a strengthening agent. It is present as a fine crystalline dispersion throughout the glassy phase that is produced by the melting of the feldspar. The feldspar fuses when it melts and then cools, forming a glass matrix.

The feldspars are mixtures of potassium alumino-silicate ($K_2O \cdot Al_2O_3 \cdot 6SiO_2$) and sodium alumino-silicate, also known as albite ($Na_2O \cdot Al_2O_3 \cdot 6SiO_2$). Feldspars are naturally occurring substances, so the ratio between the potash (K_2O) and the soda (Na_2O) will vary somewhat. This affects the properties of the feldspar, in that the soda tends to lower the fusion temperature and the potash increases the viscosity of the molten glass.

During the firing of porcelain, there is always the danger of excessive *pyroplastic flow* (flow of the molten glass) that may result in rounding of the edges and loss of tooth form. It is important that the right amount of potash is present to prevent this. These alkalis either are present as a part of the feldspars, or they may be added as carbonates to ensure the correct ratio. The typical oxide composition of a dental porcelain is presented in Table 3.4.3.

The porcelain powder used by the dental technician is not a simple mixture of the ingredients in Table 3.4.3. These powders have been fired once already. The manufacturer mixes the components, adds additional metal oxides, fuses them, and then quenches the molten mass in water. The resultant product is known as a *frit*, and the process is known as *fritting*. One consequence of the rapid cooling is the build-up of large internal stresses in the glass, resulting in extensive cracking. This material

can be ground very easily to produce a fine powder for use by the dental technician.

During the firing of these porcelains, there is no chemical reaction taking place; the glass is simply melted above its glass transition temperature when the particles fuse together by liquid-phase sintering and cooled down again. Thus all that has happened is that the individual particles have fused together by sintering to produce the final, solid item.

The particle size distribution is critical in ensuring that the particles pack together as tightly as possible, in order that the shrinkage on firing is minimized. The average particle size is generally in the region of 25 μm, with a wide distribution of other particle sizes, such that the smaller particles fill in the spaces in between the larger particles. Some porcelain powders have a multimodal particle size distribution to increase the packing density.

Several other ingredients will be present in the dental porcelain powders. These include metal oxides, which provide the wide variety of colors of the porcelain; for example, oxides of iron act as a brown pigment, copper as a green pigment, titanium alloys give a yellowish-brown, and cobalt imparts a blue color. A binder, consisting of starch and sugar, may also be present to help in the manipulation of the powders.

PROPERTIES OF DENTAL PORCELAIN

Dental porcelain is chemically very stable and provides excellent aesthetics that do not deteriorate over time. The thermal conductivity and the coefficient of thermal expansion are similar to those of enamel and dentine, so in the presence of a good marginal seal, marginal leakage is less likely to be a problem.

Although the compressive strength of dental porcelain is high (350–550 MPa), its tensile strength is very low (20–60 MPa), which is typical of a brittle solid. The material, being primarily a glass, lacks fracture toughness. The maximum strain that a glass can withstand is less than 0.1%. Glasses are extremely sensitive to the presence of *surface micro-cracks*, and this represents one of the major drawbacks of the use of dental porcelain. On cooling from the furnace temperature, the outside of the porcelain will cool more rapidly than the interior, particularly as the porcelain has a low thermal conductivity. The outside surface contracts more than the inside initially, resulting in a compressive load on the outside and a residual tensile stress on the inside as the interior is being prevented from shrinking by the outside skin.

PROCESSING

The porcelains described above are used for the creation of PJCs, which consist of an outer porcelain layer, benefiting from the mechanical and optical properties of porcelain and its resemblance to natural tooth tissue, which is mounted on an underlying metallic substructure, which is not (or should not be) visible once the crown is in place but provides support for the fragile porcelain and overall imparts the strength that the crown requires. The production of a PJC involves three technical stages:

- compaction
- firing
- glazing.

Compaction

In the construction of a PJC, the porcelain powder is mixed with water and made into a paste. This paste is applied to the die, which has been coated beforehand with a very thin platinum foil, to allow the porcelain crown to be separated from the die and transported to the furnace.

A PJC is made from more than one type of porcelain powder because it is impossible to recreate all of the aesthetic features of a tooth with the use of a single porcelain. Conventionally, three basic types of porcelain powder are used. These are an opaque shade to mask the color of the underlying structure, which may be an amalgam or a metal post and core construction. Then a dentine shade is applied and finally an enamel shade. The exact enamel shade is selected from a guide that is used to compare with the shade of the natural tooth. The final construction is as shown in Figure 3.4.3.

The powder is mixed with water and a binder to form a slurry that can be applied to the die in various ways, such as spatulation, brush application, whipping, or vibrating, all of which are aimed at compacting the powder. The objective of these condensation techniques is to remove as much water as possible, resulting in a more compact arrangement with a high density of particles that minimizes the firing shrinkage. The particle size and shape are extremely important, as they affect the handling characteristics of the powder and have an effect on the amount of shrinkage on firing. The binder helps to hold the particles together, as the material is extremely fragile in this so-called *green state.*

Firing

Initially, the crown is heated slowly in the open entrance to the furnace. This is carried out to drive off excess water before it has a chance to form steam. If the water in the mix were allowed to turn into steam, it would cause the fragile powder-compact to crack as the steam tried to escape to the surface. Once the compact has been dried, it is placed in the furnace and the binders are burnt out. Some contraction occurs during this stage.

When the porcelain begins to fuse, continuity is only achieved at points of contact between the powder particles. The material is still porous and is usually referred to as being at the *low bisque stage.* As the exposure to the elevated temperature continues, more fusion takes place as the molten glass flows between the particles, drawing them closer together and filling the voids. A large contraction takes place during this phase (~20%), and the resultant material is virtually nonporous. The cause of the high shrinkage of porcelain on firing is therefore due to the fusion of the particles during sintering, as the powder particles are brought into close contact.

The firing of the porcelain must be carried out exactly according to the manufacturer's instructions. If the crown should remain in the furnace for too long, it will lose form due to pyroplastic flow and will become highly glazed.

A very slow cooling rate is essential to avoid cracking or crazing. The furnaces available usually offer a considerable degree of automation and can be used for air- or vacuum-firing. Vacuum-firing produces a denser porcelain than air-firing, as air is withdrawn during the firing process. Fewer voids are formed, resulting in a stronger crown with a more predictable shade. Areas of porosity in air-fired porcelain alter the translucency of the crown, as they cause light to scatter. An additional problem is that air voids will become exposed if grinding of the superficial layer should be necessary, giving rise to an unsightly appearance and a rough surface finish.

Glazing

There will always be some porosity in the porcelain, with small air voids being exposed at the surface. If not dealt with, these will allow the ingress of bacteria and oral fluids and act as potential sites for the build-up of plaque. To avoid this, the surface is glazed to produce a smooth, shiny, and impervious outer layer. There are two ways in which this can be achieved:

- Glasses that fuse at low temperatures are applied to the crown after construction, and a short period at a relatively low temperature is sufficient to fuse the glaze.
- Final firing of the crown under carefully controlled conditions fuses the superficial layer to an impervious surface glaze.

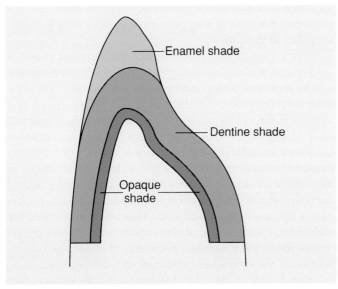

Figure 3.4.3 Porcelain build-up for a jacket crown.

Enamel shade

Dentine shade

Opaque shade

CLINICAL SIGNIFICANCE

If the differential dimensional change is sufficiently high, the internal surface layer that is under tension will rupture to relieve the stresses. This will result in the fit surface of the crown containing many minute cracks, and it is these that will ultimately cause the crown to fracture catastrophically (Figure 3.4.4). The application of a glaze with a slightly lower coefficient of expansion would potentially fill in the cracks and also place the surface under compression. Unfortunately, this is not possible on the fitting surface of the crown, as it may result in the crown not seating properly.

Over the years up until the 1960s, the composition of the dental porcelains was changed by removing the quartz as well as the kaolin. This was done for the purpose of enhancing the aesthetics (kaolin increases the opacity) and reducing the abrasiveness caused by the exposure of quartz at the surface. Thus what was generally referred to as dental porcelain is in fact a feldspathic glass.

Feldspathic Glasses

The feldspathic glasses were not strong enough to be used for the manufacture of dental restorations, and problems even arose for anterior PJCs, especially when they were used in situations of heavy occlusion. The tiny surface flaws in the interior of the crown act as initiating sites for catastrophic failure. The inherently low tensile strength of dental porcelains (<60 MPa) restricted their use to very low stress-bearing anterior applications. Thus, until things changed in the 1960s, the use of ceramics in dentistry was essentially limited to the production of porcelain teeth for removable dentures.

To overcome the problem of lack of strength and toughness of the feldspathic glasses, one solution is to provide the dental ceramic with support from a stronger, tougher substructure. It is well known that enamel is not a strong material when

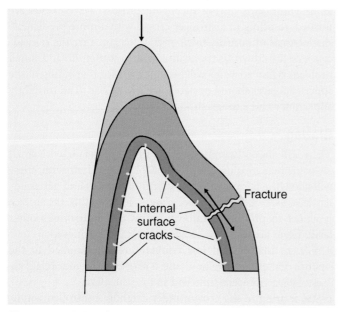

Figure 3.4.4 Palatal fracture of a porcelain jacket crown initiated from an internal surface flaw.

examined in isolation; however, because it is supported by the underlying dentine, the tooth can withstand much larger forces than might be supposed if considering the enamel alone. The tensile strength of enamel is estimated to be in the region of 30 MPa and yet it can provide a lifetime of function as long as it is supported by dentine and not eroded, abraded, dissolved, or otherwise damaged. Two developments occurred in the 1960s that gave a new lease of life to the use of ceramics in dentistry, namely the alumina-reinforced PJC and the porcelain fused to metal restorations (PFM), now more commonly referred to as metal–ceramics. For the PJC, feldspar is used as an aesthetic veneer over an alumina-reinforced feldspathic glass as detailed below. For the metal–ceramic restorations, the main issue, a recurring theme in dental biomaterials, was to achieve compatibility between two dissimilar materials within a single structure – in this case the outer ceramic and the underlying metallic support structure. It was necessary to ensure a strong and lasting bond between the two, very different, materials and to eliminate any mismatch in thermal properties between them to avoid stresses building up at this interface. This was made possible by the addition of leucite crystals to the feldspar, which allowed close control of the coefficient of expansion of the veneer in order to ensure it closely matched the metal substructure. Two further developments took place in the 1980s that extended the use of glasses in dentistry with the introduction of the glass infiltrated ceramics and the concept of the resin-bonded laminate veneer.

Alumina-Reinforced Porcelain Jacket Crown

The work by Land in the early 1900s and others since then showed that one of the problems with the all-ceramic anterior crown was that the porcelain would fracture from the fit surface outward. Some improvements in the strength of porcelain were achieved by the introduction of vacuum-firing furnaces, which helped to minimize porosity, and raised the flexural strength of the porcelain from 20–30 MPa to approximately 50–60 MPa. However, this proved not to be adequate to produce reliable ceramic restorations and thus the search was on for a core material that would provide the necessary strength and toughness to prevent fractures arising from cracks propagating from the fit surface of the crown.

Since ceramics tend to fail at the same critical strain of ~0.1%, one means of achieving an increase in fracture strength is to increase the elastic modulus of the material. If, at the same time, the propagation of cracks is made more difficult such that a greater strain can be supported, a higher-strength ceramic will result (Figure 3.4.5). The flexural strengths of some ceramics are shown in Table 3.4.4. As the tensile strength is a difficult property to measure (giving rise to a wide degree of scatter in the data), it is common practice instead to measure the flexural strength and use this to predict, to a degree, its clinical performance and ability to withstand the forces that arise within the oral cavity. Although the silicon nitrides and carbides are attractive from the viewpoint of strength, they are not suitable because of the difficulties associated with the manufacture of individual crowns: the color differences and the mismatch in the coefficient of thermal expansion.

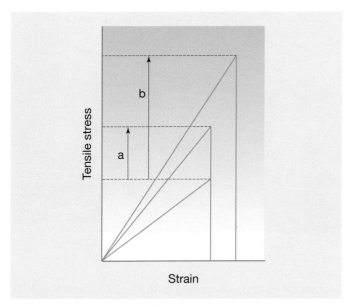

Figure 3.4.5 Improvements in the strength of ceramics by (a) raising the elastic modulus and (b) increasing the resistance to crack propagation.

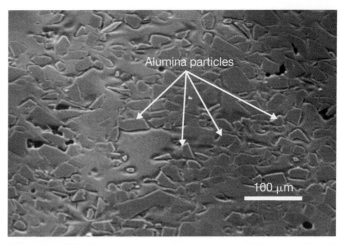

Figure 3.4.6 Scanning electron micrograph of an alumina-reinforced core material showing the alumina particles embedded in a glassy matrix composed of feldspar.

TABLE 3.4.4 **Typical Strength Values for High-Strength Ceramics**	
Type of Ceramic	**Flexural Strength (MPa)**
Hot-pressed silicon nitride	800–900
Hot-pressed silicon carbide	400–750
Partially stabilized zirconia	640
Alumina 98% pure	420–520

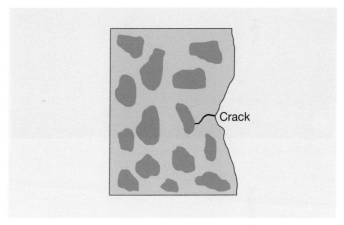

Figure 3.4.7 Alumina particles acting as crack stoppers.

CLINICAL SIGNIFICANCE

Alumina and zirconia are white and strong, and therefore these ceramics are now used in dental ceramic systems.

In the mid-1960s, McLean and Hughes developed a core material based on the reinforcement of a feldspathic glass with alumina, commonly referred to as the alumina-reinforced porcelain jacket crown (PJC). The material consists of a feldspathic glass containing 40–50% alumina particles (Figure 3.4.6). The alumina is far stronger than the glass, and the particles are more effective at preventing crack propagation than quartz, acting as crack stoppers (Figure 3.4.7). Whereas the flexural strength of feldspathic glass is some 60 MPa at best, this is raised to 120–150 MPa for the aluminous core ceramic.

In the construction of a crown the opaque shade shown in Figure 3.4.10 is made with an alumina-reinforced feldspar ceramic. It is still necessary to use the weaker dentine and enamel shades of the feldspathic glasses because it is not possible to produce alumina-reinforced feldspar ceramics with the required translucency as the alumina causes the core ceramic to appear dull and opaque.

The main application of the alumina-reinforced PJC is for the restoration of anterior teeth. Although the improvement in strength is considerable, it is still insufficient to allow its use posteriorly and the construction of even a three-unit bridge is out of the question.

Resin-Bonded Ceramics

One way in which the traditional approach of cemented restorations such as the PJC has been challenged is with the development of new adhesive techniques. These have extended the use of ceramics to areas not previously thought possible. The concept of the resin-bonded ceramic restoration could not become reality until techniques for bonding the ceramic to enamel and dentine had been developed. The idea of bonding ceramics to enamel using a combination of the acid-etch technique and resins began to be developed during the 1970s, which led, in the 1980s, to the ceramic laminate veneer restoration, a very thin sliver of ceramic material that is bonded to the tooth structure to support it (Figure 3.4.8).

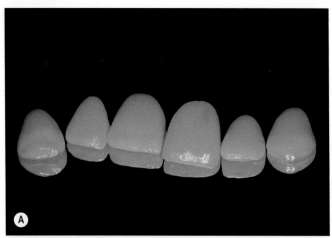

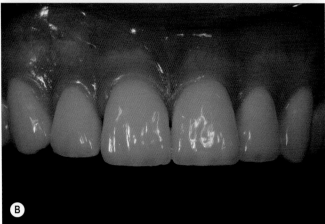

Figure 3.4.8 (a) Porcelain laminate veneers and (b) clinical result when resin bonded to the anterior teeth. Images courtesy of and copyright Dr Andrea Fabianelli, Cortona, Italy, with thanks.

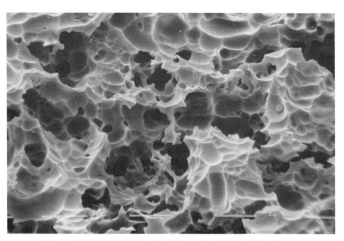

Figure 3.4.9 HF etched surface of a feldspathic glass.

etchant for veneers constructed from a leucite-containing feldspar, so as to enhance the bond between the ceramic and the resin by creating a micromechanical interlocking surface on the ceramic (Figure 3.4.9). Thus using the phosphoric acid-etch technique on enamel, he was able to bond the ceramic veneers permanently to the teeth with a resin-based composite. Bonding to ceramic has since been improved by the additional use of a silane coupling agent.

As major progress was made in the development of dentine-bonding agents, this opened up the possibility of resin-bonded crowns. The combination of adhesion to enamel, dentine, and ceramic and the improved strength characteristics of the ceramics has produced restorations with excellent mechanical integrity. In fact, the adhesive bond has the effect of eliminating the internal surface flaws and thus reduces the potential for fracture. This has led to a growth in the use of resin-bonded ceramics for crowns, veneers, and inlays.

CLINICAL SIGNIFICANCE

Before the advent of resin-bonded ceramic veneers, the only options available were the composite veneer, the porcelain jacket crown, and the metal–ceramic crown.

Ceramic veneers are considered superior to composites in terms of their aesthetics, color stability, surface finish, abrasion resistance, and tissue compatibility. They are also chemically very stable and have a coefficient of thermal expansion similar to that of enamel. The finishing of porcelain veneers is more difficult than that of composites due to their high hardness. The thin feathered margins are more easily damaged than the margins of crowns, both in the laboratory and in the surgery. The ceramic veneers have the distinct advantage over crowns in that improved aesthetics can be achieved with minimal tooth reduction, and the palatal surface of the tooth is unchanged so that incisal guidance is maintained. When the technique first developed in the 1980s, the material used for the construction of veneers was either a feldspathic glass or a leucite-containing feldspathic glass. This was simply down to an issue of availability at the time. Feldspathic glasses were readily available as these

The concept of using ceramics as veneers is not new and can be traced back to Dr. Charles Pincus of Beverley Hills, who constructed porcelain veneers in the 1930s for actors in Hollywood. The porcelain veneers were baked on platinum foil and retained on the teeth by denture powder. However, the veneers often broke because the thin porcelain was brittle and they were frequently removed from the teeth. When acrylic resin was introduced in 1937, Pincus switched to this material for the production of veneers for the acting profession. This eventually developed into the use of composite veneers, and ceramics were not used for a long time.

The advent of procedures for bonding resins to enamel using phosphoric acid etching of the enamel allowed the development of the resin-bonded ceramic veneer as a viable treatment option. This technique permitted bonding of resins to tooth enamel. In this situation the fact that the thin ceramic material is bonded to the underlying tooth structure via a resin means that the tooth itself provides the support for the weak veneering material. An early reference to supporting a ceramic restoration by resin-bonding it to enamel was published by Rochette in 1975. This idea was then extended by Horn in 1983, who proposed the use of hydrofluoric acid as a glass

were used to veneer PJCs and leucite-containing feldspathic glasses were used to veneer metal substructures. These were the ceramics of choice for the construction of veneers due to their excellent aesthetics, especially from the point of view of color and translucency, something that it is difficult for any other ceramic to match.

Although in the time of Land and Pincus the veneers were constructed on platinum foil, a variety of methods have been made available since then, which include:

- sintering on a refractory die
- hot pressing (see Chapter 3.5, which covers glass-ceramics)
- computer-aided design–computer-aided manufacture (CAD–CAM) machining from a block or disc.

Sintering Process

In the sintering process a slurry of the ceramic powder is applied to a refractory die (as opposed to a Pt-foil-coated die in the case of the PJC), dried, and subsequently fired in a porcelain furnace. Multiple layers can be built up to develop detailed characterization. Great skill is required by the dental laboratory technician to get the best aesthetics and appropriate contour. An example of a commercial leucite containing feldspathic glass using the sintering processing route is Mirage (Mirage Dental Systems, Kansas City, USA). Unfortunately, due to new developments in ceramic processing, such as pressable ceramics and CAD–CAM, the customization and high aesthetic value typically seen in feldspathic veneers is being lost.

CAD–CAM

Nowadays, the preferred route for manufacturing crowns and veneers from feldspathic glasses is the use of CAD–CAM. The VITABLOCS® from Vita Zahnfabrik are probably the most widely used feldspar-based CAD–CAM ceramics. In 1985 Vita Mark I was launched, followed in 1991 by Vita Mark II, a monochromatic feldspathic glass. In order to replicate the natural colors of the tooth, Vita then introduced a range of CAD–CAM blocks from 2003 onward that consist of multi-layers of different shade intensities, namely, VITABLOCS® TriLuxe (2003), TriLuxe forte (2007), and VITABLOCS® RealLife (2010). The latter is described as a multi-chromatic feldspar ceramic with different color intensities in three dimensions. The most recent blocks are similar to the earlier material but are produced by a different process described as extrusion molding. A plasticized ceramic mixture is pressed and extruded through a nozzle and the resultant blocks are dried for several days before being sintered.

METAL-BONDED CERAMICS

Introduction

A major limitation of the aesthetic ceramics such as the feldspathic glasses was their lack of strength. For ceramic restorations, the presence of micro-cracks on the fitting surface is a major source of weakness, and their elimination would significantly improve the strength of the crown. Glazing the internal fitting surface would achieve this end but would compromise

the fit of the crown. Another possibility is bonding the ceramic to a metal substrate, such that these microscopic cracks are effectively eliminated, with the consequence that the combined metal–ceramic structure is considerably stronger. This is the basic premise of the metal-bonded system (Figure 3.4.10). The significant breakthrough came with the publication of a patent by Weinstein, Katz, and Weinstein in 1962, where they explained how it is possible to get a feldspathic glass to bond to an alloy surface by the inclusion of leucite crystals. The latter were added so as to ensure that the coefficient of thermal expansion of the ceramic closely matched that of the metal, as explained in more detail later.

The crown consists of a cast metal coping, onto which is fired a ceramic veneer. If a proper bond is created, then the internal cracks are eliminated, as the metal presents a barrier to the propagation of cracks by virtue of its high fracture toughness. One of the most likely modes of failure with this system is the separation of the ceramic from the metal due to an interfacial breakdown of the metal–ceramic bond. The success of the system depends on the quality of this bond.

> ### CLINICAL SIGNIFICANCE
>
> From a materials perspective, the most likely cause of failure of a metal–ceramic restoration is a breakdown of the metal–ceramic bond. As long as this is secure, the longevity of these devices is generally good, with caries and periodontitis being the main potential negative outcomes as opposed to failure of the materials themselves.

An important contributory factor to the ability to bond the ceramic to the metal is the degree of mismatch between the coefficients of expansion of the ceramic and the metal. If the mismatch is too great, then stresses will build up during the cooling process after firing. These stresses can be sufficient to result in crazing or cracking of the ceramic. The issues of the bond and the coefficients of expansion both require careful consideration.

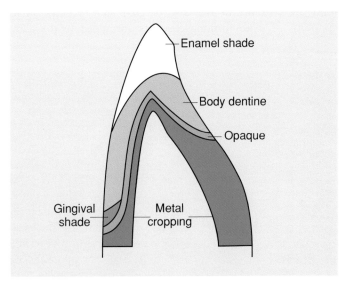

Figure 3.4.10 Construction of a metal–ceramic crown.

THE BOND

The nature of the bond between the metal coping and the ceramic has been extensively studied and it is agreed generally that there are three mechanisms involved:

- mechanical retention
- compression fit
- chemical bonding.

Mechanical retention is a form of interlocking that occurs as the ceramic flows into the microscopic spaces in the surface of the metal. The roughness of the surface is enhanced, often by applying an alumina-air abrasive or by grinding, so that the amount of interlocking is increased (Figure 3.4.11). This has the added benefit of producing a very clean surface that aids the wetting of the ceramic onto the metal.

Good bonding relies on an intimate contact between the ceramic and the metal coping, and any contaminants will jeopardize the quality of the bond. Before the ceramic is applied to the surface of the coping, the coping is subjected to a degassing cycle in the furnace, which burns off any remaining impurities and reduces the formation of bubbles due to trapped gases at the interface. The various stages in the surface preparation of the metal coping are described in more detail below. Most ceramics have a coefficient of thermal expansion that is considerably lower than that of metals (Table 3.4.5). On cooling, the metal will contract more than the ceramic due to its higher coefficient of thermal expansion. This leaves the ceramic in a state of compression. While this is potentially highly beneficial for this brittle material, it is important that the mismatch in the coefficients of thermal expansion is not too great. If the mismatch is too large, internal stresses created during cooling could cause the ceramic to fracture, with the most likely place for failure being the interface between the metal and the ceramic.

There is now considerable evidence that in addition to mechanical interlocking and compressive forces, a strong chemical bond is also created between the ceramic and the oxide coating on the metal. During firing, the ceramic is taken above its glass transition temperature such that it can flow and fuse with the oxides on the metal surface by migration of the metal oxides into the ceramic. In the case of gold alloy copings small amounts of oxide-forming elements are added to the alloy

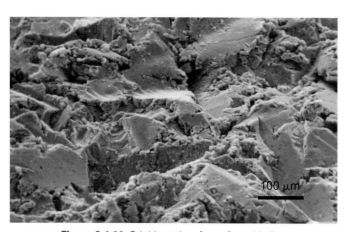

Figure 3.4.11 Grit-blasted surface of a gold alloy.

Material	α (ppm °C^{-1})
Metals	
Aluminum	23.6
Gold	13.8
Nickel	13.3
Silver	19.0
Ceramics	
Alumina	8.8
Spinel (MgAl$_2$O$_4$)	7.6
Fused silica (SiO$_2$)	0.5
Soda–lime glass	9.0

TABLE 3.4.5 Typical Values of the Coefficient of Thermal Expansion (α) of Metals and Ceramics

because gold does not naturally form an oxide. As a consequence, the strength of the bond between the metal and the ceramic is increased manyfold. This shows the importance of the presence of the surface oxides.

CLINICAL SIGNIFICANCE

The quality of the metal–ceramic bond is governed by the amount of micro-mechanical bonding, the compatibility of the coefficients of thermal expansion, and the chemical interaction between the metal oxides and the ceramic.

PREPARATION OF THE METAL SURFACE

To obtain a good bond between the metal coping and the ceramic veneer, it is important for the metal surface to be carefully prepared. This involves a series of technical stages that warrant closer examination. The main reasons for the surface preparation of the metal are to ensure the removal of any contaminants and to produce a surface oxide layer of the correct composition and character to which the ceramic will fuse. The various stages can be identified as follows:

- surface grinding
- heating under partial vacuum
- acid pickling
- heating in air.

Surface Grinding

When the metal casting is removed from the investment, there is always residual investment bonded to the surface of the casting. The surface is also contaminated with unwanted oxides, small porosities, and fine projections, especially if the investment is susceptible to fracture of the surface layer.

A grinding process is carried out to remove all of these imperfections. It also roughens the surface, and the consequently increased surface roughness is believed to aid the retention of the ceramic by micro-mechanical interlocking.

However, the grinding process can itself leave debris, such as oils, waxes, bits of skin tissue, or gases becoming trapped in undercuts. Even though the ceramic may be very effective in wetting the surface of the metal, it cannot always penetrate deep fissures.

In general, methods of grinding that do not result in the formation of deep fissures, porosities, or undercuts are preferred, and to this end, the use of fissure burs or carbide burs appears to be the recommended procedure.

Cleaning the casting in an organic solvent (e.g. carbon tetrachloride) in a sealed ultrasonic bath will remove surface contamination that has arisen during the handling of the casting.

Heating Under Partial Vacuum

In the as-cast condition the metal will not have the ideal oxide coating on its surface. Gold alloys will have virtually no oxide coating, given the noble nature of this metal. An oxide film can be formed by heating the casting at a temperature near the firing temperature of the ceramic. This has the effect of allowing the metallic elements that are incorporated in the alloy (e.g. tin, indium, zinc, or gallium) to migrate to the surface and form an oxide surface layer.

Great care must be taken to ensure that the correct heating cycle is used. Too brief a heat treatment could result in the formation of a thin or partial oxide coating, providing a poor substrate for the ceramic to fuse to. An excessively long heating cycle could result in the depletion of the oxidizing elements from the surface layer of the gold alloy. The heating duration must be balanced between these two extremes, and no bond will form if all of the oxide formed is removed during the subsequent acid pickling process and none of the oxidizing elements are left sufficiently close to the surface to allow the formation of additional oxides.

Carrying out the heat treatment under reduced pressure aids in the removal of gases that have been absorbed by the metal in great amounts during the casting process. The removal of these gases helps prevent the formation of interfacial bubbles. For this reason, the heat treatment of the alloy prior to the ceramic firing cycle is often referred to as a degassing treatment.

In the case of base metal alloys, where nickel and chromium are commonly used, the metals oxidize very readily, and the problem is generally the opposite of that for the gold alloys, in that too much of the oxide is formed.

Although oxides will naturally form during the firing of the ceramic, it has been found that it is better to preform the oxide coating, as this improves the wetting of the ceramic on the metal surface.

Acid Pickling

The heat treatment of gold alloys will produce not only tin oxide but various other oxides on the surface as well. The acid pickling procedure seeks to remove the unwanted oxides in preference to the tin oxide. There is the added advantage that the dark surface of the alloy is lightened from gray to white due to the increased concentration of tin oxide on the alloy surface. Commonly used acids are 50% hydrofluoric acid or 30% hydrochloric acid, with the latter preferred because of the hazards associated with the use of hydrofluoric acid. Neither this nor the following procedure is generally required for base metal alloys.

Heating in Air

A further heat treatment in air is frequently carried out in order to form an oxide coating of the correct thickness and quality.

The optimal oxide film on precious metal alloys should have a matte, grayish-white appearance, being composed mainly of base metal oxide. If the surface has a glossy appearance, this indicates a lack of oxide film and is usually the consequence of too many repeated surface treatments.

THE IMPORTANCE OF RELATIVE COEFFICIENTS OF THERMAL EXPANSION

The composition of the ceramic for metal–ceramic restorations needs to be different from that of the ceramic used for all-ceramic restorations. The coefficient of thermal expansion (α) of the feldspathic glasses used in the construction of the PJCs is 7–8 ppm °C^{-1}. This is far too low to be compatible with the alloys, which are typically in the region of 14–16 ppm °C^{-1}. This mismatch would give rise to serious problems due to excessive differential shrinkage on cooling. Depending on their composition, the coefficient of thermal expansion of the alloys and the ceramics can differ quite considerably.

Thermally Induced Stresses

The ceramics used in the construction of metal–ceramic restorations lose their thermoplastic fluidity once they are cooled below their glass transition temperature, which is typically in the range of 600–700°C. From this point onward, any difference in the coefficients of expansion between the metal and the ceramic will produce stresses in the ceramic as the ceramic attempts to shrink more or less than the metal substructure, depending on the type of mismatch. There are three possible scenarios that can be considered, namely:

$$\alpha_p > \alpha_m$$

$$\alpha_p = \alpha_m$$

$$\alpha_p < \alpha_m$$

where p is porcelain and m is metal. The stresses that result from each of the above conditions are shown in Figure 3.4.12.

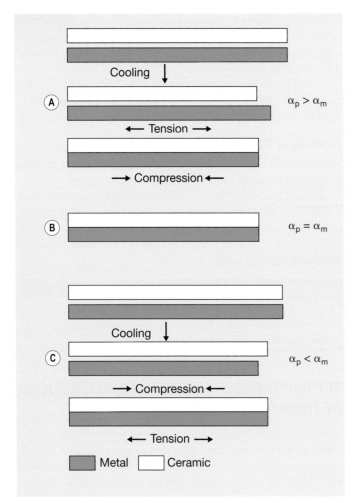

Figure 3.4.12 The effect of thermal mismatch on residual stress in the metal and the ceramic.

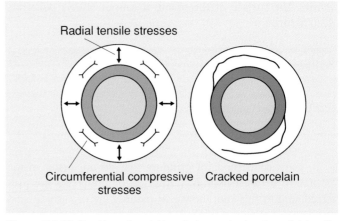

Figure 3.4.13 Cracking of metal-bonded-ceramic due to radial tensile stresses when αp << αm.

system may cause crazing or fracture of the ceramic, or debonding from the metal surface.

The reason for this is best explained by considering ceramic that is fused to a circular metal structure, especially as this is more akin to the real situation (shown in Figure 3.4.13). When the metal attempts to shrink more than the ceramic, radial tensile stresses and a circumferential compressive stress are generated. The latter are advantageous, but the former can be sufficient to cause debonding between the ceramic and the metal. If the mismatch is very large, the radial tensile stresses can cause the ceramic itself to fracture, with the fracture appearing circumferentially.

CLINICAL SIGNIFICANCE

It is extremely important that the metal and ceramic have coefficients of thermal expansion that are carefully controlled, to avoid stress and failure at the interface. The best combination of metal and ceramic is one where the coefficient of expansion of the ceramic is only slightly lower than that of the metal.

Effect of Composition of the Ceramic

The coefficient of thermal expansion of the feldspathic ceramics used in the manufacture of PJCs is incompatible with that of the metals available for ceramic bonding. To overcome this problem, the alkali content of the ceramic is increased, as indicated in Table 3.4.6. Both soda (Na_2O) and potash (K_2O) are added to increase the coefficient of expansion to be in the region of 14–16 ppm $°C^{-1}$.

Much more important is the fact that the addition of these oxides results in the formation of a crystalline phase in the glassy matrix. This crystalline phase is known as *tetragonal leucite*, which has a high coefficient of thermal expansion of 22–24 ppm $°C^{-1}$. The amount of precipitated leucite can be carefully controlled to provide a ceramic with the correct coefficient of expansion to suit a particular alloy and can be 30–40% of the volume of the material (Figure 3.4.14). The associated reduction in firing temperature has the benefit of reducing the potential for distortion due to creep of the alloy.

When $α_p > α_m$, the ceramic will attempt to contract more than the metal (Figure 3.4.12a). As the metal prevents this from happening, the ceramic will be under a state of tension when it is cooled to room temperature, with the metal being in a state of compression. The surface tensile stresses cause the formation of surface cracks and a crazed surface.

When $α_p = α_m$, the two materials will shrink at the same rate and no differential stresses are generated (Figure 3.4.12b).

When $α_p < α_m$, the metal will attempt to shrink more than the ceramic, and this places the ceramic in a state of compression (Figure 3.4.12c). This substantially reduces the potential for the ceramic to crack, since these compressive stresses have to be overcome before the ceramic is placed under tension. The metal will be in a state of tension but, since the tensile strength of the alloys used is quite high (500–1000 MPa), there is no danger of the metal failing. Thus it would appear that the best situation is one in which the coefficient of expansion of the metal is greater than that of the ceramic.

Whereas it would appear from the above discussion that the greater the mismatch, the better (as the ceramic will be under a higher compressive stress), this is in fact not the case. The mismatch should not be too large, as the stresses generated in the

TABLE 3.4.6 Typical Compositions of Metal-Bonded Ceramics as Compared With a Porcelain Jacket Crown (PJC) Porcelain

	PJC Porcelain	METAL-BONDED CERAMICS	
		(a)	(b)
SiO$_2$ (%)	66.5	66.4	59.2
Al$_2$O$_3$ (%)	13.5	14.5	18.5
Na$_2$O (%)	4.2	6.2	4.8
K$_2$O (%)	7.1	10.2	11.8
Firing temp. (°C)	960	940	900

to obtain the highest possible strength. In fact, the flexural strength of the ceramics used for metal–ceramic restorations is only of the order of 30–50 MPa. Hence the ceramic build-up on the metal framework should not be too thick, as this can lead to ceramic fractures when loaded in the mouth.

CLINICAL SIGNIFICANCE

By careful modification of the chemistry and structure of the ceramic, a highly aesthetic result can be achieved that has appropriate physical properties to suit the underlying alloy. This ensures a strong and lasting bond between the two dissimilar materials. The general recommendation is that the ceramic thickness should not exceed 2 mm.

An increase in the number and size of the leucite crystals can occur when firing the ceramic onto the metal. In the case of multiple firings this will increase the coefficient of expansion of the ceramic. Such an increase can compromise the compatibility of the metal and the ceramic. Thus excessive multiple firing of the metal–ceramic system is contraindicated. Slow cooling can also have the same effect as repeated firing, as can post-soldering, and the temperature should be raised and lowered as quickly as possible without giving rise to thermal shock effects.

The opaque shade of the ceramic when it is first laid down on the metal coping tends to contain larger amounts of metallic oxides that help to mask the color of the coping.

Great care must be exercised during the firing process, since the ceramic has a tendency to devitrify by a process of recrystallization. This results in the cloudiness of the ceramic, as the small crystals that are formed act as scattering sites for light.

CHOICE OF METAL–CERAMIC ALLOYS

The requirements for alloys used in the metal-bonded ceramic system are somewhat different from those for the all-metal constructions (Table 3.4.7). As it is necessary to fire ceramic onto the surface of the metal, its melting temperature must be higher than the sintering temperature for the ceramic. If the melting temperature of the metal is too close to the firing temperature of the ceramic, partial melting of thin sections of the coping may occur, or the coping may deform.

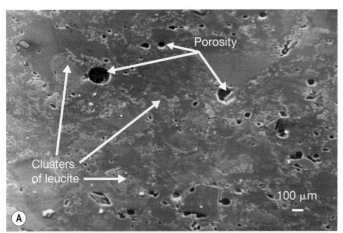

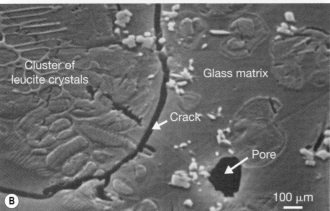

Figure 3.4.14 (a) The structure of a leucite-containing ceramic used in the construction of metal–ceramic restorations. Note the presence of residual porosity. (b) A close-up showing the detail of a leucite cluster and an associated crack, often seen in these ceramics due to the large mismatch in the coefficient of expansion of the leucite and the glass matrix

After the ceramic frit is prepared by the manufacturer, it is held at an elevated temperature for a specific time to allow the formation of leucite crystals. Thus this is a process identical to the ceramming of the glass-ceramics. Hence the ceramics used for metal–ceramic restorations are perhaps best described as leucite-containing glass-ceramics. These glass-ceramics are, nevertheless, different from the leucite-reinforced glass-ceramics, in that in this case the primary concern is to match its coefficient of thermal expansion with that of the metal and not

Table 3.4.7 Requirements of a Metal–Ceramic Alloy

1. Biocompatibility
2. Corrosion resistance
3. Ease of casting
4. Accurate fit
5. High bond strength to the ceramic
6. Absence of adverse reaction with the ceramic
7. Melting temperature > firing temperature of ceramic
8. High elastic modulus
9. Low creep
10. Low cost

TABLE 3.4.8   Typical Compositions of Metal–Ceramic Alloys

Type	Au%	Ag%	Pd%	Pt%	Ni%	Cr%	Mo%	In%, Cu%, Zn%, Ga%
High-gold	88	1	6	4	–	–	–	Balance
Au–Pd	50	10	38	–	–	–	–	Balance
High-palladium	–	–	80	–	–	–	–	Balance
Pd–Ag	–	30	60	–	–	–	–	Balance
Ni–Cr	–	–	–	–	70	20	10	–

Especially in the construction of long-span bridges, the metal must have a high elastic modulus and high yield stress. The resultant high stiffness of the bridge structure will prevent the occurrence of excessively high strains (that the ceramic cannot cope with) on occlusal loading. In addition, a low stiffness of the metal framework can result in distortion due to the differential contraction stresses that are generated on cooling after porcelain firing.

At one time, only high-gold alloys were available but, with the rising cost of gold, a variety of alternative alloys have been developed, which may be classified as high-gold, gold–palladium, high-palladium, palladium–silver, nickel–chromium alloys, or commercially pure titanium (cpTi). The compositions of some of the alloys are shown in Table 3.4.8.

High-Gold Alloys

For the high-gold alloys, the melting temperature is raised by the addition of platinum and palladium, both of which have a high melting temperature.

An immediately obvious difference between the non-ceramic–gold alloy and the ceramic–gold alloy is the omission of copper in the latter. This is done because copper reduces melting temperature and also has a tendency to react with the ceramic, producing a green discoloration. This is another feature of the alloys: they must not react with the ceramic in such a way as to spoil the aesthetics of the restoration.

The high-gold alloys have the advantage that they have been around for some considerable time and clinical experience has shown that they are extremely successful. In particular, the bond between the ceramic and the metal is very strong and highly reliable.

The main disadvantages of high-gold alloys are their relatively low melting temperatures, their susceptibility to creep at high temperatures, and their low elastic modulus. A minimum coping thickness of 0.5 mm is required with their use.

In situations of limited biological width this can give rise to aesthetic problems and often results in over-contouring to mask the metal color. In this respect the Pd–Ag and base metal alloys are more attractive.

Gold–Palladium Alloys

One reason for the introduction of the Au–Pd alloys was the rapidly rising cost of gold in the mid-late 20th century. Precious metal prices have proved very fickle over recent years and costs can swing wildly from one year to the next. Perhaps it should be remembered that the cost of the material will represent only a small component of the cost of the dental treatment.

The performance of Au–Pd alloys is comparable to that of the high-gold alloys in terms of castability, accuracy of fit, and corrosion resistance. However, there are some alloy–ceramic combinations that should be avoided due to a mismatch in thermal expansion characteristics.

High-Palladium Alloys

These alloys are primarily palladium, with small additions of other elements, such as copper, gallium, and tin; they too rose in popularity in the mid-20th century when the price of gold increased substantially. The price of palladium has since also increased and thus even these alloys are falling out of favor simply due to cost.

The copper, which can be present in amounts up to 15%, may be a surprising addition, since this might have been thought to cause porcelain discoloration. However, unlike gold alloys, the inclusion of copper in palladium alloys does not seem to have this effect. Their sag resistance can be poor due to excessive creep on ceramic firing.

CLINICAL SIGNIFICANCE

These alloys are contraindicated for long-span bridges where creep may present a particular problem.

Palladium–Silver Alloys

The Pd–Ag alloys have the most favorable elastic modulus of all of the precious metal alloys, producing castings with low flexibility and a reduced tendency to sag on porcelain firing. The alloys are somewhat less forgiving in terms of castability and fit, but as long as appropriate procedures are followed, results can be as good as with the gold alloys.

Due to the presence of high amounts of silver, there is concern that porcelain discoloration may occur. This problem appears to be more severe with certain alloy–porcelain combinations than others and can be minimized by careful selection of the metal–porcelain combination.

Multiple firings should be kept to a minimum, and overheating of the alloy avoided.

Nickel–Chromium–Molybdenum Alloys

The Ni–Cr–Mo alloys have a composition that is typically 77% Ni, 12% Cr, and 3.5% Mo, although the Mo and Cr content can rise to 9% and 22%, respectively, at the expense of nickel. The Ni–Cr–Mo alloys are very stiff, as their elastic modulus can be some 2.5 times higher than that of the high-gold alloys.

This has the advantage that the coping thickness can be reduced from 0.5 to 0.3 mm, which lessens the problem of over-contouring. It also means that this alloy is a better choice for resin-bonded bridges, especially those with a cantilever design, where the high elastic modulus helps to reduce stresses in the adhesive layer.

They would also be better for the construction of long-span bridges, as they provide greater rigidity and, because of the high melting temperature, there is less potential for sag during firing.

The disadvantages with these alloys are that casting is more difficult and the higher casting shrinkage can give rise to problems of poor fit. Also, clinical experience would indicate that the ceramic-to-metal bond is not as reliable as for the other alloys. However, as more experience is gained with these alloys, their performance may well improve. The low cost of the alloy is certainly very attractive.

The biocompatibility of alloys is always a consideration, and in particular, it is important to consider whether a patient has allergy or sensitivity to any of the component metals, as these can be released from the prosthesis, albeit usually in small quantities but sufficient to cause an allergic reaction. For instance, Ni–Cr alloys should not be used for patients with nickel allergy or sensitivity.

CLINICAL SIGNIFICANCE

Nickel-containing alloys are contraindicated in patients with known nickel allergy.

Commercially Pure Titanium

The dental use of cpTi has already been dealt with in Chapter 3.3 on casting alloys. It has also become popular for metal–ceramic restorations because of its good corrosion resistance, excellent biocompatibility, low density, and relatively low cost compared to the precious metal alloys. However, there are some additional issues that it is appropriate to address here, relating to its use with ceramics.

When titanium is cast, a reaction layer with a thickness of 50–100 μm forms on the surface of the casting due to an interaction between the titanium and the refractory investment. This reaction layer can become even more pronounced during the subsequent ceramic firing cycle. This layer, if not removed, will interfere with the bonding of the ceramic to the titanium. A variety of suggestions have been put forward to deal with this problem that include sand blasting, silicon-nitride coating, and immersion dissolution.

The casting problems can be avoided by producing the restorations using an alternative technique, consisting of spark erosion and copy-milling. However, titanium has a high chemical reactivity, and, if taken above 800°C, this gives rise to a thick oxide coating, with the consequence of a weak bond to the ceramic.

Unlike the alloys described above, titanium has a coefficient of expansion of 9.6 ppm °C^{-1}. Thus the leucite-containing

ceramics developed for the metal–ceramic alloys are inappropriate and it is important that ceramics specially designed for use with cpTi are used.

The bonding of the ceramic to cpTi is problematic and the bond strength is not as good as that obtained to the alloys.

3D-Printed Frameworks

In recent years the use of 3D-printed frameworks using metal powder bed fusion technology has become popular given their ease of manufacture and reasonably low cost. The choice of metal powders is limited, and thus these frameworks are usually manufactured using a Co-Cr alloy in fine powder form with a typical composition of Co: 63.9%, Cr: 24.7%, W: 5.4%, Mo: 5%, and Si: ≤1%. The nickel content is usually less than 0.1% and the alloy contains no cadmium or beryllium, which reduces the possibility of any adverse reaction.

MOVING ON FROM METAL-BONDED CERAMICS

The aesthetic results with the feldspathic glasses and the leucite-containing feldspathic glasses are excellent due to their high translucency, fluorescence, and opalescence. When used in combination with resin bonding to enamel and dentine, these materials are very good for veneers and inlays and are also used for low-stress-bearing anterior crowns. However, the mechanical strength is insufficient for this class of ceramic to be used in the construction of posterior crowns and all-ceramic bridges. Due to these limitations and a desire to produce ceramics suitable for use in the posterior part of the mouth, linked to a wish to extend their use to the construction of small three-unit bridges, there has been a major drive to develop new ceramics suitable for posterior use without the need of a metal substructure.

CLINICAL SIGNIFICANCE

Yet stronger core materials were needed if the use of ceramics was to be extended to the posterior teeth.

GLASS-INFILTRATED HIGH-STRENGTH CERAMICS

The addition of alumina to the feldspathic glass of the PJC core during the pre-fritting process limits the amount of alumina that can be incorporated to about 40–50 vol. %. An alternative approach has been adopted in a system called InCeram (Vita Zahnfabrik, Bad Säckingen, Germany). This material, used for cores, has an alumina content of ~85%.

A ceramic core is formed onto a refractory die from a fine slurry of alumina powder by a process known as slip-casting. After the die has dried, it is sintered for 10 hours at 1120°C. The melting temperature of alumina is too high to produce full densification of the powder by liquid-phase sintering and only solid-phase sintering occurs. Consequently, the coping thus created is only just held together at the contact points between the alumina particles

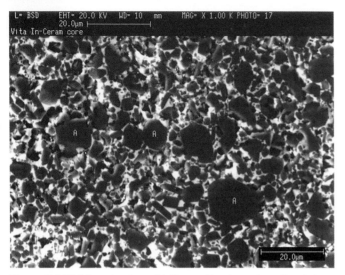

Figure 3.4.15 Microstructure of InCeram Alumina, where the dark regions are the crystalline phases and the light regions represent the infiltrated glass. Image courtesy of and copyright Dr Alvaro Della Bona, Passo Fundo, Brazil, with thanks.

and a porous structure is the result. The strength of this porous core is only about 6–10 MPa. The porous structure is then infiltrated with a lanthanum glass, which has a low viscosity when fired at 1100°C for 4–6 hours. The molten glass is able to penetrate into the pores, producing a dense ceramic (Figure 3.4.15). The aesthetics and functional form are then achieved by veneering the core with conventional feldspathic dental ceramics.

CLINICAL SIGNIFICANCE

Very high flexural strength values (400–500 MPa) have been claimed for this core ceramic, which makes this system suitable for anterior and posterior crowns, with excellent results. Several attempts have also been made at producing anterior cantilever and posterior three-unit bridges, which is a highly ambitious use of ceramics but shows considerable promise.

A similar approach has been adopted with spinel (MgAl$_2$O$_4$) replacing the alumina or a mixture of alumina and zirconia. The InCeram Spinel offers superior aesthetics over the InCeram Alumina but at a slightly reduced flexural strength (~350 MPa) and is recommended for inlays and anterior crowns. The InCeram Zirconia is based on the InCeram Alumina, but with the replacement of 33 wt % alumina by zirconia, and produces a ceramic core with a strength of up to 700 MPa (See Table 3.4.9). Its drawback is that the combination of a glass, alumina, and/or zirconia means that this core material is very opaque and thus they need to be veneered with an aesthetic feldspathic glass.

As with the feldspathic glasses, this range of glass-infiltrated ceramics is available in block and disc form for CAD–CAM processing, which makes the processing much simpler as it avoids the pre-sintering step for the laboratory technician. To produce the blocks, powder is dry-pressed by the manufacturer, which creates a denser, homogenous structure, which has a higher flexural strength after glass infiltration.

CLINICAL SIGNIFICANCE

The introduction of high-strength ceramic core restorations for crowns and bridges and resin-bonded ceramic restorations for crowns is challenging in many of the situations where traditionally a metal–ceramic crown would have been used. However, the metal–ceramic crown has provided sterling service for many years, whereas the all-ceramic restorations are still relative newcomers.

Whatever the advantages and disadvantages of the different systems, the responsibility for the choice of alloy rests with the dentist and should not be delegated to the dental laboratory technician.

SUMMARY

Metal–ceramic restorations can produce a good aesthetic outcome. The presence of a metal framework that has to be masked by the ceramic is a limitation with this system, but if given sufficient space to work in, the dental laboratory technician can produce a very good result. However, this does mean that these restorations are inherently destructive of tooth structure.

The main advantage of the metal–ceramic restoration over the all-ceramic restoration is its resistance to fracture. Until very recently, only short-span bridges could be made out of ceramics, such that metal-bonded ceramic was the only option available for anything more than a small three-unit bridge. New developments in high-strength core ceramic systems using new materials are radically expanding the options compared to a market that for decades was dominated by the metal–ceramic restoration.

TABLE 3.4.9 Typical Values for the Flexural Strength and Fracture Toughness of Glass-Infiltrated Ceramics

System	Core material	Biaxial Flexural Strength (MPa)	3-Point Flexural Strength (MPa)	Indentation Fracture Toughness (MPa·m$^{1/2}$)
InCeram Alumina	Glass-infiltrated alumina	350	450–550	3.1–4.8
InCeram Spinel	Glass-infiltrated magnesium spinel		350	2.4
InCeram Zirconia	Glass-infiltrated alumina with 35% partially stabilized zirconia	540–930	480–700	5–8

FURTHER READING

Behr, M., Zeman, F., Baitinger, T., Galler, J., Koller, M., Handel, G., et al., 2014. The clinical performance of porcelain-fused-to-metal precious alloy single crowns: chipping, recurrent caries, periodontitis, and loss of retention. International Journal of Prosthodontics 27, 153–160.

Land, C.H., 1889. Porcelain restorations. Dental Cosmos 31, 191.

Levi, L., Barak, S., Katz, J., 2012. Allergic reactions associated with metal alloys in porcelain-fused-to-metal fixed prosthodontic devices: a systematic review. Quintessence International 43, 871–877.

Pincus, C.R., 1938. Building mouth personality. Journal of California Dental Association 14, 125–129.

Sailer, I., Makarov, N.A., Thoma, D.S., Zwahlen, M., Pjetursson, B.E., 2015. All-ceramic or metal–ceramic tooth-supported fixed dental prostheses (FDPs)? A systematic review of the survival and complication rates. Part I: single crowns (SCs). Dental Materials 31, 603–623.

Wildgoose, D.G., Johnson, A., Winstanley, R.B., 2004. Glass/ceramic/refractory techniques, their development and introduction into dentistry: a historical literature review. Journal of Prosthetic Dentistry 91, 136.

Win, L.C., Sands, P., Bonsor, S.J., Burke, F.J.T., 2021. Ceramics in dentistry: which material is appropriate for the anterior or posterior dentition? Part 1: materials science. Dental Update 48, 680–688.

Zhang, Y., Kelly, J.R., 2017. Dental ceramics for restoration and metal veneering. Dental Clinics of North America 61 (4), 797–819.

Contemporary Dental Ceramics

Dental ceramics were introduced in the preceding chapter, wherein we discussed the development of ceramics in general, and dental ceramics in particular, over an extended period of over 2000 years. We also covered some of the more traditional ceramic materials and ceramic-metal devices still used in modern dentistry; the reader should note that "traditional" should not be read as "historic" or "outdated," and these are very much still in use today. In this chapter we focus on some of the most recent *versions* of dental ceramics – materials that themselves represent an evolution of the dental ceramic. We consider their composition and structure and their properties and applications, including how they differ from the conventional materials discussed already.

GLASS–CERAMICS

Introduction

The aesthetic results with the feldspathic glasses are excellent due to their high translucency, fluorescence, and opalescence. When used in combination with resin bonding to enamel and dentine, these materials are very good for veneers. However, the mechanical strength is insufficient for this class of ceramic to be used in the construction of crowns and all-ceramic bridges.

Due to these limitations and a desire to produce ceramics suitable for use in the posterior part of the mouth, linked to a wish to extend their use to the construction of small three-unit bridges, there has been a major drive to develop new ceramics suitable for use as resin-bonded all-ceramic restorations. The focus of this development has been a class of materials known as glass–ceramics.

What Are Glass–Ceramics?

Glass–ceramics were first developed by Corning Glass Works in the late 1950s. In principle, an article is formed at a high temperature while the glass is in the liquid state, and a metastable glass results upon cooling. Some glass compositions have a tendency to devitrify (see Chapter 1.3), such that during a subsequent heat treatment, controlled crystallization occurs, with the nucleation and growth of internal crystals. This conversion process from a glass to a partially crystalline glass is called *ceraming*. Thus a glass–ceramic is a multiphase solid containing a residual glass phase with a finely dispersed crystalline phase, *all derived from the one material and yet chemically identical or distinct*, as compared with a glass matrix containing particles of a different material such as in the reinforced dental glasses and glass

infiltrated ceramics discussed in Chapter 3.4. The controlled crystallization of the glass results in the formation of tiny crystals that are evenly distributed throughout the glass. The number of crystals, their growth rate, and thus their size are regulated by the time and temperature of the ceraming heat treatment.

There are two important aspects to the formation of the crystalline phase: crystal nucleation and crystal growth. The schematic in Figure 3.5.1 shows that the rate of crystal nucleation and the rate of crystal growth are at a maximum at different temperatures. The ceraming process consequently involves a two-stage heat treatment. The first heat treatment is carried out at the temperature for maximum nucleation of crystals, so as to maximize the number of crystals formed. The material temperature is then raised, after a suitable period of time, to the higher temperature to allow crystal growth. It is held at the higher temperature until the optimum crystal size is formed.

To ensure a high strength for the glass–ceramic, it is important that the crystals are numerous and are uniformly distributed throughout the glassy phase. The crystalline phase will grow during ceraming and can eventually occupy from 50% to nearly 100% of the material.

Mechanical Properties of Glass–Ceramics

The mechanical properties are believed to be greatly influenced by:
- particle size of the crystalline phase
- volume fraction of the crystalline phase
- interfacial bond strength between phases
- differences in elastic moduli
- differences in thermal expansion.

Fracture in brittle solids is nearly always initiated at a small internal or surface defect, such as a micro-crack, that acts as a stress raiser. If the crystalline phase is relatively strong, then the cracks will form in the glassy phase. The dimension of these micro-cracks can thus be limited to the distance between the crystalline particles. Therefore the critical parameter is the mean free path, in the glassy phase, L_s, which is given by:

$$L_s = d(1-V_f)/V_f$$

where d is the crystal diameter and V_f is the volume fraction of the crystalline phase.

Thus the smaller the crystals and the larger the volume fraction of the crystals, the shorter the mean free path will be, and consequently, the greater the strength of the material.

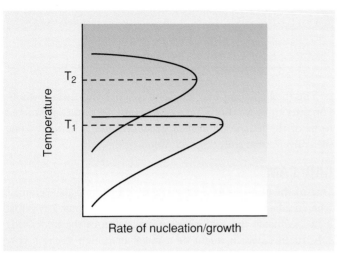

Figure 3.5.1 Rate of nucleation (T_1) and growth (T_2) of crystals in a glass–ceramic.

CLINICAL SIGNIFICANCE

A feature of glass–ceramics is that the size of the crystals and the proportion of the material in the crystalline phase can be carefully controlled during the ceraming process.

Most glass–ceramics are opaque or cloudy and would not be suitable for dental use. The first glass–ceramic employed in dentistry was introduced by MacCulloch in 1968 for the construction of denture teeth and was based on the $Li_2O \cdot ZnO \cdot SiO_2$ system. At the time, the use of acrylic denture teeth was becoming popular, and the idea of glass–ceramics was not exploited further. Now we have a wide range of glass–ceramics and processing routes for the construction of ceramic restorations.

Leucite-Reinforced Feldspar Glass–Ceramics

The ceramic used in the original experiments of Horn was a leucite ($KAlSi_2O_6$)-containing feldspathic glass, which he would have used in the construction of metal–ceramic restorations. This ceramic was optimized with regard to being able to bond to the metal surface (see Chapter 3.4).

The ceramics used presently for resin-bonded ceramic restorations are a modified version of the ceramic used by Horn. They differ from the ceramic used in metal–ceramics primarily in that the composition and microstructure has been changed in order to produce the best leucite crystalline phase distribution from the point of view of strength, since compatibility with a metal framework is no longer a consideration. The properties of a leucite glass–ceramic can be readily modified and adjusted by the careful management of the starting glass composition and control of the microstructure by heat treatment schedules. Another important feature of leucite glass–ceramics is their excellent aesthetics for dental applications. The material has a naturally white translucent appearance, which gives it the ability to match the color and translucency of the natural dentition. The leucite phase has substantially the same refractive index as the feldspathic glass forming the matrix. Consequently, the

translucency of the leucite glass–ceramic is not compromised by the crystallization of the leucite in the glass.

The stoichiometric composition of leucite is $K_2O \cdot Al_2O_3 \cdot 4SiO_2$. However, this composition has a very high melting point, so various oxides are added to achieve a low fusion leucite glass–ceramic. These additives can include Na_2O, B_2O_3, Li_2O, BaO, P_2O_3, or ZnO. Leucite crystals are created by the controlled firing of feldspar at 1150°C. Potassium aluminum silicate glass is converted into leucite and two molecules of silica as follows:

$$K_2O \cdot Al_2O_3 \cdot 6SiO_2 \rightarrow K_2O \cdot Al_2O_3 \cdot 4SiO_2 + 2SiO_2$$

Another problem with the production of leucite glass–ceramics is that the leucite is only able to crystallize by a surface and not a bulk crystallization mechanism. For this reason, the leucite glass is best crystallized via the surface crystallization mechanism from a fine glass powder, which is then sintered to produce glass bodies. When the glass is milled into a very fine powder, the total surface area of the glass becomes very high, and crystallization is achieved from the surface of the individual glass particles. The densification is carried out by sintering at a temperature where the glass phase is above its softening temperature and the glass particles fuse together.

Leucite has two crystal formations, namely tetragonal and cubic. When manufacturing a leucite glass–ceramic as a veneering material for a metal substructure, the leucite needs to be in its tetragonal form in order to raise the coefficient of expansion of the ceramic to be near that of the metal (see Chapter 3.4). No such constraint is necessary when the leucite glass–ceramic is used as a monolithic restoration. In such circumstances the cubic form of the leucite is preferable as this allows the strength to be optimized. Thus the high-strength leucite glass–ceramics are based on cubic rather than tetragonal leucite.

This explains why the leucite-containing ceramic used in metal–ceramic restorations have a flexural strength of the order of 30–40 MPa, while the leucite-reinforced glass–ceramics have flexural strengths of up to 180 MPa. A typical example of the structure of leucite-reinforced ceramic is shown in Figure 3.5.2.

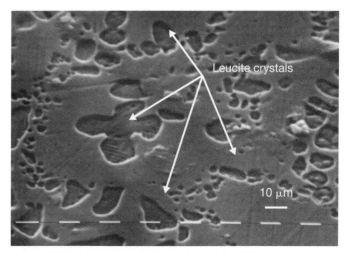

Figure 3.5.2 A scanning electron micrograph of the structure of a leucite-reinforced glass–ceramic.

What is particularly noticeable is the uniform distribution of the leucite crystals and the lack of internal cracking that is so evident in the example of the leucite-containing feldspars used in the early days for veneering a metal framework.

Processing Routes

The construction of ceramic restorations using leucite-reinforced feldspars can be done either by sintering, using a modified version of the sintering process described earlier to construct the porcelain jacket crown, by hot-pressing, or by CAD–CAM. The mechanical properties of leucite feldspar glass–ceramics are considered to be suitable for this material to be used primarily for veneers, anterior crowns, and posterior inlays.

Hot-Pressing

In order to surmount the problems of the inherent inaccuracies of fit of the sintered ceramics, which are due to the high firing shrinkage, attention has been paid to glass–ceramics that employ a casting process for the manufacture of crowns, veneers, and inlays. Hot-pressing is one such approach and is a technique that involves the heating up an ingot of the ceramic. The ingot is a solid block of the material, which is made of a leucite-reinforced feldspar, as is the case with Empress I (Ivoclar-Vivadent, Schaan, Liechtenstein). This method utilizes parts of the lost wax casting technique. As in lost wax casting, a wax pattern is produced, which is then invested in a refractory die material. The wax is burnt out to create the space to be filled by the leucite-reinforced glass–ceramic. A specially designed pressing furnace is then used to fill the mold space from a pellet of the glass–ceramic using a viscous flow process at a temperature of 1180°C (Figure 3.5.3). When the ingot is heated to a sufficiently high temperature, it will become a softened mass such that under pressure it will flow into a refractory mold. This process is also often described as transfer molding. It is distinctly different from the sintering technique since it does not rely on the fusion of powder particles.

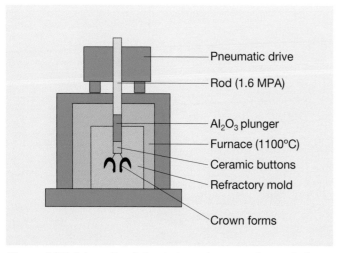

Figure 3.5.3 Schematic of the hot-pressing route for producing a leucite-reinforced glass–ceramic restoration.

The final shading may be done by applying surface stains. For anterior restorations, the veneer is cut back and a powdered form of the leucite-reinforced glass–ceramic is bonded using the conventional sintering technique.

CAD–CAM

One of the constraints on the use of leucite feldspar ceramics when used as a veneer on a substructure (see Chapter 3.4) is that it has to match the coefficient of expansion of the underlying substructure, which might be a metal or a high-strength core ceramic. If one uses prefabricated blocks of a ceramic, which are used to create the *entire* restoration, there is no such constraint. The main considerations are aesthetics, mechanical properties such as strength and toughness, and practical properties such as machinability. In order to maximize the strength, the CAD–CAM blocks consist of homogeneously distributed cubic leucite crystals (35–45 vol. %) in a glassy matrix.

Since the leucite glass–ceramics can be prefabricated into blocks, the veneers can also be constructed using CAD–CAM technology. This can be done at the chair side with an in-surgery milling machine or in the dental laboratory using discs or blocks of the ceramic. Polychromatic blocks such as those in the IPS Empress CAD range have a natural gradation of shade and fluorescence from the dentin to the incisal edge. This gives the restorations a natural appearance, even without additional characterization.

Fluoromica Glass–Ceramics

In order to be able to extend the possible use of resin-bonded ceramic restorations for posterior crowns, onlays, and bridge construction, a glass–ceramic was developed that was based on the composition $SiO_2 \cdot K_2O \cdot MgO \cdot MgF_2 \cdot Al_2O_3 \cdot ZrO_2$. The addition of some fluorides imparts fluorescence in the prostheses in a way similar to that encountered in the natural dentition. These glass–ceramics are known as fluoromicas. For this composition, the ceraming process results in the nucleation and the growth of fluorophlogopite tetrasilicic mica crystals within the glass. The crystals are needle-like in shape and arrest the propagation of cracks through this material. Unlike the leucite glass–ceramics, which are surface nucleating systems, the mica-based glass–ceramics bulk nucleate. Thus in this case a block or disc can be fabricated in the base glass and then heat-treated to encourage the formation of the mica crystals. This is much simpler than the production route for the leucite glass–ceramic. Mechanical property measurements suggest that the flexural strength is in the region of 120–180 MPa, which, when combined with the adhesion to tooth tissues, may just be adequate for posterior crowns but is probably still insufficient for the construction of all-ceramic bridges.

The passage of light through the material is affected by the crystal size and the difference in the refractive indices of the glass phase and the crystalline phase. If the crystals are smaller than the wavelength of visible light (0.4–0.7 μm), the glass will appear transparent, such that the tendency for light to scatter is lower than for the aluminous porcelains.

CLINICAL SIGNIFICANCE

The refractive index of the small mica crystals is closely matched to that of the surrounding glass phase, which produces a translucency close to that of enamel.

The processing of this glass–ceramic involves the same principles as for the lost wax casting process of metallic restorations. The restoration is waxed up on a die, using conventional materials. The pattern is removed from the die and invested in a special phosphate-bonded investment. Then an ingot of the castable ceramic material is placed in a special crucible and centrifugally cast at a temperature of 1380°C. The casting then requires a further heat treatment to create the crystalline phase and develop the strength. The desired shade is achieved by firing self-glazing shading porcelains on the surface. The concept of producing ceramic restorations using a casting technique is by no means new and was first attempted in the 1920s. It is only with the recent introduction of the castable glass–ceramics that this has become possible.

In recent years the casting route has lost its popularity with laboratories and now the main application of fluoromica glass–ceramics is in the CAD–CAM production of restorations, an example being MACOR® (Corning), which is a fluorphlogopite mica in a borosilicate glass matrix.

Lithium Disilicate and Apatite Glass–Ceramics

Some versions of glass–ceramics have the strength and toughness to be considered suitable for the production of posterior crowns and possibly even short-span bridges. However, these materials do not have the necessary aesthetics to allow the production of the restoration as a single unit. The option then is to produce a high-strength core material and veneer it with an aesthetic ceramic. The difference with the high-strength crystalline ceramic-core systems is that these core materials are still based on silica glass and therefore can be bonded to the tooth structure using a combination of silane coupling agents and resins. One such system is a lithium disilicate glass–ceramic based on an SiO_2–Li_2O. Similar to the mica glass–ceramic, this system also bulk nucleates. The lithium disilicate glass is prepared from an appropriate glass batch by melting between 1000 and 1450°C for 4 hours and cast into transparent glass ingots. With the addition of a nucleating agent such as P_2O_5, the glass will bulk nucleate so it can be cast into a block and cooled to room temperature. A process of partial crystallization is carried out that leads to the formation of 40% platelet-shaped lithium metasilicate crystals (with an average size of 0.2–1.0 μm), Li_2SiO_3, embedded in a glassy phase. This is an intermediate crystalline phase or "blue" state, with a flexural strength of 130 ± 30 MPa. In the "blue" state the blocks can easily be milled in the CAM unit. The milled restoration is subsequently heat-treated at 850°C, resulting in the formation of lithium disilicate crystals – $Li_2Si_2O_5$.

Lithium orthosilicate (Li_4SiO_4) → lithium metasilicate (Li_2SiO_3) → lithium disilicate ($Li_2Si_2O_5$).

The crystalline structure of the final restoration consists of randomly oriented, densely distributed, elongated fine-grained lithium disilicate crystals, some 1.5 μm in length. This crystalline phase makes up some 70% of the volume of the glass–ceramic. Lithium disilicate has an unusual microstructure in that it consists of many small, interlocking, plate-like crystals that are randomly oriented (Figure 3.5.4). This is ideal from the point of view of strength because the needle-like crystals cause cracks to deflect, branch, or blunt. Thus the propagation of cracks through this material is arrested by the lithium disilicate crystals, providing a substantial increase in the flexural strength. A second crystalline phase, consisting of a lithium orthophosphate (Li_3PO_4) of a much lower volume, is also present.

The mechanical properties of this glass–ceramic are far superior to those of the leucite and mica glass–ceramic, with a flexural strength in the region of 350–500 MPa and a fracture toughness approximately three times that of the leucite and mica glass–ceramics. The glass–ceramic is claimed to be highly translucent due to the optical compatibility between the glassy matrix and crystalline phase, which minimizes the internal scattering of the light as it passes through the material. Lithium disilicate blocks ready for machining are shown in Figure 3.5.5.

CLINICAL SIGNIFICANCE

The high strength of lithium disilicate glass–ceramics creates the possibility of producing not only anterior and posterior crowns but also all-ceramic bridges.

The processing route is either by the hot-pressing route described earlier, except that the processing temperature, at 920°C, is lower than for the leucite glass–ceramic or more preferable these days by CAD–CAM. Because the fully crystallized lithium disilicate glass–ceramic is very hard to machine, it is used in a two-stage process. The CAD–CAM blocks or discs are only partially crystallized to form a metastable lithium metasilicate

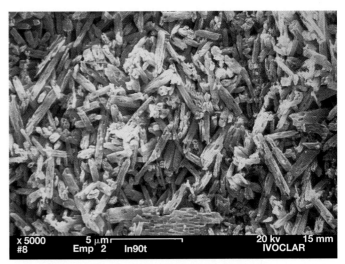

Figure 3.5.4 Scanning electron micrograph of the microstructure of a lithium disilicate glass–ceramic, showing the interlocking needle-like crystals. Courtesy of Ivoclar-Vivadent UK Ltd, Leicester, UK.

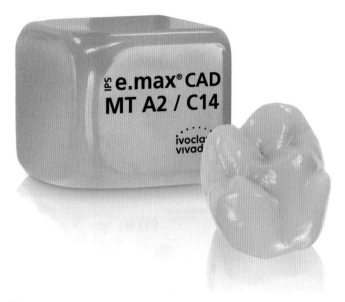

Figure 3.5.5 Lithium disilicate blocks ready for machining. Image courtesy of and copyright GC Dental Europe, with thanks.

phase, at which point they can be readily machined using a multi-axis milling machine. The final restoration is then given a further heat treatment to maximize the formation of the lithium disilicate crystalline phase.

For the alumina-based core systems described earlier, it is possible to use feldspathic glasses to provide the aesthetic surface layer, as their coefficients of thermal expansion are closely matched at ~7–8 ppm °C^{-1}. For the leucite glass–ceramics, the layering ceramic is identical to the core ceramic and so a mismatch in the coefficient of expansion does not arise. However, for the lithium disilicate glass–ceramic, the coefficient of expansion is greater than 10 ppm °C^{-1} and, consequently, a new compatible layering ceramic had to be developed. This new layering ceramic is an apatite glass–ceramic. The crystalline phase formed on ceraming is a hydroxyapatite [Ca_{10} (PO_4)$_6$ (OH)$_2$], which is the same basic constituent from which enamel is made. Thus it represents a material that, at least in composition, is the closest match to enamel that has been achieved so far. The crystals, responsible for the material's opalescence, are less than 300 nm in length and 100 nm in diameter, whereas crystals along the longitudinal axis are larger, 2–5 μm in length and less than 300 nm in diameter. IPS e.max Ceram is a nanofluorapatite layering ceramic in the form of a powder, used for the production of veneers or as veneering material for lithium disilicate glass–ceramics.

Summary

A wide range of glass–ceramics is now available to create highly aesthetic dental restorations. The leucite glass–ceramics are ideally suited to the construction of veneers, inlays, onlays, and anterior crowns; the fluoromica glass–ceramics can be used to produce anterior crowns; and the lithium disilicate glass–ceramics can be used for veneers, inlays, onlays, crowns, and three-unit bridges (up to the second premolar as the terminal abutment).

CRYSTALLINE (MONOPHASE) CERAMICS

Introduction

Solid-sintered, monophase ceramics are materials that are formed by directly sintering crystals together without any intervening matrix to form a dense, air-free, glass-free, polycrystalline structure. It would seem a natural extension from alumina-reinforced core systems (~40% Al_2O_3) and glass-infiltrated ceramics (~80% Al_2O_3) to consider the possibility of a pure alumina core. Initially the impediment to the use of pure alumina was that it was a very difficult material to process in the confines of a dental laboratory. The advent of digital processing and CAD–CAM changed all that and made it possible for dental laboratories to design and manufacture pure alumina crown and bridge frameworks, closely followed by the introduction of monophase zirconia.

Alumina

Alumina or aluminum oxide (Al_2O_3) is a white or nearly colorless, semi-translucent crystalline substance. It occurs in its natural form as the mineral corundum and its gemstone forms, sapphire and ruby. Alumina is a major engineering material, offering a combination of good mechanical properties and electrical properties, leading to a wide range of applications. It can be produced in a range of purities with additives designed to modify and enhance properties for particular applications. A wide variety of ceramic processing methods can be applied including machining or net shape forming to produce a wide variety of sizes and shapes of component. Typical alumina characteristics of relevance to dentistry include:

- Suitable strength and stiffness
- Favorable hardness and wear resistance
- Corrosion resistance
- Thermal stability

The mechanical behavior of alumina is strongly affected by its microstructure because of the propagation of cracks and secondary micro-cracks. For polycrystalline alumina to have optimum properties, it must have a high purity (99.5%), a grain size of less than 5 μm, and a density of more than 98%. Typical values for the mechanical properties are:

Compressive strength	3 GPa
Modulus of elasticity	450 GPa
Flexural strength	380 MPa
Fracture toughness	3.5 MPa·m$^{1/2}$
Vickers hardness	15 GPa
Tensile strength	267 MPa

The combination of a high flexural strength and fracture toughness makes these materials highly desirable for the construction of dental crowns and bridges. A range of oxides may be added in small amounts during the production of alumina, such as magnesium oxide (MgO), zirconium oxide (ZrO_2), and chromium oxide (Cr_2O_3) in order to improve the properties. For example, the addition of MgO and/or ZrO_2 can increase the flexural strength of alumina significantly.

Pure Alumina Cores

The first dental use of monophase alumina was with the introduction of Procera AllCeram (Nobel Biocare, Stockholm,

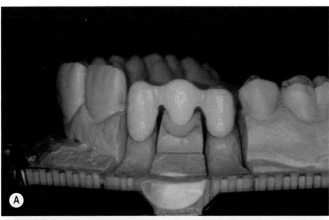

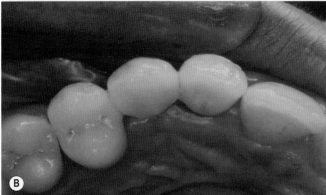

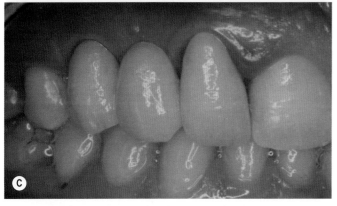

Figure 3.5.6 Procera bridge showing (a) alumina framework prior to veneering and (b and c) clinical result. Image courtesy of and copyright Derek Priestley, DP Dental Laboratories Ltd, UK, with thanks.

Sweden), which uses a densely sintered 99.5% pure alumina as the core material. The potential advantages were increased strength and superior translucency compared with the glass-infiltrated core materials. A clinical example can be shown in Figure 3.5.6.

Production of the Procera AllCeram core involves producing a die from the impression, digitizing the geometry of the desired coping using specially designed computer software, and transferring this information down a modem to a laboratory in Stockholm. This is all done by a designated dental laboratory that is a member of the Procera Network. The coping is produced by a special process, which involves sintering 99.5% pure alumina at 1600–1700°C such that it is fully densified. The coping is then returned to the dental laboratory for building on

the crown's aesthetics using compatible feldspathic glasses. The process can be quite efficient, with quoted turn-around times being 24 hours. The flexural strength of the Al_2O_3 core materials is in the region of 700 MPa and thus similar to that achieved with the glass-infiltrated InCeram-Zirconia.

> ### CLINICAL SIGNIFICANCE
>
> One of the potential benefits of producing a pure alumina core is that the translucency is considered to be better than that of the glass-infiltrated alumina composite structures.

The reason for the improved translucency of monophase alumina over glass-infiltrated alumina is due primarily to the refractive index mismatch between the glass and the alumina in the glass-infiltrated ceramic causing extensive scattering and refraction of the light, whereas this is not an issue for the monophase alumina. While this is an improvement, the translucency is still limited because of the refraction of light at the grain boundaries between the crystals and thus an aesthetic veneer is still required.

Zirconia

Zirconium dioxide (ZrO_2), commonly referred to as zirconia, is a very high-strength material (flexural strength $\sim$1000 MPa). It is also very hard (Vickers: $\sim$12.7 GPa), extremely refractory (m.p. $\sim$2690°C), and has a very high modulus of elasticity ($E \sim 210$ GPa). Zirconia is an allotropic material, which means that it can exist in a number of crystalline forms depending on the temperature: it is cubic (c) above $\sim$2370°C but tetragonal (t) below.

The transformation of c-ZrO_2 to t-ZrO_2 on cooling involves an overall increase of the bulk volume of $\sim$2.3%. The change from t-ZrO_2 to m-ZrO_2 involves an even bigger bulk volume change that can range from 3 to 5% or more, depending on the history of the material. This magnitude of change could not possibly be accommodated in any ceramic and would cause extensive cracking. Hence, on cooling, the item being manufactured would be destroyed. This problem can be overcome by suppressing the tetragonal to monoclinic transition by the addition of other metal oxides such as MgO, CaO, and CeO_2. However, the most effective method of stabilizing the tetragonal form of ZrO_2 is to add a small amount of yttrium oxide (Y_2O_3), or yttria. The addition of yttria lowers the temperature at which the potentially damaging transformation to m-ZrO_2 occurs. The idea is to add enough yttria to create a partially stabilized zirconia (PSZ), typically 3 molar %, which is then referred to as 3Y-PSZ, or alternatively 3Y-TZP: yttria-stabilized tetragonal zirconia polycrystals. The tetragonal phase is metastable and the spontaneous transformation of c $\rightarrow$ t, or t $\rightarrow$ m, will now not occur but can be triggered by stress. This has proved to be very beneficial to the performance of the zirconia.

The strength of ceramics is a function of the size, shape, and position of surface and internal cracks. The more difficult it is for these cracks to grow, the stronger the ceramic. The t $\rightarrow$ m transition can be used to good effect at the tip of a crack where the local stress is very high. The stress-induced

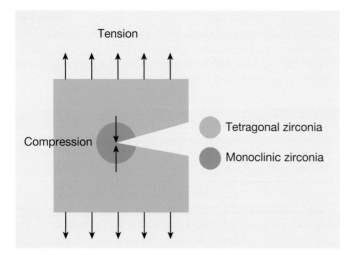

Figure 3.5.7 The stress concentrating effect at the tip of the crack causes the tetragonal zirconia crystals to transform into monoclinic crystals with an accompanying increase in volume.

t → m transition is accompanied by a significant increase in the zirconia crystals at the crack tip. This has the effect of putting the crack region in compression, effectively closing the crack and preventing it from propagating (Figure 3.5.7). This behavior is known as transformation toughening and is the reason why the flexural strength of 3Y-PSZ can be in excess of 1000 MPa.

Zirconia Core Systems

Originally, yttria-stabilized tetragonal zirconia was introduced for biomedical use in orthopedics for total hip replacements, where it was found to exhibit excellent mechanical properties and biocompatibility. Then, in the early 1990s, 3Y-PSZ was used for endodontic posts and implant abutments. All these devices were possible to be made from zirconia because they could be prefabricated in a factory setting.

The introduction of CAD–CAM technology to the manufacture of fixed partial dentures in the dental laboratory profoundly influenced the choice of materials available. Until CAD–CAM, it was not possible to consider the use of zirconia as a material for the construction of crowns and bridges, largely because a zirconia powder would not densify until reaching a temperature in excess of 1600°C, making it impractical as a dental laboratory material. This has all changed and, with the aid of CAD–CAM technology, it is now possible to manufacture crown copings and bridge frameworks from this material.

The key to being able to use zirconia was a combination of data processing and computer-aided manufacture. By using a porous, only partially sintered block of zirconia, it was possible to machine the desired restoration. Of course, on densification, it would shrink considerably, by some 20–30%. This was accounted for in the design process by machining the restoration bigger than its final size to compensate for the shrinkage that would occur during the densification firing cycle. The result is a very close-fitting, semi-translucent to white core or bridge framework.

The mechanical properties of zirconia are considerably superior, in restorative dentistry terms, than those of any other dental ceramic. This means that, for the first time, it became possible to produce a full range of anterior and posterior crowns and bridge frameworks with both short and long spans from one single ceramic material. Due to its very high strength, 3Y-TZP is suitable for all indications – from single-tooth crowns to 14-unit bridges. The high strength also meant that the core thickness could be substantially reduced, which is highly beneficial to producing good aesthetics. Nevertheless, the final restoration would still need to be veneered due to the lack of translucency of the zirconia. The veneering ceramic is made up of a leucite glass–ceramic, where the leucite content has been carefully controlled to match the properties of the veneer to those of the zirconia. Since the zirconia ceramic core is white in appearance, the overall aesthetics can be superior to that of the metal–ceramic restorations (Figure 3.5.8).

Monolithic Zirconia Restorations

While veneering the zirconia core framework solved the aesthetic problem, it did introduce another problem, which is that the veneer ceramic had a tendency to chip or delaminate. Although the reasons for this problem are not clear, it did stimulate an interest in developing a form of polycrystalline zirconia that is sufficiently translucent not to require a veneering ceramic. An example of monolithic zirconia is IPS e.max ZirCAD MT Multi, which is designed for the anterior and posterior region. In this version of y-TZP the shade and translucency have been maximized such that monolithic crowns and bridges can be produced without necessitating the application of a veneer while also introducing further efficiency to the dental laboratory. The tooth shade is reproduced by the use of polychromatic discs in the A-D shades. If necessary, restorations can be customized using the staining or cut-back technique. IPS e.max ZirCAD MT Multi is available as a disc with a diameter of 98.5 mm and as a block in different sizes. The strength is not as high as for the core zirconia ceramics (850 MPa) and therefore the indications for use include:

- Monolithic crowns and bridges (Figure 3.5.9)
- Implant-supported superstructures

While long-term clinical evidence is necessarily somewhat sparse, there is a growing body of randomized clinical trials that we can draw upon to assess the success of zirconia as a dental material, be it as a crown, bridge, or fixed partial denture. The studies primarily focus on recall periods of 5–10 years and broadly conclude that zirconia is a suitable replacement for metal–ceramic prostheses, although with sometimes higher failure of the veneering ceramic where this has been used.

BONDING OF CRYSTALLINE CERAMICS

One drawback with all the high-strength crystalline ceramic systems described above is that they are not amenable to acid etching to produce a micromechanically retentive surface, although sandblasting is effective in roughening the surface

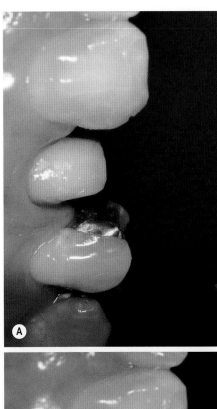

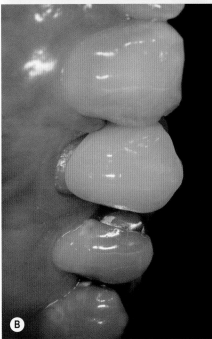

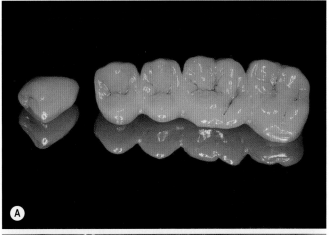

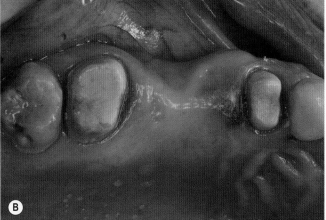

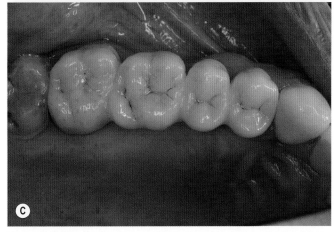

Figure 3.5.8 Example of a layered zirconium crown, with (a) showing the prepared tooth and (b) the crown *in situ*. Images courtesy of and copyright Dr Andrea Fabianelli, Cortona, Italy, with thanks.

Figure 3.5.9 Example of a monolithic zirconia posterior bridge, (a) the bridge, (b) the prepared teeth, and (c) the bridge *in situ*. Image courtesy of and copyright Dr Andrea Fabianelli, Cortona, Italy, with thanks.

suitable. Furthermore, since the fit surface is made up largely of alumina and/or zirconia rather than silica, silane agents cannot effectively bond the core, but 10-MDP primers are suitable to form an adhesive bond to resin cements.

CLINICAL SIGNIFICANCE

Care must be taken to ensure the pretreatment of the fit surface is effective to achieve a good bond; different ceramics require different approaches.

Summary

CAD–CAM technology has opened up new opportunities to use materials not previously considered to be a viable option and thus new approaches to the construction of all ceramic crowns and bridges. Robust clinical data on the long-term viability of these restorations will necessarily not be available until such materials have been in use for much longer, but what data is available to compare the survival of zirconia restorations with those of more traditional materials appear to be encouraging.

RESIN–MATRIX CERAMICS

Introduction

Resin–matrix ceramics are a comparatively new class of dental ceramic materials. They have many similarities to the resin-based composites discussed in Chapter 2.2, although they also have a few key differences. For these resin-containing materials to be classified as dental ceramics required nothing less than a redefining of the term *dental ceramic*!

Until 2013, a dental ceramic was defined by the American Dental Association Code on Dental Procedures and Nomenclature as "non-metal, non-resin inorganic refractory compounds processed at high temperatures (600°C and above) and pressed, polished, or milled, including porcelains, glasses, and glass-ceramics." Note the *non-resin* clause – prior to 2013, anything that included a resin was by definition not a ceramic (at least according to the ADA). This was revised in 2013 and a new definition was adopted wherein the terminology was adjusted to "pressed, fired, polished, or milled materials containing predominantly inorganic refractory compounds – including porcelains, glasses, ceramics, and glass-ceramics." Note this time the use of *predominantly* and the removal of reference to resin – now, as long as the greater proportion of the material is a conventional glass/ceramic/porcelain composition, there is more flexibility for other components, and this allows the incorporation of resin into what we term a dental ceramic. With this loosening of the definition of a dental ceramic, the resin–matrix ceramic was born.

Resin–matrix ceramics, as the name suggests, are composed of glass or ceramic particles embedded in a matrix of resin. If that sounds familiar, it should: the same description could, of course, be applied to our standard resin-based composite encountered in Section 2.2. The main differences include the nature of the filler (composition, particle size, form) and the polymerization conditions of the resin (in the factory, not in the mouth, thus offering a much wider range of curing conditions). The inclusion of resin in the ceramic materials has many implications for the properties of these materials when compared to all ceramic materials.

> ### CLINICAL SIGNIFICANCE
> Over the past decade, a new class of dental ceramics have been introduced: the resin–matrix ceramics. This was not so much an innovation in materials science – resin matrix ceramics were used in other industries prior to this date – as a change in definition, which has led to a new generation of indirect restorative materials.

Composition

The "filler" – the ceramic, glass, or glass–ceramic component – varies somewhat between brands in both composition and form. Silica and zirconia particles are common choices – in some instances both are used within a given material – and alumina is also used in some products. As with resin composites, other minor components may be included, such as heavy metal oxides to impart radiopacity. Also as with a resin-based composite, the filler needs to be silane coated to enable a covalent bond to the resin matrix. In some instances the individual ceramic particles may be very small – as little as a few nanometers in diameter – although they are not dispersed at this size but exist as clusters of many particles that result in an effective particle size much larger, closer to micrometers. As an alternative to a jumble of close packed but unconnected particles, there may be two inter-penetrating networks, with a porous ceramic structure – in effect, ceramic particles that have been fused together by sintering – infiltrated by resin. Both of these approaches can lead to a ceramic loading upward of 80 wt %, with the consequent strength and hardness implied by this high ceramic:resin ratio.

The resin that forms the matrix is usually similar to that used in resin-based composites – urethane dimethacrylate (UDMA) copolymerized with triethylene glycol dimethacrylate (TEG-DMA) – although some manufacturers are less forthcoming with this information, so not all may conform to this formula. The difference between these materials and the resin-based composite is that the resin is pre-cured – the polymerization takes place under carefully controlled conditions during manufacturing. This means that the limited depth of cure and the polymerization shrinkage that afflict composites are not relevant to resin–matrix ceramics – any shrinkage that takes place has done so before it is in the hands of the dentist, and the conditions required for an adequate degree of conversion can be assured in the factory and are of no concern to the clinician. Indeed, it has been found that by conducting the polymerization under increased temperature and pressure, even superior mechanical properties can be achieved.

> ### CLINICAL SIGNIFICANCE
> These materials have much in common with the resin-based composites, but some of the limitations of composites – limited depth of cure, polymerization shrinkage – are more readily mitigated in indirect materials, as the polymerization happens in the factory and not in the mouth.

Properties

The introduction of the resin–matrix ceramic structure brings with it some implications for materials properties. Compared to conventional ceramic materials, they have generally higher flexural strength and are less prone to fatigue-related failure. They have lower elastic moduli than many conventional ceramics, indicating a degree more flexibility (although they are still rigid materials in the greater scheme of things). Some have a modulus of elasticity similar to or approaching that of the dentin. Most resin–matrix ceramics have a lower hardness than conventional ceramics, which renders them less damaging to the opposing teeth – there is less wear of the enamel of the teeth that contact a resin–matrix ceramic, although potentially this could result in more wear of the resin–matrix ceramic itself. Some examples of these materials have thus far proven to be inferior in aesthetic terms, particularly in relation to the translucency of those materials with a high alumina content, but other materials seem with the limited data available to be quite satisfactory in this regard. Likewise, some laboratory studies have raised concerns about the color stability of these materials, but others have shown this to be acceptable.

CLINICAL SIGNIFICANCE

As with any relatively recent development in dental biomaterials, there is a dearth of clinical data available to support the long-term stability and suitability of these materials. On the basis of what data is available, they seem to offer useful characteristics, but only with the benefit of longitudinal studies will we see the full picture.

Handling

As described above, the pre-cured nature of the material means that it is supplied in its polymerized state, in the form of a rectangular cuboid attached to a spigot used to mount in the CAD–CAM machine. A range of shades and translucencies are available and some materials are supplied with a graded shade and translucency within the same block, to better mimic the variable color and translucency of a natural tooth. The resin–matrix ceramic does not require any firing after milling and, being generally less hard than other ceramics used for CAD–CAM, it is somewhat easier and faster to mill, causing less wear to the CAD–CAM machine parts. It has been estimated that owing to the relative ease of milling this material, a set of CAD–CAM milling burs could mill 10–20 resin–matrix ceramics for every one all-ceramic or glass–ceramic crown –not an insignificant saving in the cost of the CAD–CAM equipment. Furthermore, the resin matrix being similar or identical to that in resin-based composites raises the possibility of intraoral repair, in that a composite could be used to repair a damaged resin–matrix ceramic crown using a similar approach to a composite repairing a damaged composite, whereas intraoral repair of conventional ceramics is very challenging.

CLINICAL SIGNIFICANCE

The conveniences and favorable properties of these relatively new materials are substantial, but only over the decades to come will we see whether they stand the test of time.

FURTHER READING

de Alves Lucena, M., Relvas, A., Lefrançois, M., Azevedo, Venicio, M., Sotelo, P., Soltelo, L., 2021. Resin matrix ceramics: mechanical, aesthetic and biological properties. Revista Gaucha de Odontologia 69.

Denry, I., Kelly, J.R., 2014. Emerging ceramic-based materials for dentistry. Journal of Dental Research 93 (12), 1235–1242.

Facenda, Cadorim J., Borba, M., Corazza, P.H., 2018. A literature review on the new polymer-infiltrated ceramic-network material (PICN). Journal of Esthetic and Restorative Dentistry 30, 281–286.

Lüthy, H., Filser, F., Loeffel, O., Schumacher, M., Gauckler, L.J., Hammerle, C.H., 2005. Strength and reliability of four-unit all-ceramic posterior bridges. Dental Materials 21, 930.

Poggio, C.E., Ercoli, C., Rispoli, L., Maiorana, C., Esposito, M., 2017. Metal–free materials for fixed prosthodontic restorations. Cochrane Database of Systematic Reviews 12 (12), CD009606.

Rizkalla, A.S., Jones, D.W., 2004. Mechanical properties of commercial high strength ceramic core materials. Dental Materials 20, 207.

Ruse, N.D., Sadoun, M.J., 2014. Resin-composite blocks for dental CAD/CAM applications. Journal of Dental Research 93, 1232–1234.

Raigrodski, A.J., 2004. Contemporary materials and technologies for all-ceramic fixed partial dentures: a review of the literature. Journal of Prosthetic Dentistry 92 (6), 557–562.

Spear, F., Holloway, J., 2008. Which all-ceramic system is optimal for anterior esthetics? Journal of the American Dental Association 139 (Suppl.), 19S–24S.

Tinschert, J., Zwez, D., Mark, R., Anusavice, K.J., 2000. Structural reliability of alumina-, leucite-, mica- and zirconia-based ceramics. Journal of Dentistry 28, 529.

Win, L.C., Sands, P., Bonsor, S.J., Burke, F.J.T., 2021a. Ceramics in dentistry: which material is appropriate for the anterior or posterior dentition? Part 1: materials Science. Dental Update 48, 680–688.

Win, L.C., Sands, P., Bonsor, S.J., Burke, F.J.T., 2021b. Ceramics in dentistry: which material is appropriate for the anterior or posterior dentition? Part 2: recent clinical research. Dental Update 48, 690–696.

Cementation of Indirect Restorations

INTRODUCTION

For most of the 20th century, the only materials available for the retention and marginal seal of fixed prostheses such as veneers, inlays, crowns, and bridges, were zinc oxide–eugenol and zinc–phosphate cements. Hence the term *cementation* represented an appropriate description of the process of fixing a metallic or ceramic restoration to the teeth. In the latter decades of the 20th century things began to change with the introduction of many more adhesive materials and procedures. Now, a wide variety of cements are available to the clinician, including the more conventional zinc–polycarboxylate cements and glass ionomer cements (GICs) as well as resin-modified glass ionomer cements (RMGICs) and a substantial array of resin-based materials based on various monomer technologies. In the last decade or so there has been a rise in so-called 'universal adhesives', which can be used for indirect *and* direct restorations (see also Chapter 2.5). There is arguably almost too much choice for the modern clinician – to have many options can be good, but sometimes it can be difficult to make an objective selection. In this chapter we will seek to demystify some of the most commonly used materials and get behind the marketing to see the science, all with the intention of helping today's (and tomorrow's) clinicians choose the best material for the specific circumstance.

In the modern context the term 'cementation' hardly does justice to the range of materials now available, although it is still in common use. Another term for the process of fixing a restoration in place is *luting*. The word 'lute' dates back to the days of alchemy and in the modern sense means a cement or other material used as a protective covering or airtight seal. As this term is not specific to a cement, the term *luting agent* perhaps provides a more appropriate description of some of the materials that are used today, such as the resins. However, as cementation is probably the more commonly used of the two, we will persist with the use of the terms cement and cementation.

GENERAL REQUIREMENTS FOR CEMENTATION OF INDIRECT RESTORATIONS

Biocompatibility

When cements are used in such situations as crowns and inlays, the material will inevitably be in contact with a relatively large surface area of dentine, so their susceptibility to eliciting postoperative sensitivity or pulpal inflammation is a very important consideration. Cements will also provide the main barrier to the ingress of bacteria, such that, besides a good marginal seal, antibacterial properties may prove to be beneficial.

Retention

The primary role of the cement is to provide retention of the restoration. With the water-based cements such as zinc–phosphate cement retention is governed by the geometry of the tooth preparation, the control of the path of insertion, and the ability to provide mechanical keying into surface irregularities. In this instance the cement is not an adhesive as such, but a 'space filler' between the tooth and biomaterial. This is not always ideal and lack of retention is a major cause of failure with fixed prostheses cemented in this way. If, in addition, an adhesive bond can be created, this can enhance the retention significantly. Resin adhesive technologies have made this possible.

Mechanical Properties

It is important that the thin layer of cement placed between the tooth and the restoration is able to withstand the large forces that can be transmitted through it. In order to resist fracture, a high tensile strength, fracture toughness, and fatigue strength are beneficial. The situation can be improved significantly by ensuring that the restoration produces a good marginal fit, such that a minimal amount of the cement is required.

Although only a small amount of the cement is exposed at the surface, it is important that the material is able to resist wear. Excessive wear can lead to sub-margination, which, in effect, means that a small groove is formed around the periphery of the restoration. Such a groove can become a site for marginal staining and plaque accumulation.

Marginal Seal

The cement must provide a good marginal seal in order to prevent recurrent caries. An ideal cement should not be susceptible to dissolution in the oral environment so as to maintain the marginal seal in the long term. A low solubility in neutral and acid environments is therefore important. If the cement can provide an adhesive bond to the tooth tissues and the restoration, then this will also help to maintain the integrity of the marginal seal. Recent developments in cementation have sought to achieve exactly that but, with the wide variety of materials to be bonded (enamel, dentine, metal, ceramic), a correspondingly wide variety of adhesion promoters have also become available.

Low Film Thickness

The film thickness is important because a cement needs to be sufficiently thin both to fill the space between the crown or bridge and the tooth, and to ensure proper seating of the restoration. A thick film would be unacceptable, as the restoration may end up higher than was originally intended, causing occlusal problems and a need for it to be ground down. Also, a poor marginal fit would result in more cement being exposed at the surface than necessary, which can exacerbate the problems described above, whereby the material at the margin dissolves and leaves a space susceptible to staining and plaque accumulation.

Ease of Use

Some cements are provided as powder–liquid delivery systems and, as long as great care is exercised to make sure that the correct powder-to-liquid ratio is used on mixing, these can be very effective. However, some clinicians are in the habit of adding more of the liquid to produce a slightly more fluid mix to give rheological properties that allow the cement to flow more readily into the space between the tooth and the restoration and produce a very close adaptation. For some materials, changing the powder-to-liquid ratio even modestly can have a profound effect on its properties, especially working and setting times, and this practice is therefore not generally recommended.

The working and setting times need to be such that sufficient time is allowed to place the restoration and yet it does not take too long to set once placed. The best way to ensure the correct powder-to-liquid ratio is to follow the instructions for use carefully or to avoid the whole issue by using encapsulated delivery systems or the resin-based adhesives, which tend to employ a dual light-activated and chemically activated curing mechanism where the chemical activation is sufficiently slow to provide a more than adequate working time.

Radiopacity

It is important for the practitioner to be able to distinguish between a cement and recurrent caries under a fixed prosthesis, especially as this is one of the main failure mechanisms of indirect restorations. In order to avoid possible misinterpretation, it is beneficial if the cement is more radiopaque than dentine. It also makes it easier to detect possible excess cement and marginal overhangs, especially in those difficult-to-see proximal areas.

Aesthetics

Although not a major consideration with metal and metal–ceramic restorations, aesthetics becomes very important when using all-ceramic restoration. For some of the core-reinforced ceramics, a cement that has a white/opaque appearance is acceptable, but as the ceramic restoration becomes more translucent, the optical properties become more important. This has meant that, for the highly translucent resin-bonded ceramics, such as those used in the construction of anterior veneers, new cements with comparable color and color stability, translucency, and surface texture have had to be developed.

CLINICAL SIGNIFICANCE

No one material is capable of meeting all the stringent requirements for a cement, which is one reason why there is such a wide choice.

CHOICE OF CEMENTS

The oldest cement still in use is zinc–phosphate cement, which provides nothing more than a space filler, sometimes referred to as a grout between the restoration and the tooth, a bit like the grout that is used to hold bathroom or kitchen tiles in place. Retention depends primarily on the careful design of the tooth preparation and the quality of fit of the restoration, as the cement has no adhesive affinity for tooth tissue, metal, or ceramic. The polyacrylic acid-based cements, such as zinc–polycarboxylate cement, GICs and RMGICs, go a stage further in being able to bond to enamel and dentine and also are claimed to have some affinity for metal and ceramic surfaces. Although these water-based cements have some ability to bond to metals, in general it is considered that these materials do not provide an adequate bond to metal or ceramic restorations for some of the more demanding situations encountered. Hence, new ceramic and metal adhesives needed to be developed for it to impact on prosthetic dentistry to the same degree as new adhesive procedures and materials have changed operative dentistry. It is the advent of resin-bonding technology that most probably has had the biggest impact on the procedures used to retain indirect restorations.

In order to manage this wide diversity of cements and associated clinical procedures, for simplicity, they will be considered under two categories, namely:
- water-based cements
- resin-based cements

WATER-BASED CEMENTS

The water-based cements include zinc–phosphate cement, zinc–polycarboxylate cement, GIC, and RMGIC.

Zinc–Phosphate Cements

Zinc–phosphate cement is one of the oldest cements available and continues to be popular because of its long history of clinical success and favorable handling properties. These cements are presented as a white powder that is mixed with a clear liquid. The powder consists of mainly zinc oxide, with up to 10% magnesium oxide included, and the liquid is an aqueous solution of phosphoric acid of 45–64% concentration.

Presentation

Powder. The powder is fired at a temperature in excess of 1000°C for several hours in order to reduce its reactivity and provide a suitable working and setting time for the cements; the material would set far too rapidly without this firing process.

The magnesium oxide is added, as it helps maintain the white color of the cement. It has the additional advantages of making the pulverization process of the zinc oxide somewhat easier and also increasing the compressive strength of the cement. Other oxides such as silica and alumina may be added in small quantities of up to 5% to improve the mechanical properties of the set material and to provide a variety of shades.

Some formulations include fluorides (usually in the form of a few percentage of stannous (tin) fluoride) and are generally used in situations where fluoride release might be particularly beneficial, such as for the cementation of orthodontic bands.

Liquid. The liquid is buffered with a combination of the oxides that are present in the powder and with aluminum hydroxide, which acts to form phosphates in the liquid. The aluminum is essential to the cement-forming reaction, producing an amorphous zinc–phosphate, while the zinc helps to moderate the reaction, making sure that the cement has the appropriate working time. This control over the working time also helps to ensure that an adequate amount of the powder is incorporated into the liquid.

Setting Reaction

When zinc oxide is mixed with an aqueous solution of phosphoric acid, the superficial layer of the zinc oxide is dissolved by the acid. In the case of pure zinc oxide mixed with phosphoric acid the acid–base reaction first involves the formation of an acid zinc–phosphate:

$$ZnO + 2H_3PO_4 \rightarrow Zn(H_2PO_4)_2 + H_2O$$

This is followed by a further reaction, where, in this second phase of the process, a hydrated zinc–phosphate is produced:

$$Z_nO + Zn(H_2PO_4)_2 + 2H_2O \rightarrow Zn_3(PO_4)_2 \cdot 4H_2O(\text{hopeite})$$

This substance is virtually insoluble and crystallizes to form a phosphate matrix, which binds together the unreacted parts of the zinc oxide particles. The reaction is slightly exothermic and some shrinkage of the cement takes place.

It is thought that, in the commercial materials, the presence of the aluminum prevents the crystallization process, thus producing a glassy matrix in the form of an alumino-phosphate gel. This lack of crystallization is exacerbated by the presence of magnesium, which delays the development of any crystallinity. Some crystallization, resulting in the formation of hopeite, may occur with time.

Unbound water forms globules within the material and makes the cement highly permeable, resulting in a porous structure when the material is dry. The final structure is that of particles of unreacted zinc oxide in a matrix consisting of phosphates of zinc, magnesium, and aluminum.

Properties

As a general observation, it is worth noting that zinc–phosphate cements have been around for some considerable time and have provided excellent clinical service. This may be related to the general ease with which the material can be used, as well as the wide range of applications available. They have a well-defined working time and a rapid setting time. Although it is tempting to think that the modern materials in the shiny packaging must be in some way 'better', in fact, some of the more traditional materials can present an excellent option for the discerning clinician.

Working and setting times. The working time for most brands of zinc–phosphate cement, when used with the consistency of a cement, is usually within the region of 3–6 minutes. The corresponding setting time can vary from 5 to 14 minutes. Both of these times depend to some extent on the mixing procedure adopted.

Depending on the application, the material is mixed to either a thick consistency for cavity bases or a thinner consistency when used as a cement. The mixing process is carried out by the slow incorporation of the powder into the liquid. The recommended procedure is that, initially, only small increments are added to the powder, followed by a couple of larger increments. Finally, smaller increments are again added, as this will ensure that the desired consistency is not exceeded.

Extended working and setting times can be achieved by mixing the powder into the liquid in increments over a large area of the mixing slab. This helps to dissipate the heat of reaction that would otherwise speed up the setting process. Conversely, the rapid mixing of powder into the liquid will shorten both the working and setting times. This will result in a thick mix obtained, with a low powder-to-liquid ratio, because of the early initiation of the setting process. The low powder content will mean that an inferior material is obtained.

By using a cooled glass slab for the mixing procedure, it is possible to extend the working time without simultaneously increasing the setting time. This also has the benefit of allowing more powder to be added to the liquid, thus raising the strength and reducing the solubility. However, great care must be exercised when using this technique, as there is a danger of water contamination either from the slab not having been dried properly or due to condensation. Both will have the effect of reducing the working time. The combination of the cool glass and the incremental process ensures that an adequate working time is maintained. The mixing procedure should be completed within about 60–90 seconds.

The setting time can be extended by a process known as *slaking the fluid*, in which a small quantity of the powder is added to the liquid about a minute before the main mixing procedure is started.

The consistency of the paste depends on the powder-to-liquid ratio, and it is important that the correct powder-to-liquid ratio is used for the particular application.

For instance, too low a powder-to-liquid ratio would produce a weak and highly soluble material with an unacceptably low pH. While the manufacturers suggest optimum powder-to-liquid ratios for their products, these are difficult to adhere to in practice since the dispensing system is not very accurate. Consequently, most dentists prefer to mix sufficient powder into the liquid until a consistency is obtained that is suitable for the particular application. This makes it all the more important that a consistent and reproducible procedure is adopted.

The liquid is kept in a sealed bottle. If the lid is kept off the bottle, loss of water by evaporation will lower the pH of the liquid as it becomes more concentrated; this will slow down the setting process. If a lot of water is lost, the phosphoric acid will begin to separate out and the liquid will take on a cloudy appearance. Should this occur, the liquid must be disposed of.

When this cement is to be used, it is important that the powder and liquid are not dispensed until just prior to when they are needed, as if they are dispensed and then left in the open air, evaporation of the water may occur and this will slow down the setting reaction. Neither should the material be left for any length of time once mixed because the setting reaction takes place virtually immediately on mixing. If the paste is left for too long, the viscosity will have increased to such an extent that the material will no longer have adequate flow characteristics.

Biocompatibility. A freshly mixed zinc–phosphate cement will have a pH in the region of 1.3–3.6. This low value tends to persist for some considerable time, and it can take up to 24 hours for the cement to return to a near-neutral pH.

When placed over a heavily prepared tooth, the initial pH is sufficiently low to induce an inflammatory response in the pulp. This is especially so if a pulpal micro-exposure is suspected. It is important to remember that the thinner the mix, the lower the pH will be, and the longer it will take for the cement to return to a neutral pH.

Zinc–phosphate cement has no antibacterial properties and this, combined with the slight shrinkage on setting, means that it does not provide an ideal barrier to the ingress of bacteria. Thus the pulpal sensitivity associated with the material may be due to a combination of shrinkage, a lack of antibacterial behavior, and the high acidity when freshly mixed, rather than only the acidity as is often thought.

The patient may experience some pain during a cementation procedure. This can arise as a result of both the low pH of the cement and the osmotic pressure developed by the movement of fluid through the dentinal tubules. Such an experience is usually only transient and should subside within a few hours. If there is a persistent pulpal irritation, it may have been caused by using too thin a mix of the cement.

The hardening process for a zinc–phosphate cement takes a considerable time, and during the first 24 hours, there is a significant release of magnesium with lower amounts of zinc. Whether this has any meaningful biological effects is sometimes questioned, but the material has been used successfully for many decades.

Mechanical properties. As with other properties, the mechanical properties are very much dependent on the powder-to-liquid ratio of the final cement. The compressive strength can vary from as low as 40 MPa up to 140 MPa. The relationship between the powder-to-liquid ratio and the compressive strength is virtually linear.

The cement shows an initially rapid rise in strength, reaching 50% of its final strength within the first 10 minutes. Thereafter, the strength increases more slowly, reaching its final strength after approximately 24 hours. The cement is extremely brittle, and this is reflected by its very low tensile strength, which is of the order of 5–7 MPa. The modulus of elasticity is approximately 12 GPa, which is similar to that of dentine.

Consistency and film thickness. To ensure the proper seating of the restoration, it is important that the cement is capable of forming a very thin film.

On mixing, the powder is partially dissolved in the acid, such that the final size of the remaining powder in the set structure ranges from 2 to 8 μm. As the mix flows readily, a film thickness of less than 25 μm can be achieved. This is adequate for cementation purposes, but the thickness of the layer is very much dependent on the procedure adopted.

The viscosity of the mix increases quite rapidly with time. Within a couple of minutes, the viscosity can already be quite high, although the material itself is still quite manageable. Nevertheless, it is recommended that no undue delay is allowed to occur when cementing a restoration, as the reduced viscosity can result in a significantly higher film thickness for the cement and thus a poorly seated restoration.

Solubility. The solubility of a cement is an important consideration. Dissolution contributes to marginal leakage around the restoration and results in bacterial penetration. This may cause either loosening of the restoration or, what is more likely, the induction of recurrent caries, which may undermine the whole tooth.

Zinc phosphate cement is highly soluble in water for the first 24 hours after setting, and the loss of material can range from 0.04 to 3.3%; an acceptable upper limit is 0.2%. After this time, the solubility is much reduced. The solubility is highly dependent on the powder-to-liquid ratio achieved for the cement, with a high ratio being desirable. Once the material has fully set, it remains only slightly soluble in water (with some release of zinc and phosphates) but is still susceptible to acid attack. As the final set takes some time to achieve, it is important that the cement is not unduly exposed to the oral fluids.

The fluoride-containing cements show a continuous release of fluoride over a long period. The fluoride uptake by the surrounding enamel should reduce the likelihood of decalcification, especially when used for the cementation of orthodontic bands.

Applications. The most common application for zinc–phosphate cements is as cements for metal and metal–ceramic crowns and bridges, although it is also used in other applications such as the cementation of orthodontic bands and as a temporary restoration.

These cements exhibit several advantages in that they:
- are easy to mix
- have a sharp, well-defined set
- have a sufficiently high compressive strength to resist the forces of amalgam condensation
- are a low-cost product.

The easy handling characteristics and their adequate retentive properties have made zinc–phosphate cements highly popular with dental practitioners for over a century.

However, the disadvantages are that they:
- have a potential for pulpal irritation due to low pH
- have no antibacterial action
- are brittle
- have no adhesive qualities
- are relatively soluble in the oral environment.

These factors contribute to the incidence of recurrent caries associated with cast restorations.

CLINICAL SIGNIFICANCE

Zinc–phosphate cements have been around for over 100 years and, notwithstanding their limitations, are likely to continue to find application for the cementation of metal and metal–ceramic restorations for many years to come.

Zinc–Polycarboxylate Cements

The zinc–polycarboxylate cements were first introduced to dentistry in 1968 when a dentist from Manchester had the bright idea of replacing phosphoric acid with one of the new polymeric acids: namely, polyacrylic acid. These materials rapidly became popular with the dental profession, as they provided the first cement that was able to bond to enamel and dentine. The bonding mechanism is the same as that described for the GICs (see Chapter 2.5).

Presentation

These cements come as a white powder and a clear, viscous liquid. The constituents of the powder are zinc oxide and magnesium oxide, and the liquid is a 30–40% aqueous solution of polyacrylic acid.

Powder. The powder is based on the same formulation used for the zinc–phosphate cements, containing zinc oxide with approximately 10% magnesium oxide or, sometimes, tin oxide. In addition, there may be other additives such as silica, alumina, or bismuth salts. The powder is fired at a high temperature to control the rate of reaction and is then ground to the appropriate particle size. Some brands also contain stannous fluoride to impart the benefits of fluoride release. Pigments may be present to provide a variety of shades.

Liquid. The liquid is usually a copolymer of polyacrylic acid with other unsaturated carboxylic acids, such as itaconic and maleic acid. (The structures of polyacrylic acid and itaconic acid were presented in Chapter 2.3.) The molecular weight of the copolymer is in the range of 30 000–50 000 Daltons.

Alternatively, in some formulations the acid is freeze-dried and then added to the powder, in which case the liquid component is distilled water, an approach that is often adopted in the presentation of GICs. This method was developed to simplify the achievement of the correct ratio between the components, which was difficult beforehand because of the high viscosity of the liquid. The pH is adjusted by the addition of sodium hydroxide, and tartaric acid is added to control the setting reaction.

Setting Reaction

The basic setting reaction of these cements involves a reaction between the zinc oxide and the ionized copolymer of acrylic acid and itaconic acid.

On mixing the powder and the liquid, the acid attacks the powder and causes a release of zinc ions. This is followed by the formation of cross-links (in the form of salt bridges), in the same way as occurs for the GICs, except that, in this case, the zinc provides the cross-links rather than calcium and aluminum, as shown in Figure 3.6.1.

The result of the reaction is a cored structure in which the unreacted powder particles are bound by a matrix of zinc–polyacrylate.

Properties

Working and setting times. When compared to the zinc–phosphate cements, the setting reaction proceeds rapidly; mixing should be completed within 30–40 seconds to ensure an adequate working time.

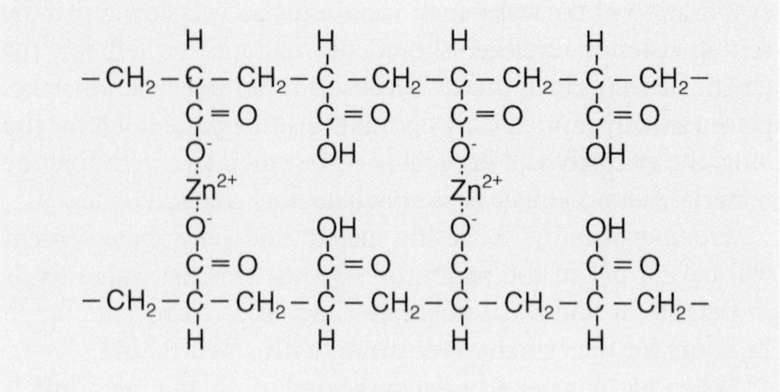

Figure 3.6.1 Zinc ions providing the cross-links between the carboxyl groups on the polyacrylic acid polymer chains.

The viscosity of these cements does not rise as rapidly as for the zinc–phosphate cements. This has the effect that, after a couple of minutes, the viscosity of the zinc–polycarboxylate cement is less than that of the zinc–phosphate cement, even though it was initially more viscous than the zinc-phosphate. In addition, the freshly mixed zinc–polycarboxylate cement has the property of being pseudoplastic and exhibits shear thinning on mixing. This means that, although the material may at first appear to be too thick to flow properly while it is being placed, the pressure that is exerted makes it flow quite satisfactorily. If this property is not appreciated by the clinician, they may be inclined to produce a thinner mix by reducing the powder-to-liquid ratio under the misapprehension that this will make the cement flow more readily. As discussed above, this is not recommended as the properties of the cement are considerably impaired.

In general, the higher the powder-to-liquid ratio or the higher the molecular weight of the copolymer, the shorter the working time will be. The recommended powder-to-liquid ratio for cementation purposes is 1.5:1 by weight, which will give a working time at room temperature of 2.5–3.5 minutes and a setting time at 37°C of 6–9 minutes.

As with the zinc–phosphate cements, the working time can be extended by using a cooled glass slab or by refrigerating the powder. It is not recommended to refrigerate those liquids that still include the polyacrylic acid, as this leads to gelation of the polymer due to the hydrogen bonding.

The ability to extend the working time is particularly useful for mixes that have a higher powder-to-liquid ratio when they are being used as cavity bases. Nevertheless, the short working times of the zinc–polycarboxylate cements have been recognized as a potential problem.

This has been overcome with more recent formulations by optimizing the amount of tartaric acid in the material. Tartaric acid has the beneficial property of extending the working time without markedly affecting the setting time of the cement, in a similar way to with a GIC (see Chapter 2.3).

Biocompatibility. Contact of zinc–polycarboxylate with either the soft or the hard tissues has been found to result in only a very mild response. Although it has a moderately low pH initially (in the range of 3.0–4.0), this does not appear to have the same adverse effect as the zinc–phosphate cements. It is suggested that this may be due to a combination of a rapid rise to the neutrality of the pH on setting and a limited ability of the polyacid to penetrate the dentine.

The zinc–polycarboxylate cements have been found to have some antibacterial properties, which means that a better barrier to the ingress of bacteria is provided than by zinc–phosphate cements; this resistance to the penetration of bacteria is augmented by its adhesive quality.

It is probably these factors that are responsible for the lack of pulpal response, rather than the higher pH and the high molecular weight of the acid compared to the zinc–phosphate cements, although these latter factors *will* contribute to the blandness of the material.

Stannous fluoride is frequently incorporated into the cements, and this does not appear to affect the biological response. The fluoride release appears to be sufficient to have a beneficial effect on the neighboring enamel and dentine.

Mechanical properties. When the cement is prepared according to the correct powder/liquid ratio, the compressive strength of the fully set cement is in the region of 55–85 MPa. This strength depends on the powder-to-liquid ratio achieved and is somewhat lower than that of the zinc–phosphate cements. The tensile strength is higher, however, being in the range of 8–12 MPa. The elastic modulus is around 4–6 GPa, which is about half that of the zinc–phosphate cement.

As already mentioned, the zinc–polycarboxylate cements set quite quickly, and this is reflected in the time it takes to reach its full strength; the cement will reach 80% of its final strength within 1 hour. Long-term storage in water does not appear to have an adverse effect on the mechanical properties.

Solubility. The solubility in water has been measured to be from 0.1 to 0.6% by weight, with higher values for solubility seeming to occur with the cements containing stannous fluoride.

As with the zinc–phosphate cements, these cements are susceptible to acid attack but, as yet, this does not appear to be sufficiently serious to be of any clinical significance, as indicated by the good clinical results obtained when using this cement. When failure has occurred, this is more often than not due to the improper handling of the material. This is usually related to the use of a powder-to-liquid ratio that is too low, possibly in an attempt to extend the working time.

Adhesion. A feature of the zinc–polycarboxylate cements that sets them apart from the zinc–phosphate and zinc oxide-eugenol cements is their ability to adhere to enamel and dentine.

The bonding mechanism is the same as that of the GICs and has already been described in Chapter 2.3. The quality of the bond is such that it is maintained in vivo and can be good enough to exceed the cohesive strength of the cement. That being the case, the bond strength is, in fact, limited by the poor tensile strength of the cement and is thus not likely to exceed 7–8 MPa.

Bonding to some metallic surfaces is possible with the zinc–polycarboxylate cements, and this can be very beneficial when it is used as a cement with cast restorations. This again involves specific ions binding to the metallic surface.

Bonding to gold alloys is not good, usually resulting in an adhesive failure of the interface due to the highly inert nature of the gold alloy's surface. This can be improved by sand-blasting or abrading the surface, thus providing some mechanical adhesion, but the benefit is small.

Superior bond strengths are obtained with the base metal alloys (giving rise to cohesive rather than adhesive failures on testing the bond strength), and this is probably related to the presence of an oxide layer that provides the necessary metallic ions. Bond strengths are not especially high because of the low cohesive strength of the zinc–polycarboxylate cements.

Applications

The zinc–polycarboxylate cements are used for the cementation of metal- or core-reinforced ceramic crowns and have also been used for the cementation of orthodontic bands.

They have the following advantages:

1. They bond to enamel and dentine, as well as some of the metallic cast restorations.
2. They have a low irritancy.
3. Their strength, solubility, and film thicknesses are comparable to that of zinc–phosphate cement.
4. They have some antibacterial action.

The disadvantages are that:

1. Their properties are highly dependent on handling procedures.
2. They have short working times and long setting times.
3. An exacting technique is required to ensure bonding.
4. Clean-up is difficult and timing is critical.

If removal of excess material is attempted too soon and the material is still in its rubbery state, the marginal seal may be compromised, while leaving it too long makes it difficult to remove due to the excellent bond to the tooth.

Although the potential advantage of fluoride release provided this cement with some popularity, the current use of zinc–polycarboxylate cements seems to be very limited and many dental practitioners prefer to use either zinc–phosphate or GICs. The perception among practitioners is that there is little to choose between the zinc–polycarboxylate and the GICs and this is supported by laboratory data on these products. If anything, the GICs described below are considered to be somewhat easier to use.

CLINICAL SIGNIFICANCE

Zinc–polycarboxylate cements are a viable alternative to the zinc–phosphate cements, with the added benefit of adhesion to enamel and dentine.

Glass Ionomer Cements and Resin-Modified Glass Ionomer Cements

Although many of the properties of the luting GICs and RMGICs, such as fluoride release and adhesion to enamel and dentine, are the same as for the filling materials described in detail in Chapter 2.3, some requirements are different when the material is used for the purpose of cementing indirect restorations. For example, since the space between the restoration and the tooth tissues is only of the order of 20–50 μm, it is important that a GIC used for luting has a very thin film thickness. For this reason, the glass powder must have a smaller particle size than that for the filling materials. Since a change in the glass powder particle size changes the working and setting characteristics, different formulations of the glass and polyacid have to be used from those used in filling materials in order to retain the optimum properties. It also means that it is not acceptable to use the restorative version of a GIC and modify its rheology by reducing the powder-to-liquid ratio.

The working time can affect the film thickness in that longer working times allow more flow and will aid the seating of the restoration. Once the material begins to set, the viscosity rises rapidly and flow becomes impossible. Thus it is extremely important that the mixing and placement of the cement is completed within 2–2.5 minutes, since, after this time, the material becomes stiff and a thicker film will result. It is a matter of preference and familiarity whether a short or slightly longer working time is desired. Of course, with the resin-modified GICs, there is less time pressure as the chemical cure is slower, since the initial cure is due to activation with blue light. The light cannot get to all areas of the RMGIC as the restoration is in the way, but it is able to reach the margins and serves to start off the curing, which can then finish via the chemical mechanism associated with the traditional GIC, and sometimes also a chemically activated polymerization of the resin, over a longer period.

It is thought that some of the newer formulations of the GIC luting cements do not need the protection of a surface coating because they have a more rapid set. The solubility, as measured by the water-leachable component at 7 minutes, has been reduced from approximately 2 to 1% in the transition from a conventional to a water-hardened cement. Nevertheless, it may be as well to continue to offer some initial protection, since the dissolution due to acid erosion will continue to be a problem. In any case it still takes some time for these materials to reach their final set.

CLINICAL SIGNIFICANCE

It is best to use a purpose-made GIC product for the cementation of indirect restorations rather than re-purpose one designed for fillings, as changing the powder-to-liquid ratio of a GIC filling material to modify the working and setting times or film thickness will result in a material with inferior properties.

Not only do the handling properties of different GIC luting cements vary, but so too do the physical and mechanical requirements. A comparison of a number of properties of two commercially available cements is presented in Table 3.6.1.

As far as the mechanical properties are concerned, the results would indicate that Aqua-Cem (Dentsply Ltd, Weybridge, UK) has a lower stiffness (which would account for the higher diametral and flexural strength), but this is at the expense of the compressive strength and creep resistance. Ketac-Cem (3M/ESPE, Seefeld, Germany) is slightly more brittle than Aqua-Cem. In both instances the materials have little resistance to fracture and need to be well supported by the surrounding structures. Clinically, it has been noted that it is easier to remove Ketac-Cem from the soft tissues than Aqua-Cem. This is probably because the former is more brittle immediately after placement.

TABLE 3.6.1 Physical and Mechanical Properties of Two Glass–Ionomer Luting Cements

	Aqua-Cem (De Trey)	Ketac-Cem (3M/ESPE)
Radiopaque	No	No
Solubility in water		
7 minutes	0.90%	1.00%
1 hour	0.46%	0.40%
Solubility in lactic acid solution	–	0.57%
Compressive strength at 24 hours	82 MPa	105 MPa
Diametral tensile strength at 24 hours	7.6 MPa	5.3 MPa
Flexural strength at 24 hours	15.2 MPa	4.1 MPa
Creep at 24 hours	1.37%	0.63%

RMGICs are another popular option for luting indirect restorations. These have all the potential advantages already discussed in relation to the GIC lining cements combined with the greater resistance to dissolution and enhanced mechanical properties associated with the resin component. In particular, the low solubility and good adhesion to enamel and dentine should help to produce a durable marginal seal and aid retention. The main difference between the restorative and lining RMGICs is that they have to rely at least in part on a chemically activated curing mechanism since it is not possible to gain access to all areas with a light source. These cements have been recommended for use with cast metal crowns, bridges and inlays, metal–ceramic crowns and bridges, and reinforced-core ceramics.

When GIC luting cements were first used, there were some reports that the use of this material resulted in a higher incidence of postoperative sensitivity. However, it is generally agreed now that there is no significant difference in postoperative sensitivity between GICs and zinc–phosphate cements. In all other respects there also seems to be no difference in the performance of GICs and zinc–phosphate cements when used for the cementation of crowns and bridges.

There have been reports of hygroscopic expansion associated with RMGICs and this expansion may increase the likelihood of fracture of all-ceramic crowns. The problem is made even more serious if RMGIC is also used as a core material. Metal posts with compromised mechanical retention may benefit from the use of RMGIC. However, clinicians should be aware that, if the post is to be removed at a later date, the removal of posts cemented with an RMGIC can be extremely difficult.

CLINICAL SIGNIFICANCE

Glass ionomer luting cements have become a popular alternative to zinc–phosphate cement, especially for reinforced-core all-ceramic restorations. The use of RMGICs for the cementation of all-ceramic restorations would appear to be contraindicated until such time that more clinical evidence is available.

RESIN-BASED LUTING CEMENTS

The resin-based luting cements can be divided into three subgroups:
1. Aesthetic light-/dual-cure composite resin cements
2. Adhesive chemical/dual-cure resin cements
3. Self-adhesive dual-cure resin cements

Aesthetic Light-/Dual-Cure Composite Resin Cements

These resins are based on conventional composite resin technology and have no intrinsic adhesive capabilities. They are used primarily for the cementation of resin-bonded ceramic restorations, where the aesthetic of the cementing medium is an important consideration. These composite resin cements need to be used in conjunction with adhesion promoters, requiring a dentine bonding agent to ensure a bond to the dentine, as well as a silane coupling agent to provide a bond to the ceramic (see below). The cement provides the all-important means of bridging the gap between the silane-treated ceramic restoration and the prepared tooth structure. For the aesthetically demanding all-ceramic veneers, a composite resin cement is often used because of the superior aesthetics and strength compared with the water-based cements, and the superior bond that is obtained to the etched and silanated ceramic surfaces. The composite resin cements are, in effect, lightly filled composites with small-sized filler particles to ensure thin film thickness. These materials are available in a wide range of shades and translucencies, which provides excellent marginal aesthetics.

Whereas the first generation of this type of resin cement was visible light activated, the tendency is now for the use of dual-cure resins. This makes the resins suitable for both veneers and inlays. The concern is that visible light curing resins may not cure properly when they are used to bond large inlays, as the light would be unable to penetrate to the full depth of the inlay. Similarly, the move toward resin-bonded all-ceramic crowns requires the use of a dual-cure resin in order to ensure that complete polymerization of the composite resin cement occurs.

Adhesive Chemical/Dual-Cure Resin Cements

In order to improve the adhesive bond of resins to the metal surface, a variety of dual-cure composite resin cements have been developed in which the resin component has been modified to provide the ability to bond chemically to suitably prepared metal surfaces without the need for any adhesion promoter. These are generally referred to as chemically adhesive resin cements to differentiate them from the variety discussed above that require a separate adhesive step. In one such system the active constituent is the carboxylic monomer 4-META (4-methacryloxyethyl trimellitate anhydride). Another approach is to incorporate a phosphorylated methacrylate monomer, such as MDP (methacryloyloxydecyl dihydrogen phosphate). Resin bonding is facilitated by the high affinity of carboxylic acid or phosphoric acid derivative-containing resins for the metal oxide on base metal alloy (Figure 3.6.2). However, these resin cements still require an adhesion promoter such as a dentine-bonding agent to bond to *enamel and dentine,* which brings us to the next group of resin cements.

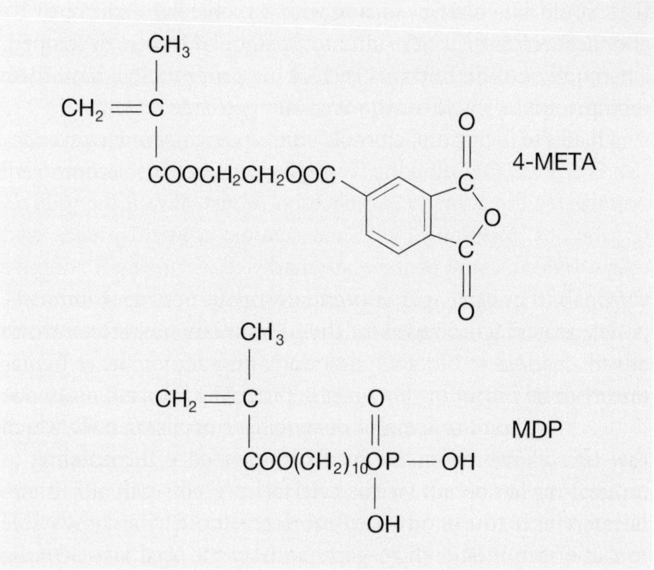

Figure 3.6.2 Structure of 4-META (4-methacryloxyethyl trimellitate anhydride) and MDP (methacryloyloxydecyl dihydrogen phosphate).

Self-Adhesive Dual-Cure Resin Cements

This group of resin cements distinguishes itself from the other resin cements used for luting described above in that no pretreatment of the tooth surface is required, yet at the same time claiming to be able to establish a bond to base metal alloys and a range of ceramics. Thus the application is carried out in a single step similar to that of the water-based cements described earlier but with the added benefit of simultaneously providing adhesion to the tooth tissue and the restoration.

One example of these self-adhesive resin cements contains a specially synthesized monomer having two phosphoric acid groups and two C=C double bonds (a methacrylated phosphoric ester), making the resin highly reactive with a very low pH of around 2.0. When the resin comes in contact with the tooth tissues, the negatively charged phosphoric acid groups react with the calcium ions (Ca^{2+}) in the enamel and dentine and form an ionic bond. By the incorporation of a slightly acid-soluble glass filler that is able to react with the acidic monomer, the pH in the body of the resin cement rapidly increases to a neutral level, with the added benefit of fluoride ion release. Conceptually, this would appear to be not so dissimilar to the compomer resin (see Chapter 2.2), except that a more reactive phosphoric acid group is grafted onto a dimethacrylate, as opposed to an acrylic acid group. Other systems are also based on the incorporation of a phosphoric acid monomer, but the acidic monomers used are ones that are commonly associated with the manufacturer's bonding agents, such as GPDM (glycerol dimethacrylate dihydrogen phosphate) or PENTA (dipentaerytritolpentacrylate phosphoric acid).

Unfortunately, it was not a simple case of adding an acidic monomer to a Bis-GMA- or urethane dimethacrylate (UDMA)–based dual-cure resin, as the acidic components interfere with the visible light and self-cure initiators. In particular, the alkaline amines used in self-cure systems become inactive in an acidic environment. In order to achieve a resin cement that would set either by curing with a visible light source or by chemical reaction, a new initiator system had to be developed. Therefore one will find that each of the products will have their own proprietary acid-resistant amine/peroxide system.

Thanks to their simplicity of use and apparently universal adhesive character, the self-adhesive resin cements have become very popular for the adhesive cementation of virtually all the indirect restorations, including metal and ceramic crowns, bridges, and inlays. Indeed, some of these are marketed as 'universal adhesive cement' as they can – with appropriate surface treatment and compatible materials – be used for the adhesion of direct restorations as well. They have become particularly popular for the cementation of posts (including fiber posts), providing good retention due to the direct bond to the root dentine. One application for which the self-adhesive resins are not recommended is the bonding of ceramic veneers because of the need for excellent aesthetics. In addition, whereas the bond to dentine is considered to be comparable to that of dentine-bonding agents, without the need for acid etching, the bond to enamel is not as good as can be achieved with the etch-and-rinse and self-etching dentine-bonding agents. For the same reason, these resin cements are not usually considered suitable for the bonding of orthodontic brackets.

RESIN-TO-CERAMIC BONDING

There was a time that all-ceramic restorations were cemented only with conventional cements, such as zinc–phosphate, zinc–polycarboxylate, and glass ionomer, and therefore relied on the strength of the ceramic core to withstand normal oral forces. This changed with the introduction of resin-bonded ceramics. As in the case of enamel, the aesthetic composite resins do not have a natural affinity for bonding to ceramic surfaces. Only with the advent of hydrofluoric acid etching of dental ceramics, introduced by Horn in 1983 for the construction of laminate veneers, did the direct bonding of resin composite to enamel become possible. The combination of adhesion provided by resin adhesion to phosphoric acid-etched enamel, dentine-bonding agents able to bond to dentine, hydrofluoric acid-etched and silane-treated resin bond to ceramic (Figure 3.6.3), and improvements in strength and toughness characteristics of dental ceramics produces restorations with excellent mechanical integrity for both anterior and posterior use. The adhesive bond has the effect of eliminating surface flaws by replacing the surface with an interface and thus reduces the potential for fracture. However, the performance of the ceramic is crucially dependent on obtaining and maintaining a strong bond to the tooth structure, which requires a full appreciation of all the aspects of the principles of adhesion. A coupling agent is used to ensure a strong chemical bond between the composite resin cement and the ceramic. Hence, the resin-to-ceramic bond is based on an acid etchant creating a micro-mechanically retentive surface and a coupling agent providing the chemical bond to the ceramic.

Hydrofluoric Acid Etching

The fitting surface of a ceramic, when constructed on a refractory die, is inherently rough due to the grit-blasting process used to remove the refractory. The application of hydrofluoric acid to the fitting surface of a ceramic, such as a leucite-reinforced

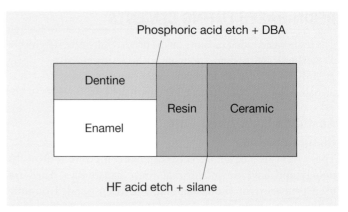

Figure 3.6.3 Schematic of the bonding interfaces when bonding a ceramic inlay. DBA, Dentine-bonding agent

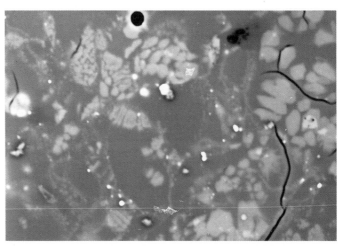

Figure 3.6.4 Back-scattered scanning electron microscope image of the surface of a leucite ceramic. The gray regions are the feldspathic glass, while the slightly lighter-shaded regions are the leucite crystals.

feldspar, enhances the surface roughness even more, due to the preferential removal of either the crystalline leucite phase or the glassy phase. An example of this is shown in Figure 3.6.4, where the back-scattered image created under the scanning electron microscope reveals the heterogeneous composition of a leucite-reinforced ceramic. This heterogeneity can be made use of by preferentially etching one or other of the components with hydrofluoric acid. The effect of this etching is shown in Figure 3.6.5, which reveals a highly micro-mechanically retentive surface due to the preferential removal of the leucite phase. The resin is able to penetrate into these microscopic spaces, resulting in a very strong bond.

In the case of an intraoral ceramic fracture the surface of the ceramic must first be etched in situ with hydrofluoric acid solution to create a micro-mechanically retentive surface. A fractured surface, even if roughened by a diamond bur, will not be as effective at providing micro-mechanical retention as an etched surface. The use of hydrofluoric acid in the mouth should be done with great care since it is a highly toxic material. Acidulated phosphate fluoride gels can also be used but the long etching time is prohibitive. Phosphoric acid is ineffectual as an etchant because the ceramic is totally resistant to attack from this acid, although it may sometimes be used as an effective surface-cleansing agent.

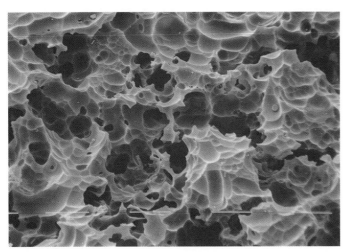

Figure 3.6.5 The surface of a leucite-reinforced ceramic seen under a scanning electron microscope after it has been etched with hydrofluoric acid. The heavily etched, angled, or re-entrant surface is a result of the more rapid dissolution of the leucite in the hydrofluoric acid than the glass matrix.

There are some general problems with hydrofluoric acid etching of which the dental practitioner should be aware:

- Hydrofluoric acid is a highly toxic substance and must be treated with great care. Every care must be taken to protect not only the patient but also the clinician and any assistant from contact with the acid.
- If the hydrofluoric acid is not neutralized completely, it may leach out and cause tissue damage at a later date.
- The hydrofluoric acid gel tends to slump, such that the lateral borders of particular veneers may not be fully etched. This can cause marginal leakage and chipping of the ceramic.

- Damage to the labial gingival margin of the veneer or inlay by the etchant can lead to plaque retention, inflammatory gingival response, and secondary caries.

Silane Coupling Agents

When two materials are incompatible, it is often possible to bring about compatibility by introducing a third material that has properties intermediate between those of the other two. Resins do not have the ability to bond chemically to a ceramic surface and yet the interface between resin and ceramic has to be able to withstand stresses generated by loads applied to the structure and polymerization shrinkage stresses. Thus a coupling agent can be used to overcome this problem (see Chapter 1.9).

The coupling agent most commonly used in conjunction with ceramic restorations is a silane, γ-methacryloxypropyltrimethoxysilane (γ-MPTS). A detailed account of how this particular silane works is provided in Chapter 2.2 – it is the same material that is used to bond the resin and filler particles together in a dental resin-based composite.

While in the composites used for fillings, it is the manufacturer who applies the silane to the material, in the case of resin-bonded ceramic restorations, the dental practitioner themselves will silanate the ceramic surface. Hence it is important to consider the method of application of a silane to the ceramic surface. Whereas, under ideal circumstances, a monolayer of the silane is all that is required to convert the ceramic surface from a Si–OH appearance to a methacrylate appearance, in reality, more than a monolayer is put down. In fact, what is formed is an *interphase*, consisting of a multiple layer of the silane containing many oligomers, which are not especially well bonded to the ceramic surface or to the resin (Figure 3.6.6); this can compromise the hydrolytic stability of the ceramic–resin bond. The

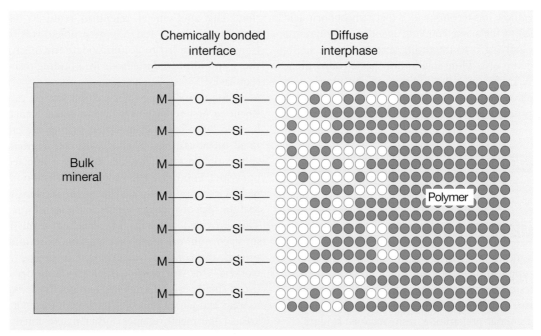

Figure 3.6.6 The interphase layer between the glass and the resin created by the application of a silane coupling agent. Adapted from Chiang C-H, Koenig JL (1982) Spectroscopic characterization of the matrix–silane coupling agent interface in fiber-reinforced composites. *J Polym Sci Polym Phys Ed* 20: 2135–2143.

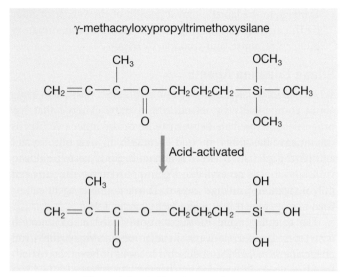

γ-methacryloxypropyltrimethoxysilane

Figure 3.6.7 Acid activation of a silane.

simple procedure of washing the surface of the ceramic after silane treatment, in order to remove the weakly bound oligomers, helps to reduce the problem. This produces a bond that is much more hydrolytically stable than if the silane were simply applied and left to dry.

Many of the resin cement kits are now provided with a silane coupling agent that can be applied directly to the clean fitting surfaces of veneers or inlays as they are received from the dental laboratory, or that can be used for the repair of fractured ceramic restorations.

Thorough cleaning of the ceramic surfaces with isopropyl alcohol, acetone, or phosphoric acid is needed after the veneer or inlay has been checked for satisfactory fit and prior to applying the silane. This is necessary in order to remove any surface contaminants such as grease or saliva that would interfere with the application of the silane coupling agent.

For some products, it is recommended that a phosphoric acid solution is added to the silane coupling agent to hydrolyze the silane prior to applying it to the fitting surface (Figure 3.6.7). Others are made up of a dilute solution of the activated silane in ethyl alcohol. In this case the addition of phosphoric acid solution is therefore not necessary because the silane is already hydrolyzed, although this will limit the shelf life of the silane coupling agent.

CLINICAL SIGNIFICANCE

The ability to bond resins to ceramics with hydrofluoric acid etching and silane coupling agents has transformed the use of ceramics in restorative dentistry.

RESIN-TO-METAL BONDING

The ability to bond resins to metals is of significant interest as there are many applications. These include:
- the use of resin instead of ceramics facings on metal substructures, especially for implant-retained prostheses
- bonding of minimal-preparation, resin-retained bridges
- resin bonding of conventional crowns and bridges where there is compromised retention

- intraoral repair of ceramic fractures on metal–ceramic restorations.

The first three of these require the adhesion of a resin to a well-defined alloy, whereas in the last case the alloy may not even be known. All represent a challenge and many new surface treatments and new resin adhesives have become available.

In order to improve the bond between the metal and the resin, a number of different approaches have been explored. Initially, these involved the use of macroscopic retentive features, but gradually, adhesive procedures involving micro-mechanical and/or chemical bonding were developed. The latter can be accomplished with a resin adhesive that has functional groups that can bond directly to the metal. Another approach is the use of adhesion promoters, such as silica coating, tin-plating, tribochemical coatings, and metal primers, which have been developed in order to improve the bond between the metal and the more conventional Bis-GMA- or UDMA-based resins. There is an added complication since the efficacy of many of these procedures depends on whether one is seeking to bond to a base metal alloy or a precious metal alloy.

Macro-Mechanical Bonding

From the 1940s, dental laboratories were using resin facings on cobalt–chrome partial dentures. At that time, the resin was polymethyl methacrylate, which was attached to the metal framework by mechanical retention. Problems arose because the resin would not adapt well to the metal due to the large polymerization shrinkage of the methyl methacrylate, resulting in the formation of microgaps, discoloration, loosening, and fracture. With the arrival of metal–ceramic restorations in the 1960s, many of these problems were overcome. It was not until the 1980s that there was a resurgence of interest in using resins as facings on metal substructures, which corresponded with the improved composite resins that had become available by then. At that time, bonding was still by mechanical retention. This mechanical retention required beads, wires, or loops in the metal design. One problem was that the bulkier framework needed to accommodate the macro-retentive features, and improved methods for bonding resin to metal were required.

In the dental clinic the situation was no different. In 1973 Rochette first reported the use of metal structures that were bonded by resins to acid-etched enamel. He used thin, perforated metal castings, bonded with cold-cure acrylic resins, to splint mobile lower incisors that were affected by advanced bone loss. Following the successful retention of these devices, he had occasion to extract one of the incisors, and it was then that the idea of adding a pontic to the splint was first conceived. This provided a means of replacing a missing tooth that involved minimal tooth preparation. As resin technology improved, the concept was explored in greater detail by other workers. One weakness of the Rochette bridge design was the use of small perforations for retention. These exposed the resin to wear and meant that the attachment was to a relatively small area of the metal retainer. Other macro-retentive features, as used on the metal frameworks produced in the dental laboratory, did not resolve the problem.

Micro-Mechanical Bonding

The problem of having to rely on macro-retentive features was overcome, to some degree, in the early 1980s, when a method of treating the Ni–Cr alloys was developed. With this method, the entire fitting surface of the retainer is rendered micro-mechanically retentive by either electrolytic or acid-gel etching. This technique is only applicable to Ni–Cr and Co–Cr alloys, which have a eutectic microstructure, as shown in Figure 3.6.8. The main alloy used for metal–ceramic restorations is Ni–Cr rather than Co–Cr alloy because of the greater difficulty of fusing ceramic to the latter. The etching process preferentially removes one of the phases, which results in a pitted and grooved surface appearance, as shown in Figure 3.6.9. This technique provides a highly retentive surface that adheres strongly to the composite resin cements due to the high degree of micro-mechanical interlocking introduced. It bonds the entire area of the retainer to the etched enamel and protects the underlying resin. Retainers can be made to a minimum thickness of 0.3 mm and can be waxed directly onto investment models, resulting in a good accuracy of fit. The bridges made using the electro-etching method were called *Maryland bridges*, as it was there that this technique was developed. However, with the advent of other methods of achieving a resin-to-metal bond, other terms such as resin-bonded bridges or minimal-preparation bridges are now commonly used.

Since electro-etching requires a high degree of skill and specialist equipment, the gel-etching process has become the more popular of the two. The gel is a high-concentration solution of hydrofluoric acid, which, as noted above, is highly toxic and needs to be handled with great care.

The main advantages of these resin-bonded bridges are:

- The minimal enamel preparation does not require local anesthetic.
- The procedure leaves the teeth largely intact, such that traditional treatment options can still be used in the future.
- Possible irritation of the pulp is prevented, as usually there is no exposure of dentine.

Disadvantages include:

- There is a high debonding rate for the retainers.
- There are color changes in anterior abutment teeth due to the shine-through of the metal retainer.
- The process is only applicable to Ni–Cr alloys.

The aesthetic problem can be overcome, to some degree, by using opaque composite resin cements for cementation. The high rate of debonding is more difficult to resolve and may require careful reconsideration of design of the retainers and the properties of the resins available.

Since the prosthesis relies on the presence of enamel for its attachment, sufficient enamel is required onto which to bond the retainers. Short crowns, extensive restorations, congenital defects, and tooth surface loss would prevent the use of these resin-retained castings. Also, for unsightly abutment teeth, conventional bridges would be a better proposition.

The composite resin cements are essentially very similar to composite restorative materials, consisting of a Bis-GMA or UDMA resin and glass filler. Where these resins differ from the restorative composites is that they are invariably two-paste chemical or dual-cure systems, since the access to light is restricted by the metal retainers. The filler particle size is less than 20 μm and the filler loading tends to be slightly lower in order to ensure a low film thickness. An optical opacifier, such as titanium oxide, may be added to prevent the shine-through of the metal.

One of the drawbacks with this restorative technique is that there is a reluctance on the part of some clinicians to use Ni–Cr alloys, as nickel is a known allergen. Some of the alloys also contain beryllium (Be), which is highly toxic in its free state. Be is usually present in order to improve the castability of the Ni–Cr alloy and to provide a superior eutectic microstructure for effective etching. However, beryllium may be released during the grinding and polishing of the castings, and therefore dental technicians are probably more at risk than either the dentist or the patient. Hence the preference of dental laboratories is for Be-free alloys, which, unfortunately, do not etch very well.

Another constraint of this approach is that it is not possible to etch precious metal alloys since they have a relatively homogeneous microstructure. Hence it is not possible to use the etching technique for resin bonding with precious metal alloys. In

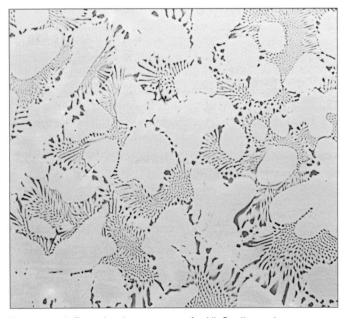

Figure 3.6.8 Eutectic microstructure of a Ni–Cr alloy as it appears under the scanning electron microscope using back-scattered imaging.

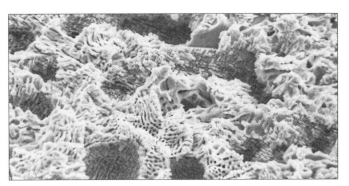

Figure 3.6.9 Scanning electron micrograph showing the surface of a Ni–Cr alloy after etching with a gel etchant

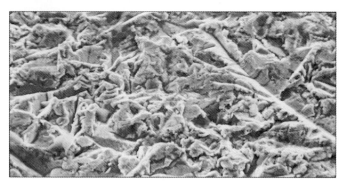

Figure 3.6.10 Scanning electron micrograph showing the surface of a Ni–Cr alloy after grit-blasting with alumina.

order to circumvent the wishes of dental laboratories that do not want to use Be-containing Ni–Cr alloys and want to avoid the etching process, some other means of bonding to the alloy had to be found. The difficulty here is that Bis-GMA- and UDMA-type resins do not adhere well to untreated metal surfaces, relying primarily on micro-mechanical and physical adhesion. The latter tends to be readily overcome by hydrolytic attack, as water is absorbed at the interface and displaces the resin. Grit-blasting of base metal alloys with 50 μm alumina grit produces some surface roughening for micro-mechanical adhesion, as shown in Figure 3.6.10. However, the surface does not have the re-entrant features associated with the etched surface and has therefore proved to be inadequate. Hence the Bis-GMA- or UDMA-based composite resin cements cannot be used directly on grit-blasted Ni–Cr alloy surfaces, as the bond to a grit-blasted metal surface is not sufficiently strong for these resin cements. In these situations the chemically adhesive resin cements are the material of choice.

Since these resins can provide a durable bond to the grit-blasted metal surface of a Ni–Cr alloy, there is no need for etching and thus no need for special laboratory equipment or the use of dangerous chemical reagents. With the advent of these resins, it is now possible to form a strong chemically adhesive bond between a grit-blasted base metal alloy and acid-etched enamel. However, while these chemically adhesive resin cements are excellent for bonding to base metal alloys, they have a relatively low affinity for precious metal alloys, such as gold and palladium alloys, due to the lack of a surface oxide coating.

Chemical Modification of the Alloy Surface

The poor quality of bonding between the precious metals and the chemically adhesive resins is a consequence of the low chemical reactivity of the surface of precious metals alloys as compared with that of base metal alloys. This problem may be overcome by surface modification of the precious metal so as to make it more amenable to forming a bond with a resin cement. Three popular options are available, namely:

- apply a coating to the surface that will create a micro-mechanical bond, for example, tin plating
- change the surface chemistry by silica coating or tribochemical coating
- apply specially formulated metal primers.

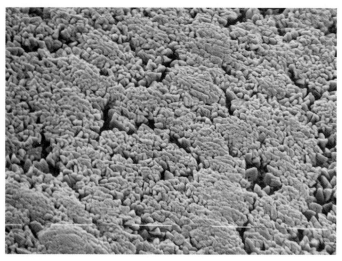

Figure 3.6.11 Scanning electron micrograph showing the surface appearance of a precious metal after tin-plating.

Tin Plating

Tin plating is based on an invention that offers a means of resin bonding to noble and precious metal alloys at the chair side. The procedure deposits a layer of tin on the alloy surface, which can be seen by the appearance of a gray discoloration. The surface layer produced is irregular in form and provides micro-mechanical retention for the resin while also being chemically attracted to the tin oxide on the alloy surface (Figure 3.6.11). This chair-side system is indicated primarily for the intraoral repair of fractured metal–ceramic restorations, where metal is exposed and is to be repaired in situ with a composite resin.

Although laboratory data suggest that there is an improvement in the bond strength of resin to a tin-plated precious metal alloy, some results suggest that the improvement is only marginal and better methods of bonding to precious metal alloys are required. Additionally, it has been suggested that the application of an excessively thick tin-plating layer can result in a low bond strength due to the oxide coating being too thick. Thus the application of the tin coating is critical and open to error. In addition, there may be clinical situations, such as in the case of intraoral repairs, when the alloy is unknown. If the exposed metal is a Ni–Cr alloy, then tin plating provides no benefit and may even be detrimental to obtaining a strong resin bond.

Silica Coating

The use of silane coupling agents to enhance the adhesion of dental ceramics to tooth structure via resin composite is well established (see above). The possibility of silanating cast metal is limited due to the lack of appropriate binding sites on the alloy surface. In contrast, these are found in abundance on a silica-based ceramic surface, such as silanols, that is, Si–OH. It is now possible to produce a silica coating on metal surfaces, making them amenable to silane coupling and successful resin bonding. Two techniques are available, one involving a special coating and heat treatment technique of the alloy, and the other involving a tribochemical approach. The coating method requires the metal surface to be passed through a propane–air

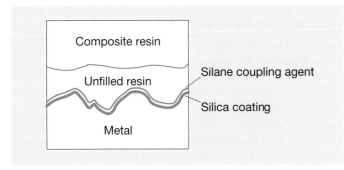

Figure 3.6.12 Metal surface with silica coating.

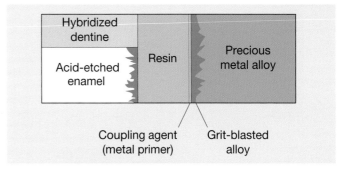

Figure 3.6.14 Schematic of metal-to-resin bond.

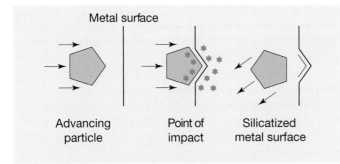

Figure 3.6.13. Tribochemical coating of metal surface.

flame, in which tetramethoxysilane is decomposed. As a result, an intermediary layer of SiO_x is formed – providing Si–OH groups for silane bonding (Figure 3.6.12). A silane coupling agent is then applied to this silicoated surface, which is then able to bond with the resin. There was a widely adopted commercial product providing this functionality, but it would appear to have been discontinued.

Tribochemical coating. In this technique the alloy surface is grit-blasted at high pressure with a special powder that contains fine alumina and colloidal silica particles. The objective is to form a thin layer of silica (SiO_x–C) that contains sufficient free hydroxyl (–OH) groups to allow coupling to resin via a silane (Figure 3.6.13). This technique is known as tribochemical silica coating, as it has been shown that high-energy colloidal silica particles impacting the alloy surface cause physical fusion of a silica layer to the metal, which is said to be stable. This pretreated surface is then silane-treated and is ready for resin bonding.

A chair-side coating system using this approach has been promoted for the *in situ* repair of fractured metal–ceramic units with exposed metal surfaces requiring improved adhesion to resin composite. In addition, the system is also claimed to be effective as a surface treatment for the repair of fractured resin composite restorations.

One drawback with these techniques is the need to purchase laboratory or chair-side equipment. In addition, the high number of steps involved potentially increases the likelihood of errors.

Metal Primers

What many dental clinicians want is a simple adhesive liquid that they can apply directly to the metal surface, requiring nothing more special than a brush (Figure 3.6.14). The use of simple chemical pretreatment techniques of the alloy surface is therefore a well-researched area. In particular, the use of coupling agents based on bifunctional monomers has attracted interest because they have been shown to be effective yet simple alternatives to most of the surface modification techniques already described. They are usually supplied as single-liquid primers composed of a polymerizable monomer in a suitable solvent. (The products are invariably called primers despite them being, in fact, coupling agents.) The monomer has a bifunctional structure, with one end carrying a methacryl or similar functional group for resin bonding, and the other end carrying mercapto or thiol (–SH) groups for bonding to the precious metal alloy. When the metal primer is applied to a grit-blasted alloy surface, it is capable of enhanced adhesion to resin composite cement because of the ability of sulfur to react with precious metal alloys. Hence the presence of the mercapto groups allows chemical adhesion to precious metal alloy surfaces. A number of commercial products, based on these bifunctional primers, are now available and include the products shown in Table 3.6.2.

The chemical structure of the primers is shown in Figure 3.6.15, from which it can be seen that these metal primers are, in fact, coupling agents. The VBATDT-containing primer works well with 4-META-based resin cements but does not work so well with the more conventional methacrylate resins, which is possibly associated with the fact that the VBATDT interferes with the polymerization reaction of the methacrylate resins. The combination of MEPS with 4-META-based resins is also deemed unacceptable. Thus there are still issues of resin-primer compatibility that need to be addressed.

TABLE 3.6.2 Examples of Metal Primers

Product Name	Primer	Manufacturer
V-Primer	VBATDT in 95% acetone	Sun Medical Co, Kyoto, Japan
Alloy Primer	VBADT/MDP	Kuraray Co, Osaka, Japan
Metal Primer II	MEPS in MMA	GC Corp, Tokyo, Japan
Metaltite	Thiouracil in 96% ethanol	Tokuyama Inc, San Mateo, USA

MDP, Methacryloxyethyl-phenyl phosphate; MEPS, methacryloyloxyalkyl thiophosphate derivatives; MMA, methylmethacrylate; VBATDT, 6-(4-vinylbenzyl-*n*-propyl)amino-1,3,5-triazide-2,4-dithiol.

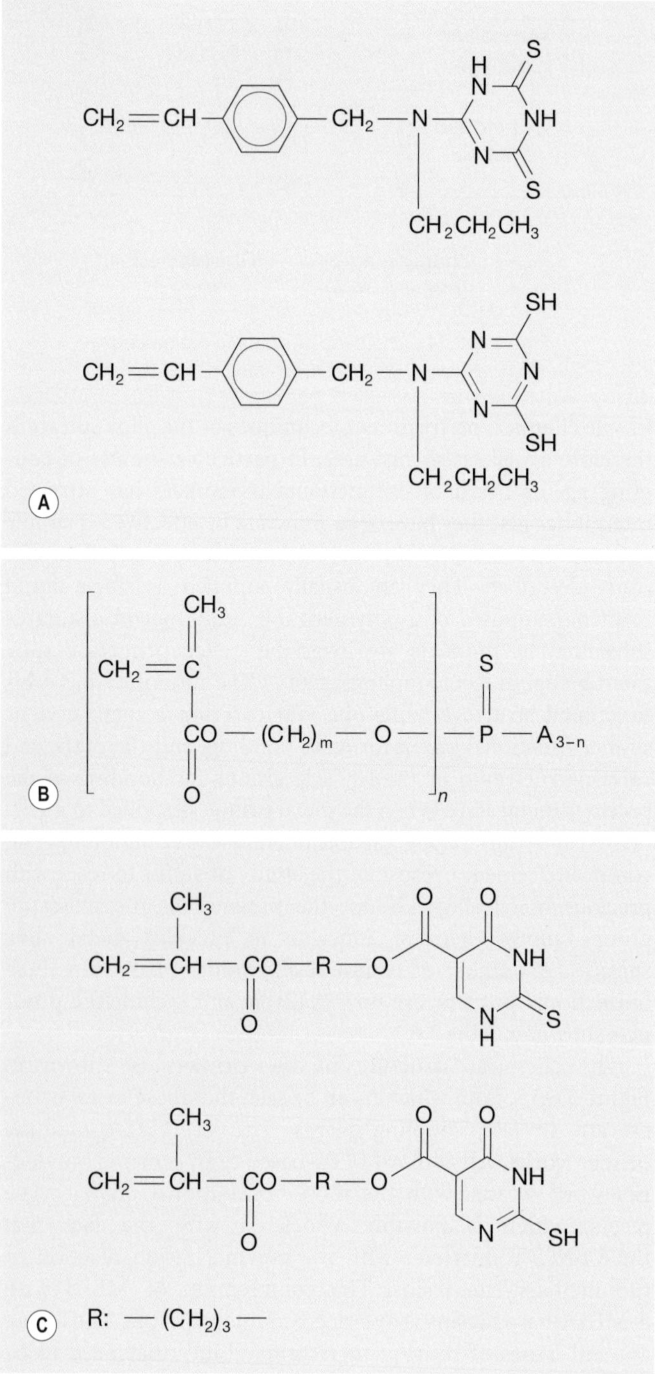

and endodontic posts. While one might imagine that resin-to-resin bonding should be free of problems, this is not the case. In particular, with composite inlays, there have been problems with debonding between the resin cement and the composite inlay.

When increments of freshly placed composite resin restorative material are being built up, the bonding of one increment to the next is helped by the fact that, after light-curing, there is still a very thin resinous surface layer of some 10–50 μm thick that has not set due to oxygen inhibition of the cure. When one deals with prefabricated resin components such as inlay and posts, this uncured surface layer does not exist. Hence, the resin cement has to bond directly to fully cured resins. This situation is similar to that encountered when considering the option of replacing the lost segment of a fractured composite restoration with new composite resin. It would seem that resins do not have any particular advantage when bonding to other resins, except that close adaptation can readily be achieved.

Various approaches to improve the resin-to-resin bond have been proposed, including grit-blasting with alumina or grinding the surface with a coarse instrument to increase the surface roughness and thus create a micro-mechanical bond. Although this helps, neither approach is particularly effective, as the retentive features created by grit blasting are not ideal, not unlike the situation encountered when bonding resins to grit-blasted metal surfaces. In the case of glass-particulate-filled composites it may be possible to remove the glass particles near the surface by hydrofluoric acid etching and to introduce more retentive features on the micron scale. However, the experience with repairs of glass-particulate-filled composites is that the best quality of bond that can be achieved is only 50–75% of the cohesive strength of the composite resins.

Chemical bonding via a silane coupling agent has also been suggested on the basis that, for glass-particulate-filled composites, there will be a large amount of exposed glass at the surface after grit-blasting or grinding, which has not been silanated. However, the problem with this is that the silane will also coat the resin part of the surface and may well impair the resin-to-resin bond while improving the resin-to-ceramic bond. Another suggestion is to use the tribochemical technique described earlier, which would embed a layer of silica into the resin surface, and then use the silane coupling agent to bond to the resin cement.

Figure 3.6.15 Chemical structure of three metal primers used in commercial products. (a) VBADT, 6-(4-vinylbenzyl-*n*-propyl)amino-1,3,5-triazide-2,4,dithiol; (b) MEPS, methacryloyloxyalkyl thiophosphate derivative; (c) Metaltite primer based on a thiouracil derivative.

CLINICAL SIGNIFICANCE

The problem of bonding resins to resins has not yet been resolved satisfactorily and thus will continue to be an area of research interest.

CLINICAL SIGNIFICANCE

Resin-to-metal bonding will continue to be an area of development and the bond is likely to continue to improve, bringing with it better clinical performance.

RESIN-TO-RESIN BONDING

There are a growing number of prefabricated resin prostheses, such as composite inlays and fiber-reinforced crowns, bridges,

FURTHER READING

Hill, E.E., Lott, J., 2011. A clinically focused discussion of luting materials. Australian Dental Journal 56 (Suppl. 1), 67–76.

Kiatsirirote, K., Northeast, S.E., van Noort, R., 1999. Bonding procedures for intraoral repair of exposed metal with resin composite. Journal of Adhesive Dentistry 1, 315.

Lad, P.P., Kamath, M., Tarale, K., Kusugal, P.B., 2014. Practical clinical considerations of luting cements: a review. Journal of International Oral Health 6 (1), 116–120.

Manso, A.P., Carvalho, R.M., 2017. Dental cements for luting and bonding restorations: self-adhesive resin cements. Dental Clinics of North America 61 (4), 821–834.

Pameijer, C.H., 2012. A review of luting agents. International Journal of Dentistry 2012, 752861.

Sindel, J., Frankenberger, R., Kramer, N., Petschelt, A., 1999. Crack formation of all-ceramic crowns dependent on different core build-up and luting materials. Journal of Dentistry 27, 175.

Teixeira, E.C., Bayne, S.C., Thompson, J.Y., 2005. Shear bond strength of self-etching bonding systems in combination with various composites used for repairing aged composites. Journal of Adhesive Dentistry 7, 159.

Yoshida, K., Kamada, K., Taira, Y., 2001. Effect of three adhesive primers on the bond strengths of four light-activated opaque resins to noble alloy. Journal of Oral Rehabilitation 28, 168.

Stainless Steel and Other Alloys

INTRODUCTION

Most of us are familiar with stainless steel as a widely used quality product for both domestic and industrial applications. However, it is also extensively used in medical and dental applications, including for the production of dental instruments such as scalpel blades and forceps, orthodontic wires, denture bases and partial denture clasps, endodontic posts, and as stainless steel crowns for the treatment of severely decayed deciduous molars. The material has generally been heavily worked to give it the desired shape and is therefore defined as a *wrought alloy*.

A wrought alloy distinguishes itself from the many casting alloys used for the construction of crowns and bridges in that it is *a cast alloy that has been formed by mechanical processing such as rolling, extrusion, or drawing to give it a new desired shape.* When this is done at a low temperature, the mechanical processing is known as *cold working*, by which the metal is simultaneously shaped and strengthened (Figure 3.7.1). The strengthening is due to the changes in grain size and shape during working, which confer a greater resistance to further shaping – that is, it becomes stronger. If the process is carried out at high temperatures, this is called *hot working* and generally involves shaping without strengthening because the metal continually recrystallizes and the grains adjust their shape, and the amount of deformation that can be performed is virtually limitless.

Many alloys besides stainless steel are available in wrought form, such as gold alloys for posts and denture clasps, Ni–Ti alloys for orthodontic wires and endodontic files, and Co–Cr–Ni alloys for denture clasps and orthodontic wires. However, stainless steel will be considered in detail in this chapter with brief consideration of nickel-titanium owing to its increasing importance in dentistry.

Steels are available in a wide variety of compositions, with each having very specific properties that are carefully tailored to suit their particular application. One feature of steels that makes them such popular materials is the enormous range of mechanical properties that can be obtained with only small changes in composition. A comparison of steel to other products is shown in Table 3.7.1. The steel wires show a wide range of strengths that the other materials cannot match.

Before the introduction of stainless steels to dentistry in the early 1930s, the only metal that was felt to have good enough corrosion resistance to allow it to be used in the mouth was gold. Stainless steel possesses a high tensile strength and is used to form springs in removable orthodontic appliances. It is also used in fixed appliances for the construction of bands, brackets,

and archwires. In fact, virtually all the components for fixed appliances used in orthodontics can be constructed out of stainless steel.

Orthodontic wire is made from what is known as austenitic stainless steel. This is a form of steel that can be readily shaped into a wire by rolling and subsequent extrusion through dies. This elongates the grains into long fibrous structures that run in the direction of the wire. More specifically, the material used for orthodontic wires is known as a *stabilized austenitic stainless steel*. The best way of describing this material is to take the raw material, iron, and develop it, step by step, into the final product. Along the way, the different types of steel will be explored and their particular applications considered.

IRON

Iron is an allotropic material, that is, it undergoes two solid-state phase changes with temperature. At room temperature, pure iron has a body-centered cubic (BCC) structure, known as the α-phase. This structure is stable up to a temperature of 912°C, where it transforms into a face-centered cubic (FCC) structure, the γ-phase.

At 1390°C, the FCC iron reverts back to BCC and retains this structure until it melts at 1538°C. These changes are accompanied by changes in the volume of the iron (Figure 3.7.2).

STEEL

Steel is an alloy of iron and carbon, in which the carbon content must not exceed 2%. Iron with a carbon content greater than 2% is classified as a *cast iron* and will not be considered here.

Carbon Steels

Carbon steel is an alloy of only iron and carbon. In its BCC form, when small amounts of carbon are dissolved in the iron, the material is known as α-iron or *ferrite*.

The solubility of the carbon in this BCC structure is very low compared with that in the FCC structure, being a maximum of 0.02 wt % at 723°C and only 0.005 wt % at room temperature. This is despite the greater unoccupied volume in BCC (packing factor 68%) compared to FCC (74%).

The FCC form of the material has a considerably higher solubility of carbon, of up to 2.11%. The reason for this is that the largest interstitial holes in BCC iron (diameter 0.072 nm) are smaller than those in FCC iron (diameter 0.104 nm). This FCC form of the steel is known as *austenite*.

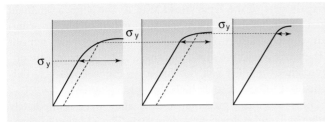

Figure 3.7.1 The effect of cold working on the mechanical properties of a metal. Note the reduction in ductility (↔) as the yield stress (σ_y) is increased.

TABLE 3.7.1 A comparison of Fracture or Yield Strengths of Steels With Other Materials	
Material	**Fracture or Yield Strength (MPa)**
Steel wire	300–2800
Bulk steel	300–800
Iron	150–200
Brass	200–400
Aluminum alloys	200–600
Copper alloys	300–600
Titanium alloys	600–1100
Glass	50–150
Carbon fiber	2200–2800

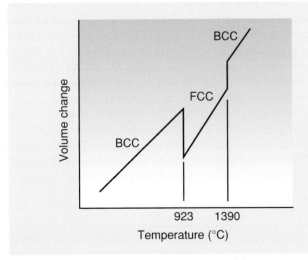

Figure 3.7.2 The volume change of pure iron with temperature. BCC, Body-centered cubic; FCC, face-centered cubic

Both of these forms of steel are relatively soft and ductile; in particular, the austenite is readily shaped at elevated temperatures by hot forging and rolling operations.

When the limit of solubility for the carbon is exceeded for either of these forms of steel, the excess carbon precipitates out as Fe_3C, which is a hard and brittle phase, given the name *cementite*. The various phases in the iron–cementite system are presented in the partial equilibrium phase diagram in Figure 3.7.3.

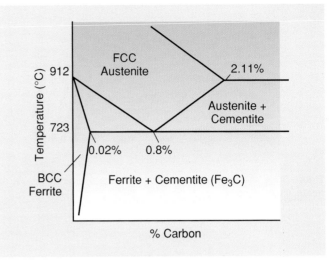

Figure 3.7.3 The Fe–Fe$_3$C system.

Hyper- and Hypo-Eutectoid Steels

At a carbon concentration of 0.8%, the alloy shows a transformation at 723°C from the single-phase austenite to a two-phase structure consisting of ferrite and cementite:

$$\gamma \rightarrow \alpha + Fe_3C$$

austenite → ferrite + cementite

This solid transformation is defined as a *eutectoid*, as distinct from a *eutectic*, which is a transformation of a single liquid phase directly into two solid phases (see Chapter 1.4).

Steels with a carbon content of exactly the eutectoid composition are called *eutectoid steels*. Those with a carbon content of greater than 0.8% are *hyper-eutectoid steels* and are used in the manufacture of burs and cutting instruments, while those with a carbon content of less than 0.8% are *hypo-eutectoid steels* and are used in the manufacture of dental instruments such as forceps.

The eutectoid transformation is very important in the production of steels because a number of interesting things can happen when a carbon steel is cooled from its austenitic high-temperature condition to room temperature.

Slow cooling. On slow cooling, the changes in structure for a 0.8% carbon steel are as predicted from the equilibrium phase diagram. The austenite is converted into a mixture of ferrite and cementite, which is described as *pearlite* (Figure 3.7.4). However, cooling is not usually carried out slowly but involves rapid cooling by immersing the object in cold water in a process that is known as *quenching*.

Rapid cooling. When austenite is quenched in water, the ferrite and cementite cannot form because there is not enough time for diffusion and rearrangement of the atoms. Instead, a very rapid transformation occurs to a body-centered tetragonal structure, which is rather like a distorted BCC. This form of steel is described as *martensite* and is extremely hard and brittle. (In fact, it is far too hard and brittle for any practical purposes.) Nevertheless, this transformation can be put to good use because, by reheating to a temperature in the range of 200–450°C and then cooling rapidly, it is possible to transform the martensite into *pearlite* (ferrite + cementite). The degree

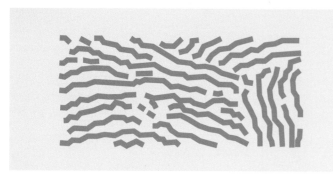

Figure 3.7.4 The structure of pearlite, which is a laminar mixture of ferrite and cementite.

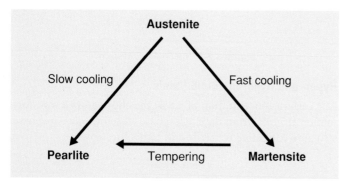

Figure 3.7.5 Heat treatment known as tempering of martensitic steels to control the mechanical properties.

of conversion can be carefully controlled by the temperature and duration of the heat treatment, a process known as *tempering* (Figure 3.7.5).

For cutting instruments, a hyper-eutectoid steel (carbon content > 0.8%) is generally used because it combines the hard martensite with a large presence of the hard cementite, such that a cutting edge can be produced which does not blunt readily. For instruments such as forceps, the brittle nature of hyper-eutectoid steel would be unacceptable and a lower carbon content is present, as in the hypo-eutectoid steels (carbon content < 0.8%). This allows the formation predominantly of the more ductile ferrite, while the hardness is controlled by the presence of martensite and much lower amounts of cementite.

> **CLINICAL SIGNIFICANCE**
>
> Excessive heating up of cutting instruments will result in a loss of hardness due to changes in the microstructure.

STAINLESS STEEL

Although many other elements can be added to the basic carbon steels to improve the properties (e.g. molybdenum, silicon, cobalt, manganese), the two of greatest importance for dentistry are chromium and nickel for the production of stainless steel.

Stainless steel is an alloy of iron that is resistant to corrosion. This was discovered accidentally in the United Kingdom during the early part of the First World War. At the time, a Sheffield metallurgist named Brearley was working on steels for armament construction. A rejected billet of a steel alloy was left out in the work's yard for some months, and he subsequently observed that the billet had not rusted in the wet weather. This turned out to be due to its high chromium content.

The possibilities presented by the alloy were immediately recognized, and it was patented in 1917. The addition of chromium to the carbon steel improves the corrosion resistance of the metal by forming a protective surface coating of chromium oxide. For this to be fully effective, the chromium content of the alloy has to exceed 11%.

> **CLINICAL SIGNIFICANCE**
>
> The chromium content of a steel must exceed 11% for it to be designated as a *stainless steel*.

Austenitic Stainless Steel

The addition of 8% nickel prevents the transformation of austenite to martensite on cooling, such that the austenite becomes stable at room temperature when cooled rapidly. Slow cooling would again allow the formation of ferrite and cementite, but, since this is a diffusion-controlled process, the rapid cooling by quenching prevents these phases from forming.

There are essentially three forms of stainless steel used for dental applications (Table 3.7.2).

The ferritic steels are used mainly for the production of tools, whereas austenitic stainless steels have a very wide application and are used in orthodontic wires, autoclaves, tabletops, and cabinets. The martensitic steels are primarily used for cutting instruments.

The attraction of austenitic stainless steel is that it is highly malleable and so can be readily shaped for a wide variety of purposes. The alloy cannot be heat-treated to change the properties in the way that martensitic and ferritic steels can, but it can be cold-worked to improve the yield stress (although this will be at the expense of the ductility). Nevertheless, it is this ability of austenitic stainless steel to be made with a wide variety of mechanical properties while maintaining its corrosion resistance in the mouth that has made it such an attractive material for orthodontic applications.

> **CLINICAL SIGNIFICANCE**
>
> For intraoral applications, we are concerned almost exclusively with the austenitic variety of steel, and the alloy most used is 18/8 stainless steel, which is composed of 18% chromium, 8% nickel, and 0.2% carbon.

TABLE 3.7.2 Three Forms of Stainless Steel that are Used in Dental Applications

	Cr (%)	Ni (%)	C (%)
Ferritic	11.5–27	0	0.2 (max.)
Austenitic	16–22	7–22	0.25
Martensitic	11.5–17	0–2.5	0.15–0.25

Stabilized Austenitic Stainless Steel

Although it is common practice for most wrought alloys to be given a stress-relief anneal, this is not possible with the austenitic stainless steels due to microstructural changes that occur at the annealing temperature.

Formation of Chromium Carbides

At temperatures in excess of 500°C, chromium and carbon react to form chromium carbides, which precipitate at the grain boundaries, causing brittle behavior. Also, the corrosion resistance is decreased due to the depletion of the central regions of the crystals of chromium, which has migrated to the boundaries to form the carbides (Figure 3.7.6).

This process is known as *weld decay,* since it was first noticed as a problem when welding sheets of steel. The problem can be overcome by adding titanium to the alloy, which has the effect that the carbon preferentially reacts with the dispersed titanium such that the chromium remains where it is at its most effective. This produces what is known as *stabilized austenitic stainless steel.*

Transformation to Ferrite and Cementite

The austenite is formed by rapid cooling from elevated temperatures so as to prevent the formation of cementite and ferrite. Raising the temperature allows diffusion of the atoms, such that these other phases *can* form.

This formation of other phases is an irreversible process unless the material temperature is raised above the eutectoid and then quenched to room temperature to reform austenitic steel.

However, the annealing process allows recrystallization and the formation of the chromium carbides, which impairs the corrosion resistance.

Recrystallization

If the temperature is raised above the eutectoid temperature, recrystallization of the metal takes place, and the long, fibrous grains that are produced by rolling and drawing during fabrication of the wire become transformed into large, equiaxed grains.

If this happens, the material will have softened and the springy properties of the wire will have been lost and cannot be restored. The rate at which this occurs is controlled by time and temperature.

Properties

Austenitic stainless steels are favored for orthodontic applications because of their excellent corrosion resistance in the biological environment, the wide range of mechanical properties available, and the ease with which they can be joined by soldering or electrical resistance welding.

Mechanical properties

Depending on the degree of cold working carried out by the manufacturer in forming the orthodontic wire, a range of mechanical properties are produced (see Table 3.7.3). It is important to select the appropriate type for the application in mind.

If little shaping, that is, cold working by bending, is needed, a hard or extra-hard stainless steel wire can be selected. If, on the other hand, a lot of shaping is required, then one needs to start with a soft alloy, as it will work-harden on bending.

Soldering and welding

Since the fabrication of appliances often requires the joining of separate components by soldering or welding, the heat produced can have an extremely detrimental effect on the properties of stainless steel. Therefore techniques must be designed to avoid prolonged exposure of the components to high temperatures.

Hard soldering. Stainless steel components are generally joined by 'hard soldering' as distinct from 'soft soldering', the latter involving the use of low melting point alloys such as Sn–Pb alloys. Hard soldering may be carried out with gold or silver alloys, which are sufficiently corrosion resistant. Since gold-alloy solders must contain at least 45% gold to ensure a low enough melting temperature, silver solders are preferred on cost grounds. The composition of silver solders used in orthodontics is approximately 50% silver; 16% each of copper, cadmium, and zinc; and 3% nickel.

There are two basic methods of producing the heat that is necessary to melt the solder: the gas blow torch and electrical

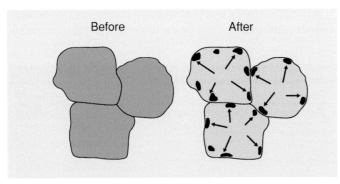

Figure 3.7.6 Weld decay due to overheating of the alloy.

TABLE 3.7.3 **Mechanical properties of a Range of Stainless Steels Used for Orthodontic Appliances**			
	0.2% Proof Stress (MPa)	Young's Modulus (GPa)	Elongation (%)	Hardness (BHN)
Soft	280	200	50	170
Hard	1050	200	6	250
Extra-hard	1450	230	1	350

BHN, Brinell hardness number.

resistance welding. Gas soldering has the advantage of requiring only low-cost equipment. The apparatus for electrical resistance soldering is considerably more expensive and requires greater skill in its use but has the advantage that the heat is much more localized.

It is important to realize that the interface between a silver solder and stainless steel is more mechanical than alloying. An adequate amount of solder must therefore be used, and excessive finishing and polishing should be avoided, as this will weaken the joint.

Spot welding. When an electrical current is passed through a metal, it causes the metal to heat up. Spot welding involves the localized application of heat to the component to be joined by the use of a high current at low voltage. If, at the same time, pressure is applied at the point where the two parts are to be joined, recrystallization occurs across the joint and the two parts are fused together.

Note that the metal does not melt. In fact, if the metal is excessively heated and melting does occur, the joint is considerably weakened. In order to avoid this problem, as well as that of weld decay, welding time is kept to 1/50 of a second.

Basically, a welder is a set of electrodes that are brought together under pressure, and that are directly connected to the secondary winding of a pulse transformer. A timer is used to limit the duration of the welding cycle.

Most of the separate components of fixed appliances are joined by spot welding, although the need for this has reduced in recent years with the introduction of complex prefabricated components. However, both spot welding and soldering are still extensively used for the repair and construction of appliances.

Coating of Archwires

Many archwire suppliers now offer coated versions of both the stainless steel wires discussed above and the nickel titanium ones discussed in the following section. While there are various reasons why one might coat a wire, two dominate: the ability to create a smooth, low-friction surface that aids the clinician's job and may make this more comfortable for the patient; and the ability to obscure the silvery metallic surface of the wire with something closer to the appearance of the teeth. Most commonly, the coating is made from polytetrafluoroethylene PTFE, which fulfills both purposes, being off-white in color and having very low friction.

OTHER ALLOYS

Other alloys that may be used for orthodontic appliances include Ni–Ti alloys, gold alloys, Co–Cr alloys, and β–Ti alloys.

The relative merits of these varieties of wrought alloy wire used in orthodontics are presented in Table 3.7.4.

The stiffness is a function of both the wire diameter and the elastic modulus of the material and determines the amount of force applied to a tooth. For materials with a high elastic modulus, thinner wires can be used than for materials with a low elastic modulus. However, the thinner the wire, the more likely it is to suffer from permanent deformation and loss of applied force to the tooth. A high stiffness is desirable when rapid large forces need to be applied to cause a tooth to move, whereas flexible wires applying a low force need to be used when slow movement of a tooth is desired.

The resilience of the wire is a measure of its ability to undergo large deflections without causing permanent deformation. It is given by the ratio of yield stress and modulus of elasticity such that a combination of low modulus and high yield strength would be ideal.

Since nickel–titanium is by far the most commonly used of these alloys, we will consider it in a little more detail.

Nickel–Titanium

What we now call Ni–Ti (out loud, this is sometimes expressed as nickel–titanium but also quite commonly 'Ni–Ti' where Ni and Ti rhyme with eye!) was originally referred to as Nitinol, short for NIckel-TItanium-Naval-Ordnance-Laboratory, reflecting the fact that it was first developed and characterized by William J Buehler and Frederick E Wang of that US military organization.

Ni–Ti is, as its name suggests, a binary alloy composed of nickel and titanium, at an atomic ratio of around 1:1; since nickel has a higher atomic mass than titanium, this results in a mass ratio of around 55% nickel and 45% titanium by weight. Ni–Ti supplemented with copper is also available for orthodontic wires, although some in vitro studies of Cu–Ni–Ti wires have suggested poorer mechanical properties and a greater propensity for corrosion than the copper-free versions.

Just as the chromium content of stainless steel is sufficient to confer passivating properties on the alloy and render the material corrosion resistant, the titanium in Ni–Ti fulfills the same purpose, and Ni–Ti has good corrosion resistance in the oral environment.

In addition to the excellent corrosion resistance, Ni–Ti orthodontic wires present two particularly interesting, and useful,

TABLE 3.7.4	**Relative Merits of Alloys for Orthodontic Applications**			
Material	**Stiffness**	**Resilience**	**Ductility**	**Ease of Soldering or Welding**
Stainless steel	High	Good	Adequate	Reasonable
Gold alloy	Medium	Adequate	Adequate	Easy
Co–Cr alloy	High	Good	Low	Difficult
Ni–Ti alloy	Low	Very high	Poor	Difficult
β–Ti alloy	Medium	High	Adequate	Difficult

properties. Ni–Ti exhibits a property known as *shape memory.* The simplest definition of shape memory is that an object made of a material exhibiting this property can be deformed at a low temperature and adopt a new shape, and when it is then *heated* to or above its *transformation* or *transition temperature,* it will return to its original shape. The transition temperatures in the case of these orthodontic wires are convenient: when the wire is at room temperature, or in some cases refrigerator temperature, it is flexible and easy to work with, but when the temperature rises to mouth temperature, it regains its engineered shape, allowing it to place the required forces on the teeth to cause the gradual realignment that is the purpose of orthodontic appliances. Furthermore, if the patient finds their appliance uncomfortable and wants a break, they can rinse with cool water to relieve the forces to an extent. In dental terminology they are often referred to as *heat activated.* This property makes them a popular, if more expensive, option for orthodontics.

The other interesting property exhibited by Ni–Ti is that of *superelasticity.* If you revisit Chapter 1.6 you will remember that a material that is said to be *elastic* is one that can be deformed and will recover – the more elastic a material, the more deformation it can handle and still return to its original shape and size (think about an elastic band that can be stretched to several times its normal size but still looks the same once you release it). A *superelastic* material, then, is one that exhibits exceptional elastic properties – one for which the degree of deformation the material can show and still return to its original shape is very large indeed. This, coupled with the temperature-dependent shape memory, makes Ni–Ti again a very convenient material for orthodontics and also makes it popular for endodontic instruments as Ni–Ti instruments can conform to any number of different root canal shapes and still straighten out again when removed.

For all their interesting properties, as is so often for dental materials, clinical data to inform a hard-and-fast choice is lacking, and the most recent Cochrane systematic review of different materials for orthodontic wires concluded that there was insufficient evidence to choose between different presentations of Ni–Ti (single-stranded, multi-stranded, coaxial, superelastic or not) and stainless steel in terms of the speed or comfort of the orthodontic process.

SUMMARY

Stainless steel and, to a lesser extent, nickel–titanium, are widely used for intraoral appliances, particularly in orthodontics. The advantages with stainless steels are high tensile strength and good corrosion resistance, along with the ability to be readily formed into complex shapes. The material has some limitations in that it is rapidly work-hardened and detrimental changes in properties can occur if excessively high temperatures are applied. The advantages of Ni–Ti include the properties of superelasticity and shape memory.

FURTHER READING

Brantley, W.A., 2020. Evolution, clinical applications, and prospects of nickel-titanium alloys for orthodontic purposes. Journal of the World Federation of Orthodontists 9, S19.

Burstone, C.J., Goldberg, J., 1983. Maximum forces and deflections from orthodontic appliances. American Journal of Orthodontics 84, 95–103.

Cohen, B.I., Penugonda, B., Pagnillo, M.K., 2000. Torsional resistance of crowns cemented to composite cores involving three stainless steel endodontic post designs. Journal of Prosthetic Dentistry 84, 38.

Fayle, S.A., 1999. UK National Clinical Guidelines in Paediatric Dentistry. Stainless steel preformed crowns for primary molars. Faculty of Dental Surgery, Royal College of Surgeons. International Journal of Paediatric Dentistry 9, 311.

Kapila, S., Sachdeva, R., 1989. Mechanical properties and clinical applications of orthodontic wires. American Journal of Orthodontics and Dentofacial Orthopedics 96, 100.

Oltjen, J.M., Duncanson Jr., M.G., Ghosh, J., 1997. Stiffness-deflection behaviour of selected orthodontic wires. Angle Orthodontist 67, 209.

Purton, D.G., Love, R.M., 1996. Rigidity and retention of carbon fibre versus stainless steel root canal posts. International Endodontic Journal 29, 262.

Soxman, J.A., 2000. Stainless steel crown and pulpotomy: procedure and technique for primary molars. General Dentistry 48, 294.

Thompson, A., 2000. An overview of nickel-titanium alloys used in dentistry. International Endodontic Journal 33, 297.

Vallittu, P.K., 1996. Fatigue resistance and stress of wrought-steel wire clasps. Journal of Prosthodontics 5, 186.

Waldmeier, M.D., Grasso, J.E., Norberg, G.J., 1996. Bend testing of wrought wire removable partial denture alloys. Journal of Prosthetic Dentistry 76, 559.

Wang, Y., Liu, C., Jian, F., McIntyre, G.T., Millett, D.T., Hickman, J., et al., 2018. Initial arch wires used in orthodontic treatment with fixed appliances. Cochrane Database of Systematic Reviews 31, CD007859.

Waters, N.E., 1975. Properties of wire. In: Von Frauenhofer, J.A. (Ed.), Scientific Aspects of Dental Materials. Butterworth, Sevenoaks, UK, pp. 2–15.

INDEX

Page numbers followed by 'f' indicate figures, 't' indicate tables.